Rural Populations and Health

Rural Populations and Health

Determinants, Disparities, and Solutions

Richard A. Crosby
Monica L. Wendel
Robin C. Vanderpool
Baretta R. Casey

EDITORS

FOREWORD BY CIRO V. SUMAYA

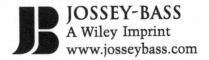

JOSSEY-BASS
A Wiley Imprint
www.josseybass.com

Copyright © 2012 by John Wiley & Sons, Inc. All rights reserved.
Published by Jossey-Bass
A Wiley Imprint
One Montgomery Street, Suite 1200, San Francisco, CA 94104-4594—www.josseybass.com

No part of this publication may be reproduced, stored in a retrieval system, or transmitted in any form or by any means, electronic, mechanical, photocopying, recording, scanning, or otherwise, except as permitted under Section 107 or 108 of the 1976 United States Copyright Act, without either the prior written permission of the publisher, or authorization through payment of the appropriate per-copy fee to the Copyright Clearance Center, Inc., 222 Rosewood Drive, Danvers, MA 01923, 978-750-8400, fax 978-646-8600, or on the Web at www.copyright.com. Requests to the publisher for permission should be addressed to the Permissions Department, John Wiley & Sons, Inc., 111 River Street, Hoboken, NJ 07030, 201-748-6011, fax 201-748-6008, or online at www.wiley.com/go/permissions.

Limit of Liability/Disclaimer of Warranty: While the publisher and author have used their best efforts in preparing this book, they make no representations or warranties with respect to the accuracy or completeness of the contents of this book and specifically disclaim any implied warranties of merchantability or fitness for a particular purpose. No warranty may be created or extended by sales representatives or written sales materials. The advice and strategies contained herein may not be suitable for your situation. You should consult with a professional where appropriate. Neither the publisher nor author shall be liable for any loss of profit or any other commercial damages, including but not limited to special, incidental, consequential, or other damages. Readers should be aware that Internet Web sites offered as citations and/or sources for further information may have changed or disappeared between the time this was written and when it is read.

Jossey-Bass books and products are available through most bookstores. To contact Jossey-Bass directly call our Customer Care Department within the U.S. at 800-956-7739, outside the U.S. at 317-572-3986, or fax 317-572-4002.

Wiley also publishes its books in a variety of electronic formats and by print-on-demand. Some material included with standard print versions of this book may not be included in e-books or in print-on-demand. If the version of this book that you purchased references media such as CD or DVD that was not included in your purchase, you may download this material at http://booksupport.wiley.com. For more information about Wiley products, visit www.wiley.com.

Library of Congress Cataloging-in-Publication Data

Rural populations and health / Richard A. Crosby, Monica L. Wendel, Robin C. Vanderpool, Baretta R. Casey, editors ; foreword by Ciro V. Sumaya. – First edition.
    pages cm
  Includes bibliographical references and index.
  ISBN 978-1-118-00430-2 (pbk.); ISBN 9781118260296 (ebk.); ISBN 9781118235485 (ebk.); ISBN 9781118221693 (ebk.)
  1. Medicine, Rural–United States.   2. Rural health services–United States.   3. Rural health–United States.   4. Health services accessibility–United States.   I. Crosby, Richard A., 1959–   II. Wendel, Monica L.   III. Vanderpool, Robin C., 1975–   IV. Casey, Baretta R., 1953–
  RA771.5.R88 2012
  362.1'04257–dc23

                              2012016810

Printed in Singapore
FIRST EDITION
PB Printing   10 9 8 7 6 5 4 3 2 1

Contents

Tables and Figures

Tables

Figures

To my friends and colleagues who have worked tirelessly to address rural health disparities—Richard A. Crosby

• • •

For my mom, one of my greatest heroes—Monica L. Wendel

• • •

To my parents, Barbara Groves Cline and Dr. Hayden Dwight Cline, both educators, who shared with me their lifelong commitment to learning and teaching—Robin C. Vanderpool

• • •

This is dedicated to my wonderful husband, Michael, for all of his support and understanding—Baretta R. Casey

Foreword

Ciro V. Sumaya

Health-related disparities remain a persistent, serious problem across the nation's more than sixty million rural residents. Although health disparities can be found across the whole of society, many of them are accentuated in rural settings, namely, increased incidence of chronic diseases, higher out-of-pocket payment for health care (compared to urban counterparts), lack of health insurance, and limited access to health professionals and health facilities, among others. Although a number of strategies and interventions have had various levels of success in addressing health disparities, these measures often lack adequate financial support, advocacy, and sustained strong political actions.

It is my perception that a greater inclusion of rural public health perspectives, approaches, and infrastructure would be helpful in tackling these recalcitrant disparities. To effect major long-term changes in our society's health and health system(s) requires a critical focus on the population in the aggregate as well as its components such as individuals, families, neighborhoods, communities, and beyond. Public health perspectives traditionally include community health assessments of disease burden and priorities, education and promotion of health through prevention measures, advocacy for appropriate health legislation and regulation, and assurance of a competent health workforce, among other essential public health services. Public health advocates recognize the significant influences on health from the environment and social settings around us, including educational levels, standards of living, and lifestyles. These social determinants of health, although complex and enormous, need to be entwined in the public debate on problem-solving strategies and interventions to improve health. Public health advocates understand the significant role that the community can play in the health enterprise, actually becoming the locus of accountability and a driving force for health improvement. Further, the steps and mechanisms to improve health need to be critically evaluated and form an evidence-based framework from which to advance and sustain the health of the people—another essential public health service.

With the current climate of health care reform (of some form), now is the time to forge additional partnerships, strategies, and effective measures around a renewed framework of rural public health to resolve rural health disparities. The Affordable Care Act, in its attempt to improve health for the American public, proposes greater access to health insurance, quality-of-care improvements that are also aligned with cost controls, removal of health care that is inefficient or of dubious merit, and expansion of prevention efforts—items relevant to "healing" rural health disparities. Now is also the time to further analyze and improve the dynamic relationships among urban, suburban, and surrounding rural communities, networking and partnering to tackle previously intractable health disparities.

The multiple areas of the current health debate should encompass—not only on paper but in action—issues of clear concern to residents of rural communities including rural economic vulnerabilities, unique rural environmental hazards, distinct agricultural and occupational injuries, economic vulnerabilities, the general lack of trained health professionals (generalists and specialists), and appropriate coordination of health facilities and staff. Priorities and interventions on these issues, particularly community-based strategies, have been clearly delineated and diffused through *Rural Healthy People 2010* among other landmark documents. Further, it is critical that the rural sector, together with its advocates and supporters, not only participate but also lead the charge for improving health disparities.

On a personal note, I am pleased to have been the founding dean of the School of Rural Public Health at the Texas A&M Health Science Center. We launched the first school of public health that explicitly adopted a mission focused on the health of rural populations. This undertaking and many more examples of innovative efforts as illustrated in this book clearly indicate that with solidarity of purpose, passion, and persistent action, we will overcome the enigma of health disparities in rural America and the nation as a whole.

The Prevention Research Centers Program

Special mention must be made of the federal Prevention Research Centers (PRCs) Program, with whom many of the contributors to this book are associated. It is administered by the Centers for Disease Control and Prevention. The program was founded in 1984 and the first three centers were funded in 1986. In the current funding cycle (2010–2014), thirty-seven centers in twenty-seven states constitute the program through which hundreds of research projects are conducted each year.

The range of public health research the centers conduct is as broad and varied as the centers themselves. The research covers all chronic diseases such as heart disease and diabetes as well as some infectious and vaccine-preventable illnesses. Research topics include sexual health, health for those who are deaf, immigrant health, school health, occupational safety, substance abuse prevention, and many, many others. All segments of the population—by race or ethnicity, age, and sex—are the subject of specific research studies. Further, the research occurs in diverse settings—clinical and community, home and school, urban and rural. In fact, consistent with the burden that rural health disparities imposes on public health, about one-third of the Prevention Research Centers devote at least a portion of their research portfolios to understanding and improving the health of people who live in rural America.

For *Rural Populations and Health*, the primary authors of the four state-specific (Colorado, Kentucky, Alabama, and Iowa) chapters on rural health systems were invited from the Prevention Research Centers located in those states. Scientists from other Prevention Research Centers, such as the Center for Community Health Development at the Texas A&M Health Science Center, were responsible for major portions of this book.

Contributors from Prevention Research Centers are particularly well suited to communicating about the health disparities addressed in this book by virtue of the type of work they do regularly—that is, they engage in community-based participatory research. In using this research approach, the scientists are embedded in the rural communities they are studying and learn from the community residents who are involved in the research. These authors have a perspective that encompasses the full socioeconomic character and distinctive cultures of rural environments in the United States. They understand the interplay of genetic, social, environmental, and other factors that contribute to health disparities. For example, rural factors such as having a family occupational history in mining can contribute to biologic risks for and very personal beliefs about health conditions and behaviors. Living in remote rural locations and lacking public transportation can exacerbate limited access to health care, which already may be compromised by low employment and associated poverty and lack of health insurance. In writing for *Rural Populations and Health*, the contributors demonstrate a mastery of this societal complexity as well as empathy for the people who must navigate through these multifaceted social and medical circumstances every day.

The support the Prevention Research Centers receive for core research multiplies in many ways. When research studies conclude, results are shared with the study group and may have immediate effects on individual lives. Results are also shared with the scientific community for replication or modification in other geographic areas. In addition, research teams often develop relationships with community organizations that build long-term capacity for independently addressing community health issues. And researchers gain knowledge, insight, and experience such as that shared in this book. *Rural Populations and Health* owes a substantial part of its richness and depth to the Prevention Research Centers Program.

Acknowledgments

The editors would like to thank Tyrone F. Borders, Maureen Mayhew, Kendall M. Thu, Michael Hendryx, and Rebecca T. Slifkin, who provided valuable feedback in the early stages of the manuscript's conception. We would also like to thank the following reviewers for their thoughtful and valuable feedback on the draft manuscript: Amy Martin, Laura Senier, and Matthew Wray.

The Editors

Richard A. Crosby, PhD, has dedicated his career to the prevention of disease, particularly HIV and other sexually transmitted diseases. He served as codirector of the Rural Center for AIDS/STD Prevention at Indiana University for ten years. He is currently the principal investigator of the Rural Cancer Prevention Center (funded by CDC) at the University of Kentucky. This center is dedicated to the prevention of cervical cancer and the promotion of the HPV vaccine in rural Appalachia. He is an author of *Research Methods in Health Promotion* and an editor of *Emerging Theories in Health Promotion Practice and Research* (first and second editions) as well as *Adolescent Health: Understanding and Preventing Risk Behaviors* (all book are published by Jossey-Bass). Although Crosby is a successful NIH and CDC researcher, his most important accomplishments have been his teaching and mentorship of graduate students at the University of Kentucky, where he currently serves as the DDI Endowed Professor and chair of Health Behavior.

Monica L. Wendel, DrPH, MA, is director of the Center for Community Health Development and is an assistant professor of health policy and management at the Texas A&M Health Science Center School of Rural Public Health. Wendel also serves as the administrator for the Program for Rural and Minority Health Disparities Research. Her work in the Center for Community Health Development, a CDC-funded Prevention Research Center, focuses on capacity building for health improvement. Wendel's research and service activities are partnered with local organizations and communities with a goal of equipping these partners to better address their own health issues with the resources available to them. She earned a bachelor of arts in English, a master of arts in communication from Texas A&M University, and a master of public health and doctor of public health from the School of Rural Public Health in College Station, Texas.

Robin C. Vanderpool, DrPH, CHES, is an assistant professor in the Department of Health Behavior at the University of Kentucky College of Public Health where she teaches graduate courses in health promotion and rural health disparities and is actively involved in cancer prevention and control research and practice at federal, state, and local levels. Vanderpool serves as the deputy director for the CDC-funded University of Kentucky Rural Cancer Prevention Center, which focuses on reducing health disparities associated with cervical, breast, and colorectal cancers among residents of the eight-county Kentucky River Health District located in Appalachian Kentucky. Prior to her work with the center Rural Cancer Prevention Center, Dr. Vanderpool served as a health educator and research coordinator for the National Cancer Institute's Cancer Information Service. Robin earned a bachelor of science degree in psychobiology from Centre College in Danville, Kentucky, a master of public health degree from Western Kentucky University, and a doctorate in public health degree from the University of Kentucky.

A native and former private practice physician from Pikeville, Kentucky, **Baretta R. Casey, MD,** received her bachelor of arts degree from Pikeville College in Kentucky and her medical degree from the University of Kentucky College of Medicine. She completed her family medicine specialty training at Trover Clinic Foundation in Madisonville, Kentucky. Dr. Casey also received her master's in public health from the University of Kentucky College of Public Health. Dr. Casey is a professor in the University of Kentucky College of Public Health, Department of Health Behavior, Health Systems Management and Preventive Medicine and a professor in the College of Medicine, Department of Family and Community Medicine. She served as the director for the University of Kentucky Center for Excellence in Rural Health in Hazard, Kentucky, from November 2005 to July 2010, and prior to that she was the program director for the University of Kentucky College of Medicine, Hazard-based East Kentucky Family Medicine Residency Program. She is a 2006 graduate of the UCLA/Johnson & Johnson Health Care Executive Program, a management development program exclusively for executive directors and leaders of community-based health care organizations. And in March 2008, she completed the prestigious Executive Leadership in Academic Medicine (ELAM) program sponsored by Drexel University. Dr. Casey is past president of the Kentucky Medical Association and the Kentucky Academy of Family Physicians. She currently holds a position as chair of the American Medical Association's Council on Medical Education and vice of the Accreditation Council for Graduate Medical Education. Dr. Casey is also a member of the Executive Committee of the National Residency Matching Program.

The Contributors

Angie Alaniz, BA, is the deputy director of the Center for Community Health Development at the Texas A&M Health Science Center School of Rural Public Health in College Station.

Britt Allen, PT, MS, is owner of Mustang Therapies in Madisonville, Texas, is a member of the Madison County Health Resource Commission, and is president of the Brazos Valley Health Partnership Board.

Andrew Anesetti-Rothermel, MPH, BA, is a graduate assistant at the West Virginia Prevention Research Center at West Virginia University in Morgantown.

Bernard Appiah, B. Pharm, MS, is a doctoral student at Texas A&M Health Science Center's School of Rural Public Health in College Station.

Jamilia J. Blake, PhD, MEd, is an assistant professor at Texas A&M's College of Education and Human Development in the Department of Educational Psychology in College Station.

Daniel F. Brossart, PhD, is an associate professor in the Department of Educational Psychology at Texas A&M University College of Education and Human Development in College Station.

James N. Burdine, DrPH., is assistant dean for public health practice, is a professor in the Department of Health Promotion and Community Sciences, and is co-principal investigator of the Center for Community Health Development at the Texas A&M Health Science Center School of Rural Public Health in College Station.

Frances D. Butterfoss, PhD, MSEd, is founding president of Coalitions Work, a consulting group that trains coalitions to build, sustain, and evaluate themselves, in addition to working as a professor at Eastern Virginia Medical School and Old Dominion University in Norfolk, Virginia.

Angela L. Carman, DrPH [C], MBA, CHE, PHR, is a doctoral student at the University of Kentucky College of Public Health in Lexington concentrating in health services management.

Linda G. Castillo, PhD, is project director and principal investigator of the Gulf Coast GEAR UP project, which prepares underrepresented students to successfully enroll and complete college, along with serving as an associate professor of counseling psychology and associate dean for research at Texas A&M University in College Station.

Heather R. Clark, MSPH, is a senior research associate at the Center for Community Health Development, associated with Texas A&M's Health Science Center's School of Rural Public Health in College Station.

Henry P. Cole, EdD, is a professor at the University of Kentucky College of Public Health in the Department of Preventive Medicine and Environmental Health in Lexington.

Sally M. Davis, PhD, is the director and principal investigator of the University of New Mexico Prevention Research Center, which works to promote physical activity in Hispanics and Americans living in Cuba, New Mexico.

Keli Dean, BS, is a graduate research assistant for the Center for Community Health Development at the Texas A&M Health Science Center School of Rural Public Health in College Station.

Wesley R. Dean, PhD, is an assistant research scientist at the Center for Community Health Development at Texas A&M University Health Science Center School of Rural Public Health in College Station.

Geri A. Dino, PhD, is the director of the West Virginia Prevention Research Center, one of the CDC's thirty-seven PRCs, along with serving as an associate professor in the Department of Community Medicine at West Virginia University in Morgantown.

Kelly N. Drake, MPH, is the center coordinator for the Center for Community Health Development at the Texas A&M Health Science Center School of Rural Public Health in College Station.

Amy L. Elizondo, MPH, is the program services vice president of the National Rural Health Association in Washington, DC.

Timothy R. Elliott, PhD, is a professor in the Department of Educational Psychology at Texas A&M University College of Education and Human Development in College Station.

Lauren Erickson, BA, is a master's student at the University of Iowa's College of Public Health, where she is also the outreach committee chair in the Department of Community and Behavioral Health.

Hon. Pam Finke, BS, is a commissioner for Grimes County, Texas, a member of the Grimes County Health Resource Commission, and a member of the Brazos Valley Health Partnership Board in Texas.

James E. Florence, DrPH, MPH, MATS, is a professor of health sciences at Liberty University.

Mona N. Fouad, MD, MPH, is the director of REACH 2010 at the University of Alabama at Birmingham (UAB) as well as professor and director of the Division of Preventive Medicine in the UAB Department of Medicine.

Whitney Garney, BS, is a graduate research assistant for the Center for Community Health Development at the Texas A&M Health Science Center School of Rural Public Health in College Station.

Teresa Harris, BS, is the former executive director of the Leon County Health Resource Center and is a member of the Brazos Valley Health Partnership Board in Texas.

L. Gary Hart, PhD, is the director of the Center of Rural Health at the University of North Dakota in Grand Forks.

Chelsie N. Hollas, BA, is a graduate student at Texas A&M Health Science Center's School of Rural Public Health in College Station.

Kimberly A. Horn, EdD, is the associate director of Population Health Research at the Mary Babb Randolph Cancer Center at West Virginia University in Morgantown, along with serving as an associate professor of Community Medicine.

Vicky Jackson, COT, CORT, is director of community and support services for Grimes St. Joseph Health Center, a member of the Grimes County Health Resource Commission, and a member of the Brazos Valley Health Partnership Board in Texas.

Cassandra M. Johnson, MSPH, is a research associate in the Program for Research in Nutrition and Health Disparities at the School of Rural Public Health at the University of Texas A&M in College Station.

Michelle C. Kegler, DrPH, MPH, is the director and principal investigator at Emory Prevention Research Center at Emory University in Atlanta, along with serving as an associate professor in the Department of Behavioral Sciences and Health Education at the Rollins School of Public Health at Emory.

Brandy N. Kelly, MA, is a doctoral graduate research assistant in the evaluation core of the Center for Community Health Development at the Texas A&M Health Science Center School of Rural Public Health in College Station.

Richard Kozoll, MD, MPH, is vice president of the New Mexico Medical Review Association and serves as chair of the New Mexico Clinical Prevention Initiative, a combined effort of the New Mexico Medical Society and Department of Health in Albuquerque, along with working in his own community health center practice.

Julie A. Marshall, PhD, is the director of the Rocky Mountain PRC at the University of Colorado School of Public Health in Aurora. The Rocky Mountain PRC is one of the CDC's thirty-seven PRCs.

Carly E. McCord, MS, is a counseling psychology doctoral student at Texas A&M University in College Station.

E. Lisako J. McKyer, PhD, MPH, is an associate professor in the Department of Health and Kinesiology at Texas A&M University, is director of the Transdisciplinary Center for Health Equity Research, and is co-director of evaluation for the Center for Community Health Development at the Texas A&M Health Science Center School of Rural Public Health in College Station.

Kenneth R. McLeroy, PhD, is a Regents Professor in the Department of Health Promotion and Community Sciences and is principal investigator of the Center for Community Health Development at the Texas A&M Health Science Center School of Rural Public Health in College Station.

Laurel A. Mills, MPH, is a doctoral student concentrating in health behavior at the College of Public Health at the University of Kentucky in Lexington.

Alan Morgan, MPA, BS, is the chief executive officer of the National Rural Health Association in Washington, DC.

Faryle Nothwehr, PhD, MPH, is an associate professor at the Department of Community and Behavioral Health at the University of Iowa's College of Public Health in Iowa City. Dr. Nothwehr is also director of the Iowa Prevention Research Center, one of the CDC's thirty-seven PRCs.

Corliss W. Outley, PhD, is an associate professor in the Department of Recreation, Park, and Tourism Sciences at Texas A&M University and is co-director of evaluation for the Center for Community Health Development at the Texas A&M Health Science Center School of Rural Public Health in College Station.

Robert P. Pack, PhD, MPH, is the associate dean for academic affairs at East Tennessee University in Johnson City, along with being an associate professor in the Department of Community Health.

Rose M. Pignataro, PT, DPT, is a graduate assistant at the West Virginia Prevention Research Center at West Virginia University in Morgantown.

Hon. Dean Player, SMSgt. USAF (Ret.), is a commissioner for Leon County, Texas, and is vice president of the Brazos Valley Health Partnership Board.

Albert Ramirez, BA, is executive director of the Burleson County Health Resource Commission and is the secretary of the Brazos Valley Health Partnership Board in Texas.

Ulrike Schultz, MD, MPH, is an assistant research scientist at the University of Iowa in Iowa City, where she teaches in the College of Public Health's Department of Community and Behavioral Health.

F. Douglas Scutchfield, MD, is a professor at the University of Kentucky College of Public Health in Lexington with appointments in the Departments of Preventive Medicine and Environmental Health, Family Practice, Health Services, along with a faculty position in the University of Kentucky Martin School of Public Policy and Administration. He is the Peter P. Bosomworth Professor of Health Services Research and Policy.

Joseph R. Sharkey, PhD, MPH, RD, is a professor in the Department of Social and Behavioral Health at Texas A&M University School of Rural Public Health in College Station, along with working with the Center for Environmental and Rural Health.

Lindsay J. Shea, MPH, is a graduate research assistant at the Center for Community Health Development, associated with Texas A&M Health Science Center's School of Rural Public Health in College Station.

Lyndsey Simpson, BS, is a graduate research assistant for the Center for Community Health Development at the Texas A&M Health Science Center School of Rural Public Health in College Station.

Jodi Southerland, MA, BA, is a doctoral student in the College of Public Health at East Tennessee State University in Johnson City.

Julie A. St. John, MA, MPH, CHW-I, is South Texas regional director and certified promotora instructor for the Center for Community Health Development at the Texas A&M Health Science Center School of Rural Public Health in College Station.

Nikki Stone, DMD, is an assistant professor in the University of Kentucky College of Dentistry and also works with the mobile dental clinic located at the University of Kentucky Center for Excellence in Rural Health in Hazard.

Hon. Mike Sutherland, BS, is the county judge of Burleson County, Texas, and is a member of the Brazos Valley Health Partnership Board.

Lisa N. VanRaemdonck, MPH, MSW, is a project manager with the Colorado Association of Local Public Health Officials and works at the Colorado Practice-Based Research Network through the University of Colorado School of Public Health in Aurora.

Camilla Viator, BBA, is the executive director of the Madison County Health Resource Commission and is the treasurer of the Brazos Valley Health Partnership Board in Texas.

Susan C. Westneat, MA, is a staff epidemiologist at the Southwest Center for Agricultural Health and Injury Prevention at the University of Kentucky in Lexington.

Randolph F. Wykoff, MD, MPH, TM, is the dean of the College of Public Health at East Tennessee State University in Johnson City.

Theresa A. Wynn, PhD, MA, BSN, is the project director of the CDC-funded Racial and Ethnic Approaches to Community Health by the year 2010 (REACH 2010) at the University of Alabama at Birmingham.

Rural Populations and Health

Part One

Rural Communities
in Context

Chapter 1

Understanding Rural America
A Public Health Perspective

Richard A. Crosby   Baretta R. Casey
Monica L. Wendel   Laurel A. Mills
Robin C. Vanderpool

Learning Objectives

- Understand the unique aspects of rural America and the key contextual influences on rural public health.
- Identify key determinants of rural health disparities in the United States.
- List and explain eight major influences on rural health disparities.
- Compare and contrast rural health disparities to those experienced in urban and suburban areas of the United States.

•••

Covering about two-thirds of the land in the United States, rural America is extremely diverse. The diversity found there exists as a function of rich cultural traditions handed down from generation to generation as well as from adaptations to the environment and the livelihood it supports. Thus, it is indeed important to know that term *rural America* is far too vague to have any practical value in this book. Instead, rural America should be thought of as a tapestry of rural cultures—shaped by geography and tradition—that spans from the rural poverty of the Mississippi Delta to the rural isolation of states like Montana and Wyoming. Rural life, and the associated challenges to public health, is therefore difficult to describe in a single chapter. Recognizing this, we urge you to remain mindful about this tapestry as you read this chapter, which by necessity will need to broadly describe rural America and its public health issues. Please also bear in mind that *rural* is not just a place. Instead, the term represents a culture of rural people who typically have tight-knit communities, strong ties to the land they live on, and a long history of shared life experiences. Despite the poverty that often characterizes rural areas, the isolation of rural places, and the growing digital divide that places rural Americans at a disadvantage in many ways, rural people may commonly perceive their lives to be of very high quality mainly because of their strong sense of community, extended families (most of whom may never leave the community), and an aesthetic beauty offered by life largely unspoiled from the trappings of urban settings.

People in rural areas of the United States do have a great deal in common: a strong sense of independence, pride in their community, and self-reliance. Although these qualities can be valuable assets to public health programs, they can also be obstacles that prove difficult to overcome. As an example of using rural assets to advance a public health agenda, consider the case of southeastern Kentucky, where a cervical cancer program known as *Faith Moves Mountains* (FMM) has been used to successfully promote and increase Pap testing among medically underserved women living in a high-incidence area for cervical cancer (see Chapter Nineteen) (Schoenberg et al., 2009). The program works through key community stakeholders—women who are well connected throughout the community. These women conduct educational sessions in churches and subsequently navigate women into screening for cervical cancer. In this rural culture (as is common in rural America), churches are a focal point of communities, serving as a mechanism for the creation and maintenance of social capital. **Social capital** can be thought of as sense of cooperation, reciprocity, and trust among community members (Putnam, 2000). As such, social capital is widely recognized as one the principle factors in any organized effort to promote public health (Kreuter & Lezin, in press). The FMM program tapped into this local source of social capital, thereby using the asset of the rural tight-knit community as a method of diffusing innovations (e.g., Pap testing) in public health. The FMM investigators are now extending their successful faith-based approach to improve eating and exercise behaviors of community residents as well as to achieve reductions in tobacco use. At its heart, FMM is about using rural social capital to catalyze the adoption of health-protective behaviors among people otherwise at-risk of morbidity and early mortality.

Rural "assets" can also be a barrier to public health efforts. For example, in many of the tight-knit rural communities across the United States, a sense of independence can be taken to the level of actively avoiding assistance from people who are not part of the community. In these modern times, this pioneer mentality can be quite limiting in terms of public health. In the absence of outside assistance, residents may create alternative beliefs and practices regarding health and healing. A rural community that is resistant to outside influences thus becomes figuratively isolated from the diffusion of public health innovations such as improved dietary practices, screenings for the early detection of cancer, cholesterol-lowering drugs, occupational safety measures, the use of contraceptives, cervical cancer vaccines, the use of infant car seats, and improved dental hygiene practices.

A Few Basic Principles

In addition to understanding the concept of rural assets, we urge you to keep the following principle in mind: geography is critical—it shapes culture and practices of people. In many ways, geography determines something that scholars have termed *context* (Phillips & McLeroy, 2004). Context includes infrastructures such as roads and bridges, social structures such as community leadership and key opinion leaders, physical topography such as mountains and deserts, and community structures such as common values and history. Rural health disparities are often an outgrowth of contextual issues. For example, consider a typical rural Appalachian community set in steep mountains that are far too covered in timber and rocks to build roads on. Consequently, the roads are all built in between the mountains; these narrow valleys are called *hollers*. Hollers are the same places that rainwater runoff filters into creeks. People build their homes (or place their mobile homes) in the hollers because the cost of doing so is far less expensive than building on mountain sides. Building in the hollers also prevents the concern of not being able to get off the mountain at times of inclement weather from late autumn to early spring. A holler may house several extended families in thirty or more dwellings. In the spring, hollers are prone to flooding and the low-lying homes can be damaged or even swept away. In the winter, driving out of the hollers into the steep mountains may be impossible because of snow and ice. This same geography does not support farming, so people are forced to travel to towns or cities for gainful employment or work literally within the mountains as coal miners. As you can imagine, the geography described in this brief example has a profound influence on the context of rural life in Appalachia.

Rural health disparities are often an outgrowth of contextual issues.

It is also important to understand that rural cultures' interactions with race and ethnicity have a profound influence on public health. This is known as *composition* (Phillips & McLeroy, 2004). In essence, the disadvantages that US minority members so often experience are compounded by the disadvantages created by the lack of employment and educational opportunities in rural areas as well as historical policies such as slavery and the creation of Indian reservations. Indeed, minorities in the rural parts of the United States have been referred to as a forgotten population (Probst et al., 2004).

Finally, as you read this chapter (and this entire book), please understand that health care and public health are two very different concepts. Public health is about prevention and its focus is always on entire populations. An all-too-frequently-held belief is that health care is the key to improving the health of the public. In actuality, this idea is arguably false. Ample evidence suggests that the key to improving public health lies in reversing the actual causes of death such as tobacco use, overeating, sedentary living, alcohol use, and other behaviors that lead to morbidity and early mortality (Farley & Cohen, 2005; Mokdad et al., 2004). Thus, we will use the phrase *rural public health* to represent the combined efforts to prevent the actual causes of disease and death (behaviors and environmentally driven causes) as well as issues pertaining to a lack of health care. The combination of prevention approaches and health care improvements are the very reasons we decided to create this textbook. Indeed, this is the first book to take this combined approach to rural public health. Unfortunately, despite a great deal of published papers on public health very little attention has been devoted to rural public health. As suggested by Phillips and McLeroy (2004) rural public health focuses on reducing population morbidity and mortality through multilevel, tailored, prevention efforts (primary, secondary, and tertiary) accounting for the unique context and composition of rural communities. Rural public health also takes an ecological perspective, meaning that the prevention approach works within the context of families, communities, culture, societal norms, and public policy.

An Overview

Galambos argued that rural health disparities have been a "neglected frontier." This reality is indeed unfortunate given that significant numbers of people live in rural areas (Galambos, 2005). Depending on how *rural* is defined, the total rural population accounts for between 10 and 28 percent of the entire US population (Hart, Larson, & Lishner, 2005); however, the land mass occupied by rural residents is approximately twice that occupied by urban residents.

This book is dedicated to the illumination of public health issues and challenges for this often-neglected population of Americans. In this chapter, you will learn about eight key factors that profoundly influence disparities in rural public health. We will then provide you with key principles that can be applied to improving rural public health. Throughout the chapter, we will provide you with case studies, vignettes, visual displays, and photographs designed to help you learn the concepts easily. Chapter One is an overview and many of the concepts you learn in this chapter will be discussed in subsequent chapters to aid the learning process. Chapter Two is then quite specific as it describes various systems of measuring **rurality** (what constitutes being rural) in the United States. Chapter Three then provides a succinct history of rural public health and further elaborates on a few of the concepts introduced in Chapter One. Chapter Four expands on the concept of overlapping disparities by describing the problems and issues faced by rural minorities. With these four chapters firmly behind you, the book then introduces the concept of rural public health systems, including health policy and efforts directed toward population-level change. After an introduction to rural public health systems (Chapter Five) you will learn about these concepts by reading chapters focused on specific rural states: Colorado (Chapter Six), Kentucky (Chapter Seven), Alabama (Chapter Eight), and Iowa (Chapter Nine). You will then be ready to learn about three key skills in conducting activities toward improving rural public health: (1) assessment (Chapter Ten), (2) coalition building in rural areas (Chapter Eleven), and (3) capacity building in rural areas (Chapters Twelve). The book will finally take you through a series of applied chapters (Chapters Thirteen through Twenty), each devoted to specific health issues such as adolescent health, food disparities, oral health, physical activity, farm injuries, mental health, cancer prevention and control, and tobacco prevention.

Eight Key Factors

Understanding rural public health requires that you first understand some key factors that influence this broad construct. In essence, any given rural community can be said to possess certain characteristics that affect its ability to promote and maintain health. A spidergram is a simple way of providing a snapshot of all factors of such a complex idea at one time. Each factor in a spidergram is represented as a "leg" of a spider, with incremental measures along its axis. In this instance, factors associated with a rural community's ability to improve and maintain public health is the purpose of the spidergram:

- Geography
- Occupation
- Infrastructure
- Demographics
- Digital divide
- Access to care
- Social capital
- Political voice

The factor being assessed of any community can be "measured" along each spider leg and then plotted. After all of the legs are plotted the connected dots form a polygon. In turn, the area of the resulting polygon represents the degree of the community's ability to promote and maintain the health of its residents. Thus, a small polygon represents poorer ability and larger polygons reflect more advanced capability. Clearly, a critical goal then is to increase the size of the polygon for a rural community. Figure 1.1 provides an example of a spidergram that plots the areas of three hypothetical rural communities.

As shown in Figure 1.1, each of these three rural communities requires a substantial degree of intervention given the very small size of their polygons. Figure 1.1 also illustrates potential priorities for intervention by graphically showing which legs (factors) of the spidergram are the shortest, thus implying greater potential for expansion. It is indeed quite fair to say that no two rural communities are likely to have the same shape polygon. Thus, the size and the shape of the polygon are important features. As is true for any spider, the movement of each leg affects the other legs and thus it is important to grasp that each leg is somewhat related to the others. To help you better understand the spidergram shown in Figure 1.1 we will systematically describe each of the eight legs.

Geography

As described earlier in this chapter, features of the land provide a variety of environmental and natural resources affecting the ways communities and their residents sustain themselves. For example, fertile farmland, minerals, oil, natural gas, and bodies of water all enable communities to incorporate farming, mining, drilling, fishing, and tourism, respectively, into their local economies. These economies also influence the rate of development and population growth. The most obvious characteristic of rural communities is the relationship between the population and its geography—a primary determinant of population density. However, in addition to population density, geography contributes to several other factors influencing rural public health.

Rurality and geographic isolation have been identified as contributing to poorer access to care (see Chapter Three), lower rates of preventive screening, decreased treatment for chronic diseases and mental health problems, and higher rates of morbidity from acute and chronic conditions (Eberhardt & Pamuk, 2004; IOM, 2005). Natural boundaries such as mountains, deserts, and rivers, as well as historic human-created boundaries such as railroad tracks, bridges, interstates, and dams, serve to connect and divide communities, thereby creating geographic isolation. In turn, this geographic isolation also presents challenges in developing and sustaining services because there is inherently less demand and fewer resources.

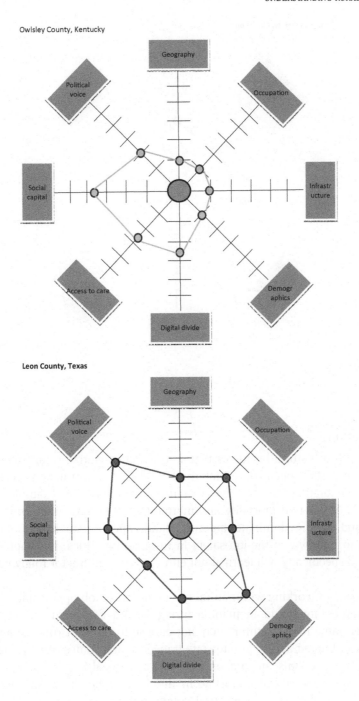

Figure 1.1. Spidergram Examples: Owlsley County, Kentucky; Leon County, Texas; Issaquena County, Mississippi

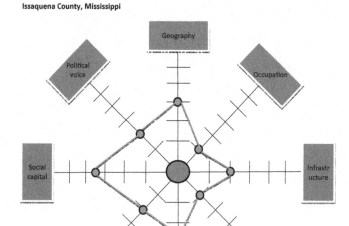

Figure 1.1. (*Continued*)

Occupation

The wealth of natural resources that so often characterize rural America also creates important occupations for rural residents. Unfortunately, these same revenue-generating jobs are often extremely hazardous. For example, Ricketts (2000) indicates that mortality and morbidity due to agriculture, mining, forestry, and fishing dominate the rural landscape. Public health efforts are needed to improve on-the-job safety in rural communities; in Chapter Seventeen, you specifically will learn about efforts to prevent tractor rollovers among farmers.

Outside of working with natural resources, other job opportunities in rural communities are found in manufacturing, health care, and service sectors. However, large manufacturers may not choose to build in rural communities because of limited access to interstate transportation routes or major railways. Small rural hospitals are not only a source of local employment, but also an economic and social mainstay. In the 1980s when rural hospitals were closing at a rapid pace, many rural communities were significantly affected. In order to stay competitive, rural hospitals must provide inpatient, outpatient, home health, skilled nursing, and long-term-care services. Unfortunately, service-related jobs often pay only minimum wage and come without benefits such as health insurance and paid sick leave. All four employment areas are sensitive to the national economic environment, particularly recessions, which often lead to less demand for consumer products, less health care use, layoffs, and closures. Furthermore, imagine how an independent, small farmer might be affected by skyrocketing gasoline prices when crop subsidies are flat or decreasing or how a rural hospital can compete with an urban hospital, which can offer a higher salary and benefit package.

Infrastructure

Infrastructure is best defined as the degree to which various structures (physical, political, social, legal, etc.) and systems (governmental and nongovernmental) within a given community have been developed. A vignette is useful as a starting point here. In a rural county in east Texas, there was an effort to expand local mental health services through the use of telehealth technology. Very simply, the community planned to use a secure network connection, high-definition cameras, and large monitors to provide mental health services over long distances. Although the health care providers and the community were fully ready to implement the services, it took two years to establish a secure connection due to the community's difficulties with physical infrastructure. Getting a simple connection for telehealth was less of an issue but getting the necessary bandwidth for the encryption needed for security was challenging simply because these services were not available in that rural area.

Building infrastructure obviously requires financial and personnel resources that are often limited in rural communities. In addition, federal and state resources are often distributed based on population, which further disadvantages rural communities and perpetuates the lack of needed infrastructure.

Demographics

In addition to geography, occupation, and infrastructure, public health practitioners must take note of the demographic characteristics of their rural communities. Due to the out-migration (leaving rural counties to move to urban areas) of younger individuals, rural communities are typically made up of older populations that in turn have higher rates of chronic conditions; this places a heavy strain on local public health resources (IOM, 2005).

As discussed previously, many rural communities have large concentrations of minority populations creating a synergistic effect of "race and place," leading to pronounced health disparities (Probst et al., 2004). One of the most stunning examples of rural health disparities was provided by Murray and colleagues who dissected the US population into "eight Americas" based on socioeconomic factors such as race, income, and place of residence (by county).

These different Americas have distinctly diverse mortality rates, highlighting huge disparities among different subpopulations such as southern, low-income blacks, low-income whites in Appalachia and the Mississippi Valley, western Native Americans, and northland low-income rural whites (Murray et al., 2006). Similarly, in 2007 the *New York Times* published a feature story on the increased infant mortality rates in Mississippi, which reached 17 deaths per thousand live births compared to 6.6 deaths for white women in 2005 (Eckholm, 2007). And in southern Arizona, the Pima Indians are recognized for having some of the highest rates of diabetes in the world; 50 percent of adult Pima Indians have diabetes and 95 percent of those with diabetes are overweight (NIDDK, 2002).

Additionally, poverty rates in rural areas are higher compared to urban areas (Blumenthal & Kagen, 2002; IOM, 2005). More than one in four non-metropolitan Hispanics, African Americans, and Native Americans live in poverty. In 2002, nonmetropolitan poverty rates for non-Hispanic African Americans and Native Americans were 33 percent and 35 percent, respectively, which was more than three times the rate for non-Hispanic whites (11 percent). The rate for Hispanics (27 percent) was more than twice as high (ERS, 2004).

Finally, education is interrelated with an individual's health status and is directly related to future job opportunities. Whereas upwards of 80 percent of all rural Americans complete high school, far less (16 percent) receive a college education compared to their urban counterparts (27 percent) (IOM, 2005).

Digital Divide

The term *digital divide* refers to a growing disparity between rural and nonrural Americans—one that involves access to and use of the Internet. Broadband access is an important issue in rural America. Evidence suggests that a significantly smaller number of rural homes have broadband access compared to suburban or urban homes. The term *access* is critical here because it is certainly not the case that simply having access always translates into an affirmative decision for people to adopt broadband (or other high speed Internet) technology. Some evidence suggests that adoption of this technology is a function of two key demographic factors: age and socioeconomic status, with younger age and higher socioeconomic status being predictive of broadband adoption. Thus, because rural Americans have a higher mean age than nonrural Americans and because collectively they have a lower socioeconomic status, it is quite likely that adoption once access is available is also slower among rural Americans. We will briefly discuss the issues affected by access and adoption.

Broadband access is an important issue in rural America.

Access to broadband technology is an unfortunate function of economics. Simply stated, the physical construction required to bring this technology to rural homes is often deemed (by the companies providing service) too expensive given the low population density. Stated differently, the potential number of customers (best case scenario) is not large enough to justify the initial outlay of money to provide the service. This may be an intractable problem. Unfortunately, this specific economic problem translates into much larger problems when thinking about the consequences of this digital divide. For example, one likely and long-lasting consequence is that rural children and adolescents will lack the same daily opportunities afforded to their nonrural counterparts relative to the vast number of websites that offer ways to advance educational opportunities. To the extent that commerce has become intimately linked with the Internet, rural Americans may also lack some of the employment opportunities afforded their nonrural counterparts. This same dynamic may also apply to purchasing given the ever-expanding number of companies that offer price reductions for products and services purchased online.

With regards to broadband adoption, rural Americans can behave quite differently from their nonrural counterparts. For example, the concept of paying yet another "utility bill" may be quite unacceptable for rural folks living in poverty. The access issue previously described did not include the notion of costs—the two constructs are indeed quite distinct. Thus, even when a company does invest in a broadband infrastructure for a rural area, it is not fair to assume that this service will be provided at a price equivalent to the same service offered in suburban and urban areas (in fact, a logical assumption is that price would be much higher to compensate the company for the greater cost of building the needed infrastructure). Adoption of broadband access in rural areas may also be affected by cultural norms suggesting that communication with "outside cultures" is not necessary or even desirable.

Access to Care

Considering all the factors discussed up until this point, it is not difficult to conclude that rural residents also face access to health care problems. Access to care can have multiple meanings. For example, distance and lack of transportation serve as barriers to care. Patients may have to travel hours and many miles to receive health care, especially in frontier communities. Additionally, public transportation is not readily available in rural communities and patients without their own form of transportation must rely on family members, friends, or social service agencies to take them to their appointments. See Figure 1.2 for a map showing areas with high proportions of carless households in the United States.

Compounding distance and transportation barriers, there may be a limited number of health care providers available in rural communities. Almost 80

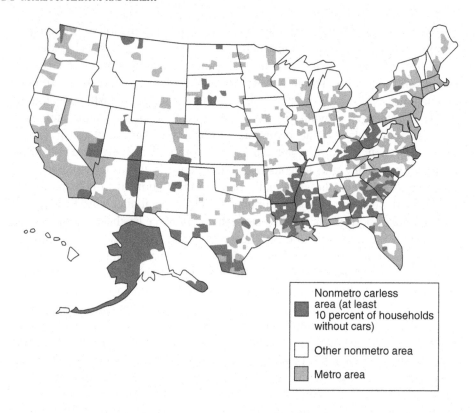

Figure 1.2. Nonmetro Areas with High Proportions of Carless Households, 2000
Source: United States Department of Agriculture Economic Research Service (2005, January).

percent of nonmetro US counties are in a whole or partial primary care health professional shortage area (HPSA), 60 percent are in dental care HPSAs, and 87 percent are in mental health care HPSAs (RUPRI, 2006). The majority of health care in rural communities is provided by local health departments, small private practices, rural health clinics, and federally qualified community health centers (FQHCs). Even though there are over two thousand rural-based hospitals, 70 percent of them have one hundred beds or less and must triage complicated or severe cases to larger facilities (IOM, 2005). In addition to health care provider shortages, approximately one in five rural residents are without health insurance and uninsured rates are over 30 percent in more isolated rural communities (Bolin & Gamm, 2003; Probst et al., 2004; Schur & Franco, 1999). Related, a higher proportion of rural individuals are enrolled in Medicaid and Medicare compared to their urban counterparts (IOM, 2005).

Primary care providers (e.g., physicians, nurse practitioners, physicians' assistants) are many times the first entry into the health care system for rural individuals. Almost 75 percent of medical visits in rural communities are to a primary care provider (Schur & Franco, 1999). Due to the lack of medical specialists in rural communities, primary care providers are required to cover a multitude of health problems: episodic care, preventive medicine, chronic disease management, pediatrics, gerontology, obstetrics and gynecology, mental health, and emergency services, to name a few (IOM, 2005). For the most part, providers practicing in rural areas do so because of their desire to live and care for rural residents; in fact, providers who were raised in rural areas are more likely to train in primary care and return to practice in rural communities (Brooks et al., 2002; Gamm, Castillo, & Pittman, 2003; Rosenblatt & Hart, 1999). However, these providers may feel professionally isolated. They have fewer of their colleagues in the community to consult with on difficult cases and are frequently on call. It is easy for these rural providers to get burned out due to longer work hours, more patient visits, cultural and professional isolation, lower net annual incomes, and a stressful role in caring for human life (Pathman et al., 2004). Further exasperating the retention of rural health care providers is the difficulty of recruiting new providers to rural America. In a position paper by the American Academy of Family Physicians (AAFP, 2009) the top five reasons new physicians give when choosing their first practice site include significant other's wishes, medical community friendly to family physicians, recreation and culture, proximity to family and friends, and significant other's employment. These reasons further illustrate this difficulty in recruiting providers to geographically isolated communities. Health care providers are traditionally trained in treating the symptoms and causes of disease in individuals. However, in rural America these symptoms are often indicative of a larger, systemic community circumstance. Thus, it is important that providers practicing in rural America have the necessary skills to address the depth of public health needs in the community.

Social Capital

Although definitive studies have not been conducted, it may be quite fair to speculate that rural communities have a greater degree of social capital compared to urban communities. As noted previously in this chapter, **social capital** is broadly conceived of as reciprocity, cooperation, and trust among community members in pursuit of a common goal (Putnam, 2000). In contrast to the negative health and sociodemographic characteristics that are often used to describe rural communities, rural residents have multiple strengths and assets that can be optimized to improve health outcomes and these assets are indeed consistent with the concept of social capital. Again, for example, rural communities are often recognized for their tight-knit, long-standing familial and social networks resulting in shared life experiences. These networks can serve as dissemination mechanisms for health information, health innovations, and positive health behaviors. As a public health professional, you will want to identify key influential members of these networks not only to collaborate on program planning, implementation, and evaluation, but also to serve as role models for others in the network through endorsement and practice of a particular protective health behavior (e.g., cancer screening, influenza immunization, healthy diet).

Related to these strong family and social networks, rural residents typically value and are committed to their community and its members. A strong sense of community can be used to rally rural communities to promote and protect the health of their fellow residents, whether it is an environmental health issue such as mountaintop removal (a method of coal mining) or smoking prevention among school students. It is important to note that the definition of *community* can vary from an entire county, to a faith-based community, to the residents of an isolated village in the Great Plains. Many rural individuals want to give back to their communities, which may have supported them during difficult times such as unemployment, a cancer diagnosis, or the death of a loved one. This notion of reciprocity serves as a foundation for engaging rural communities in public health programs and interventions that in turn are more likely to be more successful and sustainable.

Rural communities are also recognized for strong faith, spirituality, and religious beliefs (each being a powerful form of social capital). Because rural individuals regularly participate in faith-based or spiritual activities, venues such as the church or powwow become potential programmatic intervention and message dissemination points. Historically, African American communities such as those found in the Mississippi Delta have significant ties to local churches, which serve as places of worship, locations for social gatherings, and political center points. Incorporating faith-based or spiritual messages (i.e., your body is a temple; do not pollute it with alcohol, tobacco, drugs) into rural-based public health programs is thus likely to increase the salience of the health protective behaviors you may attempt to promote. Additionally, by engaging these entities, programmatic activities can be held in their facilities, which brings the familiar and comfortable to the congregations.

Interestingly, rural residents also consider themselves to have a high quality of life despite the unfavorable epidemiological and demographic data that may suggest otherwise. As an example, although many rural families may not be financially wealthy, they may consider their lives rich in family, friends, community, and faith. Additionally, land is an invaluable resource to many rural communities due to its provision of food, livestock, livelihood, and history. Consider the fact that land in the Southwest has been passed on through generations of families, the mountains of Appalachia hold mineral and timber resources vital to the local economy, and Native Americans have spiritual connection to their ancestral lands. Thus, it is important for public health professionals to identify what rural residents value in order to incorporate these assets into our outreach activities and messages.

Finally, as a public health professional, you should recognize the creativeness, resourcefulness, independence, and resiliency of rural residents. Many rural communities have struggled with economic downturns, natural and human-made disasters, corporate bullying, political strife, lack of resources and infrastructure, and other challenges inherent to their geographical isolation, which has in turn made these communities stronger, inventive, and innovative. For instance, the Frontier Nursing Service, founded in 1925 by Mary Breckinridge, was created to address the high rates of maternal and infant mortality in eastern Kentucky, a region that at the time had no physicians and few roads. Through the provision of prenatal care, birthing assistance, and general family health care services by nurse midwives, Ms. Breckinridge's innovative outreach program—much of which was delivered via horseback—contributed to significant declines in maternal and infant mortality in area. Today, some eighty-five years later, the Frontier Nursing Service operates five rural health clinics, a critical access hospital, a home health service, and a world-renowned midwifery and family nursing training program (http://www .frontiernursing.org/).

The idea of heightened social capital in rural communities has empirical support. For example, in a study testing the theory that social capital is related to health status, Folland (2007) found the relationship between the two variables to be robust for multiple variations in analysis and that rural or urban status reduced the effect of social capital on the prevalence rates of some diseases. A study examining differences in social capital between rural and urban families found that rural residents are more likely to receive social and material support from their relatives (kin) residing in close proximity than their urban counterparts (Hofferth & Iceland, 1998). Although the study primarily focused on economic exchanges, the authors concluded that persistent rural-urban differences in social capital remained and may be linked to cultural norms and the presence or absence of mediating structures to facilitate social engagement.

Focusing on broader economic issues, Israel and colleagues (2001) attributed rural-urban variations in social capital largely to structural attributes of community social capital, including "socioeconomic capacity, isolation, instability, and inequality" (p. 46). They hold that highly skilled jobs cluster in urban areas and foster a cycle in which rural communities persistently lag behind urban communities in economic capacity, leading to communities where the overall education, skill, and income levels remain lower, and expectations, opportunities, and achievement spiral downward (Israel, Beaulieu, &

Hartless, 2001). This perpetuates poverty and poor social capital in the communities where there is no intervention to interrupt the cycle. Thus, for a variety of reasons, social capital varies between rural and urban populations (Wendel, 2009).

Political Voice

An important principle of public health is that people can empower themselves to improve the influences that directly affect their health and well-being. Again, a brief vignette may be very useful here. In the State of Texas, incorporated cities have an extraterritorial jurisdiction (ETJ) that extends beyond their city limits proportional to the size of the population. Smaller cities under five thousand residents have half a mile of extra jurisdiction; cities over one hundred thousand have up to five extra miles. The ETJ can reach into contiguous counties but not into another city's ETJ. This is one example of how rural communities lack political voice. In an area of Texas where one larger city's ETJ reached into a neighboring rural county, the city purchased land in that county within their ETJ with the intention of building a landfill. They presented this information to the county commissioners' court after the fact to let them know that it would be happening; although they were outraged, the rural county could not halt the process.

Another vignette is also quite helpful in understanding the spidergram leg of **political voice**. In a specific instance, many Iowa residents had advocated against the presence of concentrated animal-feeding operations in their communities by blocking construction permits, signing petitions, holding courthouse rallies and protests, and filing nuisance lawsuits (Osterberg & Wallinga, 2004). As a community, their active belief in their own ability to correct an otherwise unhealthy and undesirable influence on the environment was indeed the key to their action, which eventually created change, thereby protecting the health and well-being of their residents.

Yet one more vignette is quite applicable to the concept of political voice. Leon County in rural east Texas is the county home to a predominately white population of close-knit people tightly tied to the community (through churches and schools) with some employment, ranching, and very few health resources. One school nurse serves five school districts. Obesity is rampant, as is substance abuse, domestic violence, elder abuse, and mental health issues (depression and anxiety). The county has a high degree of income inequality. Education levels are relatively low, with 13.9 years of school being the mean. As is common in rural areas, out-migration has created an older-than-average population in this county; 27 percent are sixty-five or older, 28 percent retired, and the median income is $50,000. Strikingly, 24 percent of people surveyed said no one in the household earned money (CCHD, 2010). The primary challenges to public health in this county once involved a lack of government support for basic services to its residents. However, this began to change in 2005 when a county health resource commission was formed. This commission slowly helped people develop and use their political voice and brought people to hold health care providers accountable and have a better sense of being health care consumers.

Conclusion

Rural communities often have a strong community identity and a great deal of local pride. Although this can sometimes impede progress in health promotion, strategically employed, these characteristics can also be an asset. For example, rural communities are more likely to have a greater proportion of older adult residents. Although this can create a greater demand for specialty care and human services, it can also provide a strong pool of volunteers for community-based initiatives. Another example relates to a sense of independence that many rural communities uphold—valuing the ability to "pull yourself up by your bootstraps" and not needing (or wanting) help from outsiders. Admittedly, this can inhibit some efforts to assist local communities. However, framed the right way, this mentality can also facilitate capacity building. In essence, rural health promotion efforts should capitalize on this type of independence by framing change as a challenge that only "locals can handle." Framing interventions so that a rural community can build their capacity to conduct them on their own and so that they will not need help excessive from the government or outsiders may create an environment that invites technical assistance in planning and development.

Summary

- Rural America is extremely diverse; it is far from being homogenous.
- Rural health disparities are vastly unexplored and improved efforts to rectify these problems are greatly needed.
- At least eight dimensions can be used to describe rural health disparities in any given area or community (represented by a spidergram).
- Rural social capital is one example of a rural asset that can be used to improve intervention capacities.
- Rural public health is affected by a host of contextual factors ranging from individual beliefs to culture and geography.

For Practice and Discussion

1. In this chapter you have learned about various rural assets. The rural assets that we have described are certainly not inclusive of all the strengths of rural communities. We challenge you to consider additional characteristics of rural areas that can be capitalized on to reduce rural health disparities. Working with colleagues from your class, please identify three additional rural assets and compose a brief justification for each that provides the logic you used to arrive at your choice.

2. One leg of the spidergram is the digital divide. Carefully read this chapter again and (while doing so) ask yourself the question, "Is access to broadband Internet a desirable priority for rural America?" Consider the following points as you reflect on this issue. First, is it possible that many rural Americans are better off being unexposed to the multiple influences of the Internet? Second, are various rural cultures always compatible with the mainstream (corporate) culture that pervades the Internet? Third, to what degree will the future demand high-speed (at home) Internet to compete in an increasingly demanding domestic and global economy? Finally, to what degree is rural Internet access a necessity to rural public health (now and in the future)?

Key Terms

infrastructure

political voice

rurality

social capital

References

AAFP. (2009). Rural practice, keeping physicians in. Retrieved from http://www.aafp.org/online/en/home/policy/policies/r/ruralpracticekeep.printerview.html

Blumenthal, S. J., & Kagen, J. (2002). The effects of socioeconomic status on health in rural and urban America. *Journal of the American Medical Association, 287*(1), 109.

Bolin, J., & Gamm, L. (2003). Access to quality health services in rural areas-insurance: A literature review. *Rural healthy people 2010: A companion document to Healthy People 2010* (Vol. 2). College Station: The Texas A&M University System Health Science Center, School of Rural Public Health, Southwest Rural Health Research Center.

Brooks, R. G., Walsh, M., Mardon, R. E., Lewis, M., & Clawson, A. (2002). The roles of nature and nurture in the recruitment and retention of primary care physicians in rural areas: A review of the literature. *Academic Medicine, 77*(8), 790–798.

CCHD (Center for Community Health Development). (2010). *Brazos Valley health assessment: Regional report.* College Station, TX: The Texas A&M University System Health Science Center, School of Rural Public Health.

Eberhardt, M. S., & Pamuk, E. R. (2004). The importance of place of residence: Examining health in rural and nonrural areas. *American Journal of Public Health, 94*(10), 1682–1686.

Eckholm, E. (2007, April 22). In turnabout, infant deaths climb in South. *New York Times.* Retrieved from http://www.nytimes.com/2007/04/22/health/22infant.html

ERS (Economic Research Service). (2004). Retrieved from http://www.ers.usda.gov/

Farley, T., & Cohen, D. A. (2005). *Prescription for a healthy nation.* Boston: Beacon Press.

Folland, S. (2007). Does "community social capital" contribute to population health? *Social Science and Medicine, 64*(11), 2342–2354.

Galambos, C. M. (2005). Health care disparities among rural populations: A neglected frontier. *Health and Social Work, 30*(3), 179–181.

Gamm, L., Castillo, G., & Pittman, S. (2003). Access to quality health services in rural areas—primary care: A literature review. *Rural healthy people 2010: A companion document to Healthy People 2010* (Vol. 2). College Station: The Texas A&M University System Health Science Center, School of Rural Public Health, Southwest Research Center.

Hart, L. G., Larson, E. H., & Lishner, D. M. (2005). Rural definitions for health policy and research. *American Journal of Public Health, 95*(7), 1149–1155.

Hofferth, S. L., & Iceland, J. (1998). Social capital in rural and urban communities. *Rural Sociology, 63*(4), 574–598.

IOM. (2005). *Quality through collaboration: The future of rural health.* Washington, DC: National Academies Press.

Israel, G. D., Beaulieu, L. J., & Hartless, G. (2001). The influence of family and community social capital on educational achievement. *Rural Sociology, 66*(1), 43–68.

Kreuter, M. W., & Lezin, N. A. (in press). Social capital theory: Implications for community-based health promotion. In R. J. DiClemente, R. A. Crosby, & M. C. Kegler (Eds.), *Emerging theories in health promotion practice and research.* San Francisco: Jossey-Bass.

Mokdad, A. H., Marks, J. S., Stroup, D. F., & Gerberding, J. L. (2004). Actual causes of death in the United States, 2000. *Journal of the American Medical Association, 291*(10), 1238–1245.

Murray, C.J.L., Kulkarni, S. C., Michaud, C., Tomijima, N., Bulzacchelli, M. T., Iandiorio, T. J., et al. (2006). Eight Americas: Investigating mortality disparities across races, counties, and race-counties in the United States. *PLoS Med, 3*(9), e260.

NIDDK. (2002). *The Pima Indians: Pathfinders for health.* Retrieved from http://www.diabetes.niddk.nih.gov/dm/pubs/pima/index.htm

Osterberg, D., & Wallinga, D. (2004). Addressing externalities from swine production to reduce public health and environmental impacts. *American Journal of Public Health, 94*(10), 1703–1708.

Pathman, D. E., Konrad, T. R., Dann, R., & Koch, G. (2004). Retention of primary care physicians in rural health professional shortage areas. *American Journal of Public Health, 94*(10), 1723–1729.

Phillips, C. D., & McLeroy, K. R. (2004). Health in rural America: Remembering the importance of place. *American Journal of Public Health, 94*(10), 1661–1663.

Probst, J. C., Moore, C. G., Glover, S. H., & Samuels, M. E. (2004). Person and place: The compounding effects of race/ethnicity and rurality on health. *American Journal of Public Health, 94*(10), 1695–1703.

Putnam, R. D. (2000). *Bowling alone: The collapse and revival of American community*. New York: Touchstone.

Ricketts, T. C. (2000). The changing nature of rural health care. *Annual Review of Public Health, 21*, 639–657.

Rosenblatt, R. A., & Hart, L. G. (1999). Physicians and rural America. In T. C. Ricketts (Ed.), *Rural health in the United States*. New York: Oxford University Press.

RUPRI. (2006). *Demographic and economic profile: Nonmetropolitan America*. Columbia, SC: Author.

Schoenberg, N. E., Hatcher, J., Dignan, M. B., Shelton, B., Wright, S., & Dollarhide, K. F. (2009). Faith moves mountains: A cervical cancer prevention program in Appalachia. *American Journal of Health Behavior, 33*(6), 627–638.

Schur, C. L., & Franco, S. J. (1999). Access to health care. In T. C. Ricketts (Ed.), *Rural health in the United States*. New York: Oxford University Press.

United States Department of Agriculture Economic Research Service. (2005, January). *Agriculture Information Bulletin Number 795*, p. 3. Retrieved from http://www.ers.usda.gov/publications/aib795/aib795_lowres.pdf

Wendel, M. L. (2009). *Social capital and health: Individual measures, community influences, and persistent questions* (dissertation). College Station, TX: The Texas A&M University System Health Science Center, School of Rural Public Health.

Chapter 2

Defining Rurality

L. Gary Hart
Baretta R. Casey

Learning Objectives

- Understand the many definitions for rurality.
- Identify the most used taxonomies and their use by various agencies.
- Understand the role of geographical taxonomies when allocating federal and state resources.
- Develop use of appropriate taxonomies to ensure reliable, valid, and unbiased data to address disparities.

•••

The term *rural* suggests many things to many people, such as agricultural landscapes, isolation, small towns, and low-population density. However, defining *rural* for health policy and research purposes requires researchers and policy analysts to specify which aspects of rurality are most relevant to the topic at hand and then select an appropriate geographic **taxonomy** (i.e., definition or classification). Rural taxonomies often do not characterize important demographic, cultural, and economic differences across rural places, which is necessary for effective health policy and research. Factors such as **geographic** (i.e., having to do with the earth's surface and distributions on it) scale (e.g., cities, counties, and states) and region also must be considered. Several useful rural taxonomies are discussed and compared in this chapter. Careful attention to the **definition** of *rural* and what it means is required for effectively targeting policy and research aimed at improving the health of rural Americans (see Hart, Larson, & Lishner, 2005).

Only by defining *rural* appropriately can we discern differences in health care issues and outcomes across rural areas and between rural and **urban** (i.e., densely populated city) locales. The definition of rurality used for some purposes may be inadequate for other purposes (Hart, Larson, & Lishner, 2005). Inappropriate definitions may bias research findings and policy analyses. Inappropriately conceived and applied rural taxonomies can mask important health care delivery and disease disparities and thus handicap ameliorative policies.

The United States has evolved from a rural agricultural society to a society dominated by its urban population. Depending on which definition is used, roughly 20 percent of the population resides within rural areas. Approximately three-fourths of the nations' counties are rural, as is about 97 percent of its landmass. Although the rural population is in the minority, it comprises the size of France's total (rural and urban) population. As important as the rural population and its resources are to the nation, there is considerable confusion as to exactly what rural means and where rural populations reside. This chapter will define *rural* and describe why it is important to do so in the context of health care policy and research (Hart, Larson, & Lishner, 2005).

Approximately three-fourths of the nations' counties are rural, as is about 97 percent of its landmass.

Key Concepts

Geographic taxonomies are critical to the governmental allocation of scarce resources. They act as eligibility criteria for a cornucopia of federal and state programs. Good geographic taxonomies coupled with additional information can be employed to better target the allocation of resources to those in most need, which reduces waste and pinpoints where resources will do the most good. These cases and others regarding the importance of geographic definitions of rural, urban, frontier, and intrarural are well portrayed by Hewitt (1989) and are also available from many other sources (e.g., Coburn et al., 2007; Cromartie & Bucholtz, 2008; Hart et al., 2005; Isserman, 2005, 2007; Morrill, Cromartie, & Hart, 1999; Ricketts, Johnson-Webb, & Taylor, 1998).

Although many policy makers, researchers, and policy analysts would prefer one standardized definition, *rural* is a multifaceted concept about which there is no universal agreement. Defining rurality can be elusive and frequently relies on stereotypes and personal experiences. The term suggest pastoral landscapes, unique demographic structures and settlement patterns, isolation, low population density, extractive economic activities, and distinct sociocultural milieus. But these aspects of rurality fail to completely define *rural*. For example, rural cultures can exist in urban places. Only a small fraction of the rural population is involved in farming, and towns range from tens of thousands to only a handful of residents. The proximity of rural areas to urban cores and services may range from a few miles to hundreds of miles. Generations of rural sociologists, demographers, and geographers have struggled with these concepts (Hart, Larson, & Lishner, 2005).

Health care researchers focus great attention and time on statistical methodologies but geographic methodologies are often neglected. Deciding which rural definition to apply to a research or policy analysis topic depends on the purpose at hand, the availability of data, as well as the appropriate and available taxonomy. There is no perfect rural definition that meets all purposes. Researchers much be deliberate and insightful when defining rural and when applying the appropriate definition and its associated taxonomy to program targeting, intervention, and research (Hart, Larson, & Lishner, 2005).

An overview of the literature suggests that a fairly small group of factors are included in most of the rural taxonomies. The Census Bureau used population density (areas of fewer than two people per square mile) exclusively in its nineteenth-century definition. In contemporary applications, geographic remoteness has been equally emphasized. For instance, McGranahan and Beale (2002) identified a set of frontier counties based on two measures applied to nonmetropolitan counties: population density (fewer than 10.1 persons per square mile) and nonadjacency to a metro area as a proxy for remoteness. Many other measures attempt to capture these overlapping but distinct concepts of sparseness and remoteness (in no particular order): population size, distance to urban areas (measured in linear miles, travel miles, or travel time), and degree of urbanization. Hewitt (1989) provided a basic description of these factors and others (such as type of economic specialization) and the apparent reasoning behind their use.

Many of the listed factors have a face validity that is quite obvious. For instance, society's perception of rural areas is that they are places where the population settlement pattern demonstrates low density (i.e., sparsely settled areas). In addition to the monograph by Hewitt, there are several other journal articles and monographs that address the differences in selected rural definitions (e.g., Coburn et al., 2007; Cromartie & Bucholtz, 2008; Hall, Kaufman, & Ricketts, 2006; Hart, Larson, & Lishner, 2005; Isserman, 2005; Ricketts, Johnson-Webb, & Taylor, 1998; Vanderboom & Madigan, 2007). Most rural and frontier geographic taxonomies use a subset of the listed factors in combination to create their geographic taxonomies.

In addition to taxonomies that attempt to measure rurality, there has been a history and an increased interest in defining frontier areas. This is a geographical concept meant to delineate areas characterized primarily by remoteness from population centers that have larger populations and high population density. It is appropriate to adopt the term in this context because it has always been used to describe distinctive aspects of America's population as Europeans expanded into remote areas of North America, and its meaning has always shifted with the times (Prescott, 1978; Turner, 1921).

Most of the rural definitions are based on counties as the geographic unit. The most important reasons for using counties are as follows:

- They have much available data.
- They are significant political entities.
- They seldom change boundaries.
- They are traditionally used in many reporting systems and data sets.
- They are well known to the populace, program managers, researchers, and politicians.

However, there are significant problems with using counties. Counties were created by means of political processes and often are extremely heterogeneous units whose aggregate averages on data items end up being representative of nowhere within the county. Furthermore, the urban-rural character within many counties differs dramatically. For instance, Pima County, Arizona, ranges from an urban city of over half a million population near its northeast corner to large remote areas that are extremely sparsely populated along its southwest Mexico–United States border. Likewise, many counties or groups of counties underbound their built-up areas (i.e., small parts of the actual built-up urban area cross the county lines into predominantly rural counties). Some large states such as Arizona (114,006 square miles—significantly larger than the United Kingdom) have few counties (17 counties), and smaller states such as Virginia (42,769 square miles) have many smaller counties (134 counties). Counties vary in size from state to state, with the counties in the West generally being much larger than those in the East.

Use of different rural definitions can make far-reaching differences in estimates of important factors. The choice of definition for *rural* that is used to present demographic and health data can make a substantive difference. For example, whether a disproportionate number of rural residents are elderly depends on how rural is defined. Furthermore, wide variations in health status indicators within nonmetropolitan areas will not be apparent unless nonmetropolitan data are disaggregated by region, urbanization, proximity to urban areas, or other relevant factors (Hewitt, 1989). When the two most used taxonomies are compared (the Metropolitan of the Office of Management and Budget [OMB] and the Census Bureau's Urbanized Areas–Urban Clusters) 17.9 percent of the US population is categorized as being either metro-rural or nonmetro-urban. Thus, depending on how these categories are handled, the rural population of the United States can be estimated at anywhere from 10.3 percent to 28.2 percent of the nation's total population. Such variation results in vastly different reported information depending on which definition is employed. Although having rural definitions that fluctuate in geographic units and criteria is not inherently bad because they may be used for different purposes, this example demonstrates that choice of definitions is important. It often leads to confusion when estimates based on two different taxonomies yield considerably different results. Clearly, the choice of existing geographic taxonomies and the development of new taxonomies are limited by the availability of data at various geographic scales (e.g., county, census tract, and residential zonal improvement program [ZIP] code area, block, and phone number codes). The confidentiality of data for small geographic units often makes access to these data either difficult or impossible.

The rural population of the United States can be estimated at anywhere from 10.3 percent to 28.2 percent of the nation's total population.

Some taxonomies are based on subcounty units, with interest increasing in subcounty units since the early 1990s (Dahmann & Fitzsimmons, 1995). The oldest and most-used geographic taxonomy is that of the US Census Bureau. The census tract data defines urbanized areas and urban clusters. The other taxonomy that has gained significant use, especially related to health care, is rural-urban commuting areas (RUCAs). In this taxonomy, census tracts are grouped using some of the Census Bureau's urban place size information coupled with Census Bureau work-commuting information. This taxonomy has thirty-three categories that can be aggregated in various ways to meet specific needs. There is also a ZIP code approximation of the RUCAs.

Geographic Taxonomy Development Concerns

An appropriate rural and urban geographic taxonomy (and frontier definitions) should accomplish the following:

- Measure something explicit and meaningful
- Be replicable (reliable)
- Be derived from available, high-quality data
- Be quantifiable and objective and not subjective
- Have on-the-ground validity
- Be practical and straightforward

- Be policy relevant but independent of specific program biases
- Be considered one of several toolkit geographic taxonomies

The concepts of *rural* and *urban* exist as part of a continuum but federal policies generally rely on dichotomous urban-rural differences based on designations of the OMB or the Census Bureau (Hewitt, 1989). Many of the rural definitions use a single rural classification and fail to distinguish subcategories of rural. Rural areas are not homogeneous across the nation and aggregating rural areas of differing sizes and levels of remoteness frequently obscures emerging problems at the local level. As a result, policies may fail to include appropriate intrarural targeting (Hart, Larson, & Lishner, 2005).

In the health care field, the monograph entitled *Defining "Rural" Areas: Impact on Health Care Policy and Research* by Maria Hewitt (1989) stands as a milestone work. It summarizes the literature, contrasts the most-used taxonomies, characterizes those factors most often employed in rural-related taxonomies, and describes the consequences such taxonomies play in health care policy.

Each of the most frequently used and recent geographic taxonomies are briefly discussed in the following sections. The first five are most frequently used in public health and health care.

Office of Management and Budget Metropolitan Taxonomy

The federal government most frequently uses the county-based OMB metropolitan and nonmetropolitan classifications as policy tools. These county-based definitions are the foundation for other, more detailed taxonomies and are used when determining eligibility and reimbursement levels for more than thirty federal programs, including Medicare reimbursement levels, the Medicare incentive payment program, and programs designed to ameliorate provider shortages in rural areas. Metropolitan areas were defined in 2003 as central counties with one or more urbanized areas (cities with a population greater than or equal to fifty thousand) and outlying counties that are economically tied to the core, which were measured by commuting to work. Of the 3,141 US counties, there are 1,100 metropolitan counties (in 366 metropolitan statistical areas) and 2,041 nonmetropolitan counties (686 micropolitan in 573 micropolitan statistical areas and 1,355 noncore areas).

Per 2009 Census Bureau estimates, there are 239 million metropolitan and 49 million nonmetropolitan residents, of whom 29 million lived in micropolitan counties and 20 million lived in noncore counties. Micropolitan counties are those nonmetropolitan counties with a rural cluster with a population of ten thousand or more. Noncore counties are the residual (the remainder). The most significant problem with this taxonomy is that county boundaries overbound (i.e., urban county boundaries extend past urban built-up areas and include rural areas) and underbound their urban cores. The metropolitan and nonmetropolitan taxonomies were most recently updated in 2003 in accordance with the 2000 census data.

This definition has changed names over the decades. They were originally called standard metropolitan statistical areas (SMSAs) and then metropolitan statistical areas (MSAs). They are now called metropolitan areas (MAs). The 2000 census methods were especially different than they were in 1980 and earlier (Hart, Larson, & Lishner, 2005; Slifkin, Randolph, & Ricketts, 2004). Micropolitan counties were added to the definition for the 2000 census data.

US Census Bureau Urbanized Area, Urban Cluster, and Rural Taxonomy

The Census Bureau partitions urban areas into urbanized areas and urban clusters. The same census tract–based criteria are used for both; however, the urbanized areas have cores with populations of 50,000 or more and the urban clusters have cores with populations that range from 2,500 to 49,999. All other areas are designated as rural. The nation has more than 65,000 census tracts that are made up of blocks and block groups. In 2000, fifty-nine million residents—21 percent of the US population—were deemed rural by the Census Bureau taxonomy. The Census Bureau's rural and urban taxonomy is the source of much of the available demographic and economic data. A weakness of this system with regard to health care policy is the paucity of health-related data at the census tract level. The Census Bureau and others often aggregate urban clusters with urbanized area data. Depending on the purpose at hand, this may be misleading for rural health policy makers. For example, a town with a population of three thousand in a very remote area is considered urban under the Census Bureau definition but that same town is often nonmetropolitan under the OMB definition.

Economic Research Service (ERS) Rural-Urban Continuum Codes (RUCCs)

This county-based taxonomy (often referred to as the Beal codes after its lead developer) distinguishes metropolitan counties by the population size of their metro area. Nonmetropolitan counties are characterized by degree of urbanization (size of their urban population—living in places of 2,500 or more) and adjacency to a metropolitan area or areas that have at least 2 percent of their workforce commuting to the metropolitan area. The RUCCs were first created in 1974 and were last updated in 2003. The ten categories (i.e., four metro and six nonmetro) are as follows:

Metropolitan

0. Central counties of metro areas of one million population or more
1. Fringe counties of metro areas of one million population or more

2. Counties in metro area of 150,000 to one million population

3. Counties in metro areas of fewer than 250,000 population

Nonmetropolitan

4. Urban population of 20,000 or more, adjacent to a metro area

5. Urban population of 20,000 or more, not adjacent to a metro area

6. Urban population of 2,500 to 19,999, adjacent to a metro area

7. Urban population 2,500 to 19,999, not adjacent to a metro area

8. Completely rural or fewer than 2,500 urban population, adjacent to a metro area

9. Completely rural or fewer than 2,500 urban population, not adjacent to a metro area

The split between the metropolitan and nonmetropolitan codes is the same as for the OMB metropolitan taxonomy. The most rural of the codes can be considered frontierlike.

ERS Urban Influence Codes (UICs)

This twelve-code county-based taxonomy is similar to the RUCC taxonomy. It distinguishes metropolitan counties by the population size of their metro area. Nonmetropolitan counties are characterized by degree of urbanization (number of population living in the largest urban place) and adjacency to a metropolitan area or areas that have at least 2 percent of their workforce commuting to the metropolitan area. Versions of the UICs are available for 1993 and 2003 (the coding criteria has changed between these code versions—specifically, there were only nine codes in 1993). The twelve categories (i.e., two metro and ten nonmetro) are as follows:

Metropolitan

1. Large metro with population of one million or more

2. Small metro area of less than one million population

Nonmetropolitan

3. Micropolitan area adjacent to large metro area

4. Noncore area adjacent to large metro area

5. Micropolitan area adjacent to small metro area

6. Noncore adjacent to small metro area and contains a town of at least 2,500 residents

7. Noncore adjacent to small metro area and does not contain a town of at least 2,500 residents

8. Micropolitan area not adjacent to a metro area

9. Noncore area adjacent to a micropolitan area and contains a town of at least 2,500 residents

10. Noncore area adjacent to micropolitan area and does not contain a town of at least 2,500 residents

11. Noncore area not adjacent to a metro or micropolitan area and contains a town of at least 2,500

12. Noncore area not adjacent to a metro or micropolitan area and does not contain a town of at least 2,500 residents

Rural-Urban Commuting Areas (RUCAs)

This taxonomy uses census tract-level demographic and work-commuting data to define thirty-three categories of rural and urban census tracts. The RUCAs were developed and are maintained by the Economic Research Service (John Cromartie) and through funding from the Federal Office of Rural Health Policy to Gary Hart and Richard Morrill (Cromartie, Morrill, & Hart, 1999; http://depts.washington.edu/uwruca/index.php; http://www.ers.usda.gov/briefing/rurality/ruralurbancommutingareas/).

The RUCA categories are based on the size of the settlements and towns as delineated by the Census Bureau and the functional relationships between places as measured by tract-level work-commuting data. For example, a small town where the majority of commuting is to a large city is distinguished from a similarly sized town where there is commuting connectivity primarily to other small towns. Because thirty-three categories can be unwieldy, the codes were designed to be aggregated in various ways that highlight different aspects of connectivity, rural and urban settlement, and isolation, aspects that facilitate better program intervention targeting. The census tract version of the RUCAs has been supplemented by a ZIP code–based version. There are more than thirty thousand ZIP code areas.

RUCAs range from the core areas of urbanized areas to isolated small rural places, where the population is less than 2,500 and where there is no meaningful work commuting to urbanized areas. Although the ZIP code version of the RUCAs is slightly less precise than the census tract version, the RUCA ZIP codes are advantageous in the health field because they can be used with ZIP code health-related data. The RUCAs are widely used for policy and research purposes (e.g., by the Centers for Medicare and Medicaid Services, the Federal Office of Rural Health Policy, and many researchers). RUCAs can identify the rural portions of metropolitan counties and the urban portions of nonmetropolitan counties. RUCAs are flexible and can be grouped in many ways to suit particular analytic or policy purposes.

Veterans Health Administration Office of Rural Health Classification

This 2009 classification is a modification of the Census Bureau's urbanized area, urban cluster, and rural taxonomy. It is based on census tracts. The classification has three categories. Urban is defined the same as the Census Bureau's urbanized areas. Rural is defined as those places not located within urbanized areas. The highly rural category is those places that qualify as rural and that are located within counties that have fewer than seven civilians per square mile. The use of this classification results in veterans being divided as follows: urban, 62.2 percent; rural, 36.3 percent; and highly rural, 1.5 percent.

National Center for Frontier Communities Frontier Consensus Definition

This National Center for Frontier Communities county-based definition was developed through a consensus process started by the Frontier Education Center in 1997 and was most recently updated in 2007. A matrix of weighted elements was developed based on density, distance, and travel time. The consensus group created a typology in which density of counties was coded as fewer than twelve, twelve to sixteen, and sixteen to twenty persons per square mile. Distance to a service or market was coded greater than ninety, sixty to ninety, twenty to sixty, and less than thirty miles. Travel time to service or market was coded greater than ninety, sixty to ninety, thirty to sixty, and less than thirty minutes. A unique aspect of the application of the consensus definition is the involvement of states throughout the process. The matrix and a list of potential counties are provided to a state, which could then analyze local conditions and provide a list of frontier areas therein. This final definition was developed to be inclusive of extremes of distance, isolation, and population density (National Center for Frontier Communities, 2012).

Federal Community Health Center Frontier Taxonomy (Six Persons per Square Mile)

In the mid-1980s, the federal Community Health Centers program decided to consider as frontier those counties with a population less than or equal to six persons per square mile located at considerable distance (greater than sixty minutes' travel time) to a medical facility able to perform a caesarian section delivery or handle a patient having a cardiac arrest. These latter criteria were forgotten through the years and programs began to define frontier counties with only the single criterion—population density of less than or equal to six persons per square mile. This county-based definition has endured and been used in myriad federal programs to identify "frontier" counties for the purposes of resource allocations of assorted types. Nearly all the designated frontier counties are west of the Mississippi.

Isserman Urban-Rural Density Typology

Recently a county-based taxonomy entitled the Urban-Rural Density Typology was introduced by Andrew Isserman (2005). The taxonomy, based on 2000 census data, has four categories of counties (number of counties): rural (1,790), urban (171), mixed rural (1,022), and mixed urban (158). The categories are differentiated by overall county population density and the percentage of the county population residing within high-density areas of various population numbers and density thresholds.

Telehealth Frontier Definition

This definition was developed by the University of North Dakota's Center for Rural Health (2006) through the use of an expert panel and associated analyses for the federal Office for the Advancement of Telehealth (OAT). The definition was specifically targeted for the needs of the OAT. It designates as telehealth frontier ZIP code areas that meet the following criteria: ZIP code areas whose calculated population centers are more than sixty minutes or sixty miles along the fastest paved road trip to a short-term nonfederal general hospital of seventy-five beds or more and are not part of a larger rural town with a concentration of more than twenty thousand population (Center for Rural Health, 2006). The definition was based on various data sources from 1998 to 2002 data and was subsequently updated to data from 2002 to 2005. The definition has not been approved for OAT use by Health Resources and Service Administration (HRSA).

Index of Relative Rurality (IRR)

This index is scaled from zero to one (zero equals most urban and one equals most rural) and has four data components: population, population density, extent of urbanized area, and distance to the nearest metro area (Waldorf, 2006). The IRR uses counties as the unit of analysis. However, the IRR could be applied to different geographic units such as aggregations of counties or census tracts. The IRR is the result of dividing the unweighted mean rescaled to a zero-to-one scale for each factor and then the sum is divided by four.

Island Geographic Taxonomies

A review of the literature dealing with island taxonomies related to frontier-remote status was performed. Although there were some materials that deal with culture, race and ethnicity, histories, and the like, no taxonomies associated with frontier-remote status were located. One document that was obtained in the literature search was a policy statement by the Hawaii Primary Association entitled *Island Designation* (2008). The advocacy brief argued that an island designation is necessary because of the following:

- The ocean is a significant barrier to accessing services.
- Air transportation is expensive and often not frequent; in bad weather air and ferry traffic stop.
- The Pacific island populations are scattered over an immense area.
- Many of the islands have few health care services (e.g., primary care providers, hospitals, and pharmacies—along with dependable electricity and water).
- There's a lack of well-prepared administrators.
- Many islands and jurisdictions significantly have underfunded health care services.
- Many of the islands are extremely culturally diverse.
- Health status on many of the islands is extremely poor.
- Many serious infectious diseases remain significant health threats.
- The costs of medical supplies and facility construction and upkeep are expensive.

Conclusion

Deciding which rural definition to apply to an area depends on the purpose at hand, the availability of data, and the appropriate and available taxonomy. There is no perfect rural definition that meets all purposes. Researchers must be deliberate and insightful when defining *rural* and when applying the appropriate definition and its associated taxonomy to program targeting, intervention, and research. It is recommended that researchers familiarize themselves with various rural definitions and geographic methodologies and then carefully weigh the pros and cons of available definitions (see a table comparing many of these definitions in Hart, Larson, & Lishner, 2005).

Defining rural and urban must be a methodological priority at the start of any program, project, or research examining health-related concerns associated with the rural and urban dimensions. Grappling early and systematically with the problems of defining rurality will significantly enhance the validity and the utility of health research work, which is essential in rural-focused health research (Hart, Larson, & Lishner, 2005).

Summary

- Appropriately defining rurality for a targeted individual and unique rural community is imperative to avoid issues such as biased research findings and policy analyses when addressing health disparities in program interventions, projects, and research.

- There is no single standardized definition of *rural*; it is a multifaceted concept about which there is no universal agreement.
- There is no perfect rural definition that meets all purposes. Determining the appropriate rural definition to apply to a research or policy analysis topic depends on the goals and objectives, available data, and appropriate taxonomy.
- Geographical taxonomies play a key role when allocating federal and state resources and should meet specific criteria in reliability, validity, and other requirements for appropriate and effective use.

Key Terms

definition(s)	taxonomy(ies)
geographic	urban
rural	

For Practice and Discussion

1. Working in a group of three or more students, discuss the strengths and weaknesses of each taxonomy presented in this chapter. After this discussion, see if the group can come to a consensus regarding which one would be the best choice if your purpose was to investigate rural health disparities.

2. Go online to determine the classification of the county you reside in currently. Determine how many different classification systems have been applied to your county and list how your county is classified by each of these systems. As a resident, describe which taxonomy best captures the true urban-rural location of your home county.

References

Center for Rural Health, University of North Dakota. (2006, May). *Defining the term "frontier area" for programs implemented through the Office for the Advancement of Telehealth*. Grand Forks: Center for Rural Health, University of North Dakota.

Coburn, A., MacKinney, A., McBride, T., Mueller, K., Slifkin, R., & Wakefield, M. (2007, March). Choosing rural definitions: Implications for health policy. Issue brief #2. Columbia, MO: Rural Policy Research Institute.

Cromartie, J., & Bucholtz, S. (2008). Defining the "rural" in rural America. *Amber Waves, 6*(3), 28–34.

Dahmann, D., & Fitzsimmons, J. (1995). *Metropolitan and nonmetropolitan areas: New approaches to geographical definition.* Working Paper No. 12. Washington, DC: US Bureau of the Census.

Hall, S., Kaufman, J., & Ricketts, T. (2006). Defining urban and rural areas in U.S. epidemiologic studies. *Journal of Urban Health, 83*(2), 162–175.

Hart, G., Larson, E., & Lishner, D. (2005). Rural definitions for health policy and research. *American Journal of Public Health, 95*(7), 1149–1155.

Hewitt, M. (1989). Defining "rural" areas: Impact on health care policy and research. Washington, DC: United States. Congress, Office of Technology Assessment.

Hawaii Primary Care Association. (2008). Island designation. Honolulu: Author.

Isserman, A. (2005). In the national interest: Defining rural and urban correctly in research and public policy. *International Regional Science Review, 28*(4), 465–499.

Isserman, A. (2007). Getting state rural policy right: Definitions, growth, and program eligibility. *The Journal of Regional Analysis & Policy, 37*(1), 72–79.

McGranahan, D., & Beale, C. (2002). Understanding rural population loss. *Rural America, 17*, 4, 2–11.

Morrill, R., Cromartie, J., & Hart, G. (1999). Metropolitan, urban, and rural commuting areas: Toward a better depiction of the United States settlement system. *Urban Geography, 20*(8), 727–748.

National Center for Frontier Communities. (2012). Retrieved from http://frontierus.org/index-current.htm

Prescott, J. (1978). *Boundaries and frontiers.* Lanham, MD: Rowman and Littlefield.

Rickets, T., Johnson-Webb, K., & Taylor, P. (1998, July). *Definitions of rural: A handbook for health policy makers and researchers.* Chapel Hill: Cecil G. Sheps Center for Health Services Research, University of North Carolina.

Slifkin, R., Randolph, R., & Ricketts, T. (2004). The changing metropolitan designation process and rural America. *The Journal of Rural Health, 20*(1), 1–6.

Turner, F. (1921). *The frontier in American history.* New York: Holt.

Vanderboom, C., & Madigan, E. (2007). Federal definitions of rurality and the impact on nursing research. *Research in Nursing & Health, 30*(2), 175–184.

Waldorf, B. (2006, July 24–27). *A continuous multi-dimensional measure of rurality: Moving beyond threshold measures.* Paper prepared for and presented at the American Agricultural Economics Association Annual Meeting, Long Island, California.

Selected Relevant Websites

Census Bureau Urbanized Area, Urban Cluster, and Rural: http://www.census.gov/geo/www/ua/ua_2k.html

Department of Agriculture Rural Information Center: http://ric.nal.usda.gov/

ERS Measuring Rurality: 2004 County Typology Codes: http://www.ers.usda.gov/Briefing/Rurality/Typology/

ERS Measuring Rurality: Commuting Zones and Labor Market Areas: http://www.ers.usda.gov/Briefing/Rurality/LMACZ/

ERS Rural-Urban Commuting Area Codes (RUCA): http://www.ers.usda.gov/Data/
RuralUrbanCommutingAreaCodes/

ERS Rural-Urban Continuum Codes (RUC): http://www.ers.usda.gov/Data/
RuralUrbanContinuumCodes/

ERS Measuring Rurality: Urban Influence Codes (UIC): http://www.ers.usda.gov/
Briefing/Rurality/UrbanInf/

Federal Office of Rural Health Policy (ORHP): http://www.hrsa.gov/ruralhealth/

HRSA Rural Health Grants Eligibility Analyzer: http://datawarehouse.hrsa.gov/
RuralAdvisor/

*Index of Relative Rurality (IRR) and Regional Cluster (Department of Agricultural
Economics, Purdue University, Lafayette, Indiana; et al.):* http://
www.ibrc.indiana.edu/innovation/data.html

National Advisory Committee on Rural Health and Human Services (NACRHHS):
http://ruralcommittee.hrsa.gov/

National Center for Frontier Communities: http://frontierus.org/index-current.htm

National Organization of State Offices of Rural Health (NOSORH): http://
www.nosorh.org/

National Rural Health Association: http://www.ruralhealthweb.org/

OMB Metropolitan and Micropolitan Statistical Areas: http://www.census.gov/
population/www/metroareas/metroarea.html

Rural Assistance Center (RAC)—Am I Rural: http://maps.rupri.org/circ/racrural/
amirural.asp

Rural Assistance Center (RAC): http://www.raconline.org/

Rural Health Research Gateway: http://www.ruralhealthresearch.org/contact/

Rural Policy Research Institute (RUPRI): http://www.rupri.org/

*West Virginia Rural Health Research Center: A Rural Socioeconomic Vulnerability and
Resiliency Index and Associated Health Outcomes:* http://wvrhrc.hsc.wvu.edu/
docs/2009_halverson_policy_brief.pdf; http://wvrhrc.hsc.wvu.edu/docs/
2009_halverson_final_report.pdf

WWAMI RHRC Rural-Urban Commuting Areas (RUCAs): http://depts.washington.edu/
uwruca/

Chapter 3

History of Rural Public Health in America

Amy L. Elizondo
Alan Morgan

Learning Objectives

- Describe the history of rural public health in the United States.
- Explain how rural public health evolved and why rural areas are still lacking in public health infrastructure and services.
- Articulate how demographics, chronic disease prevalence, and geography contribute to health disparities in rural communities.

•••

Living and working in rural America should not have dire or significant implications for health status. The reality, however, is that rural health disparities exist and many organizations are dedicated to ensuring that rural residents are afforded the best possible health care irrespective of their location. We now know more about the degree to which rural health disparities exist than we did ten to fifteen years ago. That notwithstanding, what is known today indicates that rural residents still lag in health status, in some cases alarmingly so, in comparison to their urban counterparts. This knowledge lends itself to a great urgency for addressing rural health disparities, above all, to improve the quality of life for those who choose to call rural America home.

As described in detail in Chapter Two, defining rural America is a complex and a challenging task for policy makers and health care experts alike. For the purposes of this chapter, rural America can be characterized as being an expansive and sparsely populated geographic location where the population at large experiences avoidable "differences in the incidence, prevalence, mortality, and burden of diseases and other adverse health conditions" (Minority Health and Health Disparities Research and Education Act, 2000, p. 2498).

To best understand rural health disparities, one must first understand that being rural is not merely a smaller version of being urban. Rural America has specific history and defining characteristics that represent a unique health care delivery environment.

Key Concepts

This chapter examines the rural health disparities in light of the history of rural public health. The key concepts explored include population demographics, prevalence of chronic disease, and the geographic challenges that work to impede addressing health disparities.

Development of Rural Public Health Systems

Early in America's history, population centers grew up as a function of trade, many around ports or major routes of transit. Public health then focused largely on sanitation and control of communicable disease. The germ theory had not yet been developed but there was an understanding that the movement of people from place to place also moved illness from place to place. Because outbreaks of disease were most common in more populous areas, rural public health was less of a concern. Notably, the first cities to establish formal public health entities—boards of health—included Philadelphia, Baltimore, Boston, Washington, DC, New Orleans, and New York City, all between 1794 and 1805. State boards of health were established later, with Louisiana in 1855 and Massachusetts in 1869. The National Board of Health was not formed until 1879 and focused on developing state boards of health and standard measures for enacting quarantines; this board was soon subsumed by the Marine Hospital Service in 1882.

These government bodies sought to improve public health by targeting diseases thought to spread by poor sanitation and close living quarters. The context of transmission was observed and efforts to control the spread of disease were based on these observations. Because crowded, unsanitary conditions were seen as key to the spread of disease, living in rural areas was equated to cleanliness and good health. As the population grew and became more mobile during the Industrial Revolution, the country witnessed even greater spread of disease including to rural populations, and the need for rural public health emerged.

Much of the early public health services provided in rural communities were offered by nurses. Sometimes organized through voluntary associations and sometimes on their own, these nurses provided care to sick residents within their homes. This informal delivery of public health—urban and rural—was ultimately formalized as local boards of health began to employ public health nurses in the early 1900s. Unfortunately, local boards of health existed only within urban centers, so this formalization did not improve conditions in rural communities; nurses serving rural areas continued to do so on a voluntary basis.

Only as more disease was witnessed as being spread between urban and rural communities did there become a motivation for creating local health departments in rural areas. Outbreaks of typhoid fever in rural areas as well as other conditions such as hookworm and pellagra brought attention to the need for services in geographically isolated communities. County health departments were born from urban hubs, radiating out into less populous areas, and did not have public funding. Financial assistance to support these small health departments often came from private sources including foundations such as Rockefeller, W. K. Kellogg, and the Commonwealth Fund among others.

Although the movement to establish county health departments found traction relatively quickly, the Great Depression made financial viability difficult, and rural Americans were still left without adequate public health services. The flurry of programs immediately following the Depression, however, spurred on rural public health by making new funding streams available. It was also during this time that communicable diseases began to come under control through sanitation and immunization, and the role of local health departments shifted to delivery of basic health care services, which had been lacking in rural communities.

In 1945, Congress passed the **Hill-Burton Act,** which funded states to systematically create hospitals and health centers in rural areas, and became the foundation of rural public health in the United States. Whereas many rural communities still do not have a county health department, local health organizations such as these hospitals and clinics serve as critical anchors of public health for local residents.

Additional legislation that has promoted rural public health since the Hill-Burton Act includes Section 330 of the Public Health Service Act (1975) and the Rural Health Clinic Act of 1977. These acts sought to improve infrastructure and availability of clinical services within rural areas. In 1987, the Office of Rural Health Policy (ORHP) was created within the Health Resources and Services Administration to address problems for rural hospitals related to reimbursement for services. Since then, ORHP has expanded its assistance to rural communities through a series of grants, support for rural health research, policy advocacy, and coordination of border and international health commissions.

This brief account of the history of rural public health provides a context for understanding how rural health disparities in the United States have emerged and have been perpetuated over time. In light of this, the following sections describe the way rural community characteristics have since evolved and their influence in the production and maintenance of health disparities.

Population Demographics

Health care disparities in rural areas are well documented and are much higher than in urban or suburban areas. Rural areas are confounded by factors that include education and poverty levels. Rural populations on average have relatively more elderly and children, unemployment and underemployment, and poor, uninsured, and underinsured residents.

Rural populations on average have relatively more elderly and children, unemployment and underemployment, and poor, uninsured, and underinsured residents.

There are several factors that lead to health disparities in rural areas. A comprehensive research report released by the South Carolina Rural Health Research Center on rural minorities in 2002 provided further insights on what **population demographics** (characteristics such as the distribution of age, race, ethnicity, education, and income) looked like in rural areas. Geography, poverty, and health care infrastructure were some of the main factors that were assessed. The distribution of rural minorities shows that 70 percent of poor, nonmetro African Americans live in six southern states: Mississippi, Georgia, North Carolina, Louisiana, Alabama, and South Carolina; 73 percent of all poor, nonmetro Hispanics live in five southwestern states: Texas, New Mexico, California, Arizona, and Colorado; and 57 percent of all poor, nonmetro Native Americans inhabit five western states: Arizona, New Mexico, Oklahoma, South Dakota, and Montana (Probst et al., 2002).

In terms of poverty, 34 percent of rural African Americans are poor compared to 13 percent of nonmetro whites; 25 percent of the rural Hispanic population is poor; 34 percent of the rural Native American population is poor; with rural Asian and Pacific Islanders serving as the exception at 11 percent of this population is poor versus 13 percent of the white population (Probst et al., 2002). These findings are significant given the high proportion of minorities in rural areas and the high incidence of health disparities occurring in these areas.

It is important to recognize the range of health care resources available in rural areas and the extent to which these resources are available to multi-cultural and multiracial groups. Twelve percent of rural African Americans (compared to 10 percent of whites) reside in a county without a hospital. There

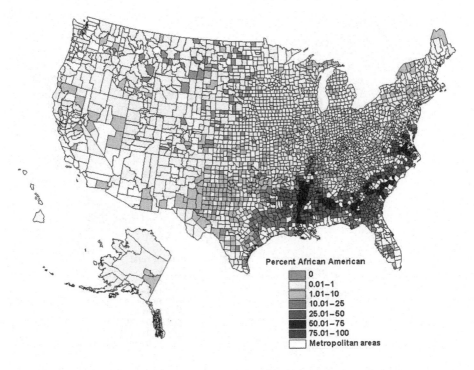

Figure 3.1. Percent of African Americans in Rural US Counties, 1999
Source: Probst et al. (2002), p. 38.

are 6.2 physicians for every ten thousand rural African Americans. For Hispanics residing in rural areas there are roughly 5.3 physicians per ten thousand residents. Additionally, 76 percent of Hispanics live in counties designated as **health professional shortage areas** (HPSAs)—a designation by the Health Resources and Services Administration related to the number of physicians per population. For Native Americans living in rural areas, there are 8.1 physicians for every ten thousand residents; however, 73 percent of rural Native Americans live in HPSA areas. See Figures 3.1 through 3.4 for an illustration of population demographics in rural areas (Probst et al., 2002).

Population demographics related to race and ethnicity, poverty levels, and health care infrastructure all affect the health status of rural residents. Disparities within these factors also lead to increased prevalence of chronic disease.

Prevalence of Chronic Disease

Once a clear understanding of population demographics in rural areas is established, one can then explore how these factors lead to impaired health status for rural individuals. The nation's private sector health insurance system is an

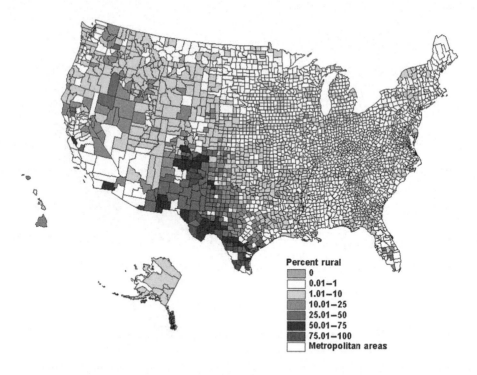

Figure 3.2. Percent of Each US Total Rural County Population That Is Hispanic, 1999
Source: Probst et al. (2002), p. 47.

employer-based system, thus posing a financial barrier for many rural residents who are not able to access insurance through their employer. This creates a challenge for rural residents who are self-employed, work for small businesses that do not provide health insurance, or are unemployed because they are less likely to have coverage.

Rural adults are also more likely to be uninsured than urban adults, with uninsurance rates among rural Hispanic adults at more than 50 percent. As a result, rural residents often delay seeking care due to cost. The average per capita income is $7,000 lower in rural than in urban areas, and rural Americans are more likely to live below the poverty level (Gamm & Hutchinson, 2005). Uninsured individuals, when compared to those who are insured, will rarely have a designated doctor they routinely see and tend to be hospitalized more often for conditions that are otherwise preventable. This is most apparent of rural minorities (Kaiser Commission on Medicaid and the Uninsured, 2006).

Uninsured individuals, when compared to those who are insured, will rarely have a designated doctor they routinely see and tend to be hospitalized more often for conditions that are otherwise preventable.

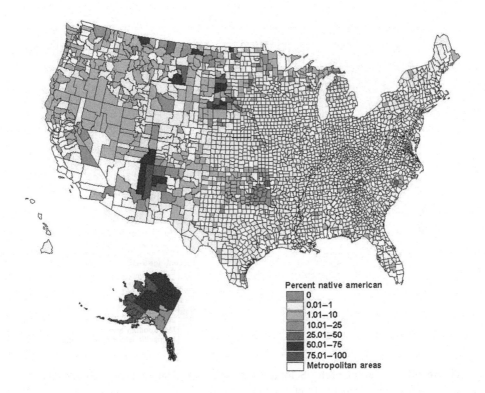

Figure 3.3. Percent of Each US Total Rural County Population That Is Native American, 1999
Source: Probst et al. (2002), p. 57.

Compromised access to health care in rural areas often directly results in higher rates of chronic diseases for rural residents. Small rural hospitals are typically the main source of care for rural residents. Many of these are critical access hospitals (CAHs) and have twenty-five beds or fewer. These are vital to rural communities because they are the first line of care for residents living in remote areas. However, these facilities are also challenged because of their size and case mix of patients. There are approximately 1,500 of these rural hospitals (Agency for Healthcare Research and Quality, 2009).

Although these CAH facilities are available to rural residents, this population is still less likely to access care because of costs even when faced with a critical illness. As a result there are chronic illnesses that are often perpetuated by this lack of access. Health care workforce shortages are also heightened in rural areas, adding to the increased challenge of access to care. Residents in rural areas tend to report their health as fair to poor (Bennett, Olatosi, & Probst, 2008).

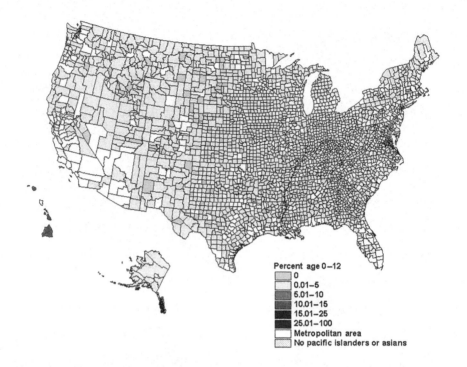

Figure 3.4. Percent of Each US Total Rural County Population That Is Pacific Islander or Asian and Ages 0 to 12, 1999
Source: Probst et al. (2002), p. 64.

Rural residents are also more likely to be obese compared to their urban counterparts, 27.4 percent compared to 23.9 percent (Bennett et al., 2008). Infant mortality, heart disease and stroke, cancer, mental health, diabetes, and HIV and AIDS are all disease conditions related to health disparities. Table 3.1 shows a breakdown of these health conditions with an index of selected populations to further highlight the prevalence of these diseases.

Other findings regarding prevalence of chronic diseases in rural areas include the following:

- Rural adults were more likely to report having diabetes than were urban adults.
- Native Americans reported having more limitations in their activities as a result of physical, mental, or emotional problems.
- Rural African Americans were particularly at risk for obesity.
- Rural residents are less likely to receive an annual dental exam.
- Rural women are less likely than urban women to be in compliance with mammogram screening guidelines.

Table 3.1. Health Disparities of Certain Diseases in Selected Populations

Health Condition and Specific Example	White	African American	Hispanic or Latino	Asian/ Pacific Islander	American Indian/ Alaska Native
Infant mortality rate per thousand live births	5.9	13.9	5.8	5.1	9.1
Cancer mortality rate per hundred thousand	199.3	255.1	123.7	124.2	129.3
Coronary heart disease mortality rate per hundred thousand	206	252	145	123	126
Stroke mortality rate per hundred thousand	58	80	39	51	38
Diabetes diagnosed rate per hundred thousand	36	74	61	DSU	See note.
End-stage renal disease rate per million	218	873	DNA	344	589
AIDS—diagnosed rate per hundred thousand female	2	48	13	1	5
AIDS—diagnosed rate per hundred thousand male	14	109	43	9	19

Note: Available data on American Indian/Alaska Native underestimates the true prevalence of diabetes; 40 to 70 percent of the forty-five- to seventy-four-year-old age group was found to have diabetes. DSU = data are statistically unreliable; DNA = data have not been analyzed.
Source: National Rural Health Association (2006).

- The death rate for people between the ages of one and twenty-four is 25 percent higher in rural areas than in urban areas (Bennett et al., 2008).

Geographic Challenges

Terrain, transportation, and distance pose additional barriers for many rural residents. Rural areas vary all across the country, and a common adage in this field is "if you have seen one rural area, you have seen one rural area." For example, frontier parts of Montana are different from rural parts of Arizona.

Frontier areas are the most remote and desolate areas found in some of the larger states. These areas, such as those in Alaska as well as other rural parts of the country, rely on telehealth technologies to help provide access to residents who are far removed from larger health facilities. The terrain found in states such as Alaska and Montana poses great challenges in trying to improve access to care. Physicians in some of these frontier areas have been known to acquire a pilot's license to help provide direct care in remote locations when driving is not an option during critical emergencies. Mountainous terrain and tundra found in some of these areas also make it difficult for rural residents to travel to the nearest hospital, especially when confounded by dramatic weather changes. There are roughly one thousand frontier counties in the country, with most having limited health care services and others having none at all (Agency for Healthcare Research and Quality, 2009).

Actual transportation to the nearest clinic or hospital is not always feasible. In addition to physicians' trying to personally fly to patients in need in the most frontier areas of the country, some programs are often tailored to offer mobile health units to bring care to rural residents who would otherwise not be able to physically travel to a health facility. Advances in technology are enabling some types of clinical care to be offered through telehealth—a secure, closed circuit, live teleconference feed with a provider on one side of the connection and a patient on the other.

Legislation over the years has improved the availability of health care facilities in many rural areas. However, travel time still poses a significant barrier when time is of the essence. Some residents face up to two hours travel time to seek care, which in emergencies is particularly staggering. Access to specialty care is also scarce because this type of care is more readily available in urban areas. Also, there is a great shortage of specialty physicians practicing in rural areas.

Conclusion

In summary, the history of rural public health in the United States provides a foundation for understanding the current context and composition of rural communities, including contributing factors that produce persistent health disparities. Just as the US Department of Health and Human Services has used *Healthy People* as a planning tool to address disparities on the national level, *Rural Healthy People* serves as a companion document to focus in on rural health priorities and models of practice. Using effective models of practice that were developed within rural communities holds significant promise for addressing similar issues in other communities. This includes efforts to improve the health care infrastructure of rural residents and enhancing community resources. These resources increase the capacity of communities to emphasize prevention, address chronic disease, and overcome geographic barriers by increasing health care services and new technologies.

Summary

- Rural public health is a relatively new phenomenon in the United States, initiated with the development of county health departments in 1908 and formally starting with the Hill-Burton Act of 1945.

- Many rural communities do not have county health departments and rely on local organizations such as hospitals and clinics to provide public health infrastructure.

- Population demographics, prevalence of chronic disease, and geographic challenges in rural communities perpetuate health disparities.

- Rural minorities experience poorer health outcomes, are less likely to seek care due to cost, and are often uninsured.

- Treating chronic illnesses that are initially preventable is a true challenge in rural areas when there is currently a health care workforce shortage in these areas.

- Terrain, distance, and geographic obstacles create a large barrier for rural residents in remote areas of the country.

- Advances in technology, the availability of health care resources, and empowering communities are important for addressing rural health disparities.

For Practice and Discussion

1. Working with one or two of your colleagues from class, identify and describe several factors in addition to population demographics that could contribute to the increased prevalence of chronic diseases in rural areas.

2. Describe the challenges to rural health care presented by the great diversity within rural America.

3. Go online or make a phone call and investigate the current services of any rural health department in your state. Then compare the services offered by that rural health department to services offered by an urban health department in the same state. Finally, compare the services offered by the rural health department to the services you think should be offered as a consequence of what you now know of the disparities experienced by rural Americans. What are the barriers

that preclude rural health departments from being able to offer a full complement of services?

Key Terms

health professional shortage areas   population demographics

Hill-Burton Act

References

Agency for Healthcare Research and Quality. (2009). *National healthcare disparities report* (pp. 266–267). Rockville, MD: Author. Retrieved from http://www.ahrq.gov/qual/nhdr09/nhdr09.pdf

Bennett, K., Olatosi, B., & Probst, J. C. (2008). *Health disparities: A rural-urban chartbook*. Columbia: South Carolina Rural Health Research Center. Retrieved from http://rhr.sph.sc.edu/report/SCRHRC_RuralUrbanChartbook_Exec_Sum.pdf

Gamm, L. D., & Hutchinson, L. L. (Eds.). (2005). *Rural healthy people 2010: A companion document for Healthy People 2010* (Vol. 3). College Station: The Texas A&M University System Health Science Center, School of Rural Public Health, Southwest Rural Health Research Center. Retrieved from www.srph.tamhsc.edu/centers/rhp2010/Volume_3/Vol3rhp2010.pdf

Kaiser Commission on Medicaid and the Uninsured. (2006). *The uninsured: A primer. Key facts about Americans without health insurance*. Washington, DC: Kaiser Family Foundation.

Minority Health and Health Disparities Research and Education Act, United States Public Law 106–525. (2000).

National Rural Health Association. (2006). *Racial and ethnic health disparities*. Kansas City, MO: Author. Retrieved from www.ruralhealthweb.org/go/left/policy-and-advocacy/policy-documents-and-statements/issue-papers-and-policy-briefs/

Probst, J. C., Samuels, M. E., Jespersen, K. P., Willert, K., Swann, R. S., & McDuffie, J. A. (2002). *Minorities in rural America: An overview of population characteristics*. Columbia: South Carolina Rural Health Research Center. Retrieved from http://rhr.sph.sc.edu/report/%281-1A%29Minorities%20in%20Rural%20America.pdf

Chapter 4

The Depth of Rural Health Disparities in America

The ABCDEs

James E. Florence   Jodi Southerland
Robert P. Pack   Randolph F. Wykoff

Learning Objectives

- Describe rural health disparities in terms of availability and access to health services.
- Explain behavioral patterns in rural communities that contribute to health disparities.
- Describe how certain elements of rural culture relate to health disparities.
- Articulate the relationship between poverty (and its determinants) and poor health status.
- Explain environmental influences on the production and maintenance of health disparities in rural communities.

•••

This chapter examines the depth of health disparities with respect to the domains of *a*vailability and access to health care in rural America, *b*ehavioral patterns, *c*ultural influences, *d*eterminants of socioeconomic origin, and *e*nvironmental factors affecting health in rural areas. The aim of this chapter is to provide a simple mnemonic device for public health practitioners to reference when planning a public health intervention in a rural setting: the ABCDEs of rural health in America.

Schroeder (2007) used somewhat similar domains in his explanation of the proportional influence of each on premature death. In his analysis, he found that access (ability to obtain) to care accounts for about 10 percent of premature deaths, behavior for about 40 percent, genetics for about 30 percent, social determinants for about 15 percent, and the environment for about 5 percent. Although these proportions may not demonstrate the same distribution for rural populations, they are instructive in identifying some of the key factors that produce and maintain health disparities in US communities.

Key Concepts

A variety of public health programs focus on different aspects of these factors in an attempt to reduce very specific disparities (e.g., education, occupation and economic status). Systematically evaluating these factors collectively will allow public health practitioners to take a comprehensive approach to understanding and addressing the unique health challenges of rural communities in which they serve.

Access to Health Care in Rural America

Many of the health and social problems faced by people living in rural and isolated communities are aggravated by lack of access to affordable health care. Although multiple factors contribute to reduced rural access, the primary challenges are as follows:

Many of the health and social problems faced by people living in rural and isolated communities are aggravated by lack of access to affordable health care.

- Shortages of health care professionals
- Lack of affordability of health care
- Geographic, cultural, and historic factors that affect the willingness or the ability of an individual to seek health care

Health Care Professional Shortages in Rural Areas

The shortage of physicians and other health care providers serving in rural communities is a well-documented, long-standing, and pervasive concern (Council on Graduate Medical Education, 1998; Ricketts, 1999). Although the number of people living in rural America is about 25 percent of the total population, less than 10 percent of US physicians practice in rural areas (Gamm et al., 2003). The primary care physician–to–patient ratio in rural areas is only three-fourths that of urban areas (fifty-five per hundred thousand population versus seventy-two per hundred thousand, respectively). In the most isolated rural areas this ratio drops to only half of urban areas (thirty-six per hundred thousand; Fordyce et al., 2007). Further limiting the ability of rural residents to access appropriate health care services is the fact that there are about half as many medical specialists in rural areas as compared to urban areas (Fordyce et al., 2007). Despite the acute and growing need for rural medical practitioners, only a handful of US medical schools consistently turn out more than one-fifth of their graduates who go on to practice in rural areas (Chen et al., 2010).

The Health Resources and Services Administration (HRSA) within the US Department of Health and Human Services maintains a variety of designations for communities to identify shortages in health facilities and providers. These designations include medically underserved areas (MUAs), medically underserved communities (MUCs), and health professional shortage areas (HPSAs); HPSAs are also broken down into primary care, mental health, and dental.

Not unexpectedly, HPSAs are much more likely to be located in rural areas. Over two-thirds of HPSAs for general providers are in rural areas (National Rural Health Association, http://www.ruralhealthweb.org/go/left/about-rural -health) and almost 90 percent of mental health professional shortage areas are in nonmetropolitan counties (Bird, Dempsey, & Hartley, 2001). The difficulty in recruiting and retaining primary care providers to work in rural areas of the country has been widely reported (Coffman, Rosenoff, & Grumbach, 2002; Rosenblatt et al., 2006). Rural physicians tend to be older than their urban counterparts and more likely to be approaching retirement age (Doescher, Fordyce, & Skillman, 2009).

Rural areas also report shortages of nonphysician providers. For example, in 2008, rural areas reported one-third fewer dentists per one hundred thousand people than urban areas (Doescher et al., 2009). The current situation follows a long-standing trend of reduced oral health services with decreasing urbanization (Eberhardt et al., 2001). In addition, small rural areas report less than half the number of registered nurses per one hundred thousand people than work in urban areas (Skillman et al., 2005). The percentage of nurses living in the most isolated areas has seen a slight but steady increase from 1 percent in 1980 to 4 percent in 2004, and the overall percentage of nurses in all rural areas has increased from 14 percent to 18 percent over the same period (Skillman et al., 2007).

To a large extent the number of health care professionals working in any area is driven by the existing job market. Because large hospitals and other major employers are clustered in and around major metropolitan areas, there are fewer jobs for health care professionals in rural areas. Those health care professionals that do locate their practices in rural areas may face increased call schedules, less ability to take vacations, greater demands on their time, and overall less income (Berk et al., 2009).

As the US population continues to grow, with a disproportionately greater percentage of the elderly living in rural areas, the demand for physicians, dentists, nurses, and other health care professionals will continue to rise. An approach that has seen some success in increasing the likelihood of health professions' students electing rural practice sites involves early and longitudinal rural community exposure during the students' educational programs (Halaas, 2005; Lang et al., 2005). Among the most successful are those that combine interprofessional experiences along with discipline-specific training (Florence et al., 2007), such as those funded by the Bureau of Health Professions' Quentin N. Burdick Program for Rural Interdisciplinary Training.

Affordability of Health Care

Health care is less affordable for many people living in rural areas for two main reasons: (1) higher levels of poverty and (2) lower rates of health insurance coverage. The higher rates of poverty in rural America are well documented as a pervasive problem. More than 15 percent of rural residents live in poverty compared to 12.5 percent of urban residents (Jensen, 2006), and 90 percent of the persistently poor counties in the United States are located in rural areas (Ganong et al., 2007).

Persistent poverty, whether in rural or urban settings, often forces people to make choices between basic human needs, such as shelter or food, and seeking health care. Poverty makes health insurance costs prohibitive (Agency for Healthcare Research and Quality, Center for Financing, Access and Cost Trends, 2008). This problem, like poverty itself, is exacerbated by rural residence, minority status, and lack of educational achievement (Jolliffe, 2004).

Rural residents are less likely to have employer-provided health insurance, less likely to have private insurance, and more likely to be uninsured (Coburn et al., 2009) than their urban counterparts (King et al., 2007). Self-employed workers in rural areas are less likely to have insurance and more likely to pay more for similar insurance policies than self-employed workers in urban areas (The Access Project, 2007). Those who are insured are more likely to be covered by a publicly funded program, such as Medicaid, which offers poor reimbursement for provided services, further skewing the economic equation in health service delivery and disadvantaging rural communities.

There is one major exception to the typically lower rates of insurance for those living in rural areas. Around 2000, the rural-urban health insurance disparity existed for children as well as adults (Rogers, 2005). In the past several years, however, increased Medicaid coverage, coupled with innovative state child health insurance programs, have all but erased this disparity (Coburn et al., 2009).

As a result of the combination of these factors, people living in rural areas on average spend 20 percent more out of pocket on health care than their urban counterparts (Ziller, Coburn, & Yousefian, 2006). Additionally, rural adults are slightly more likely to report that they have deferred health care because of costs (Bennett, Olatosi, & Probst, 2008). According to the same source, this problem is worse among rural minority populations.

Geographic Factors Affecting Entry to Health Care

A variety of factors affect the ability or willingness of rural residents to seek health care services. On the most basic level, because of geographic isolation, rural residents usually need more time to travel to a health care provider; rural residents are 40 percent more likely than their urban counterparts to have to travel thirty minutes or more to access health care (Seshamani et al., 2009). Costs associated with this travel, superimposed on the background levels of poverty and limits in public transportation, may result in unwillingness or actual inability of rural residents to seek care. The cost of traveling greater distances for services is even higher for residents whose livelihood depends on being present during business hours. Additionally, it is difficult to quantify the impact of the increased danger of road travel in rural areas on the willingness of residents to seek care. Two-thirds of all motor vehicular deaths occur on rural roads in spite of the fact that only one-third of the motor vehicle accidents occur there (National Highway Traffic Safety Administration, 2008).

Summary of Access Challenges

Rural Americans face shortages of health care professionals, treatment facilities, and the means to pay for health care when it is available. Access to existing health care options is often challenged by geographic, cultural, and historic factors. Rural residents have greater "all causes" and motor vehicular mortality than urban residents and the gap is widening.

Behavioral Patterns: Lifestyles and Health in Rural America

Human behavior is greatly influenced by context and environment. As such, major differences exist in health behavior patterns between rural residents and their urban counterparts (Eberhardt et al., 2001). Different risk behaviors have been linked to rural and urban settings (Bennett et al., 2008; Diez Rouz & Mair,

2010). This section explores health behavior with respect to rural environments and socioeconomic status (SES).

Health Risk Behaviors

The diverse effects of demography, culture, access to health care, education, income, and the physical environment contribute to differences seen in health behaviors and associated health status from one region to another (Williams et al., 2010). Health behaviors influenced by age and race, for example, are not cleanly divided between rural and urban settings but are unevenly distributed across the United States due to cultural differences, SES, and a host of other regional influences.

Greater proportions of non-Hispanic blacks, persons aged sixty-five and older, and low-income households, for example, are found in the rural South than other parts of the country. All of these factors, and more, must be considered when one seeks to understand differences in health behaviors and related health disparities in rural areas.

A more accurate understanding of the causes of health disparities may be gained when **health behaviors** (actions individuals take that directly or indirectly affect their health) are described in geographic and demographic terms, as well as the economic impact of these behaviors. As such, the behaviors that follow will be described not only along the rural-urban continuum, but also between racial and ethnic groups. Although race is sometimes used as a surrogate for SES in sociological research—albeit not without criticism (Contributing factors to racial and ethnic gaps in health, 1999; Whaley, 2003)—it is used in the context of this chapter simply to add a contextual dimension to rurality. Many of these data come from Behavioral Risk Factor Surveillance System (BRFSSP) surveys of 2005 and 2006, reported by Bennett et al. (2008). They determine rurality on the basis of county UIC codes designated by the United States Department of Agriculture (USDA).

Distinct rural-urban differences appear in self-reported health status, with rural residents being more likely to describe their health as *fair* or *poor* than urban residents (19.5 percent versus 15.6 percent, respectively). The proportion increases to 21.9 percent in remote rural counties. In those counties furthest removed from urban amenities, nearly one-third of minorities rate their health as *fair* or *poor* (Hispanics, 32.1 percent; blacks, 29.2 percent; Native Americans, 27.6 percent).

Obesity (body mass index ≥30) is a behavioral health outcome and a potent health determinant that affects self-reported health status. Not only is obesity more prevalent in rural than urban areas (27.4 percent versus 23.9 percent), but it also generally increases with increasing rurality. Blacks have the highest percentage of obesity across all levels of rurality, with a high of

40.7 percent in remote rural counties. Although Asians have the lowest percentage of all racial groups, rural Asians are over twice as likely to be obese as their urban counterparts (13.6 percent versus 6.4 percent). Among whites, 22.4 percent of urban, compared to 26.3 percent of rural, residents are obese.

Citing National Health and Nutrition Examination Survey (NHANES) data from 1999 to 2006, Liu et al. (2010) described childhood obesity as a problem that is growing disproportionately in rural America. Over one-third (35.5 percent) of rural children ages two to nineteen are overweight compared to 29.5 percent of those living in urban areas. Similarly, more rural than urban children are obese (18.5 percent versus 15.2 percent). Physical inactivity, a major contributing factor to childhood obesity, is a common and growing concern for most American children. Although rates of physical activity vary by region of the country, race, and SES, they are typically slightly lower in rural compared to urban areas (Liu et al., 2007). Among all rural residents, blacks tend to be the least physically active and Native Americans the most.

Among adults, several other lifestyle behaviors that contribute to obesity also differ markedly between rural and urban areas, including dietary consumption of fat, fruits, and vegetables. Food intake patterns for adults and children show that rural residents consume more calories, more fat, and fewer fruits and vegetables than urban residents, contributing to overall risk for overweight and obesity (McIntosh & Sobal, 2004). Greater proportions of calories and fat are consumed by rural children outside the home (frequently in fast-food restaurants) than by urban children (Lin, Guthrie, & Blaylock, 1996).

Although significant reductions in tobacco use have occurred nationally since the 1980s, prevalence of smoking remains higher among adults in rural areas than urban areas (Doescher et al., 2006; Rahilly & Farwell, 2007; Ricketts, 1999). Rural residents smoke more cigarettes per day (Schoenborn et al., 2004) and adolescent smoking prevalence continues to be higher in rural than in urban areas (Eberhardt et al., 2001).

As mentioned, health behaviors among rural populations are influenced by economics and also have economic effects. Although every individual and family can be described as balancing competing demands regardless of the community in which they reside, rural residents' demands are distinct because of the dearth of local resources and services they often encounter. Thus, in the example of healthy diet, what a rural family can afford is affected by its limited budget for groceries as well as the local availability of healthy food. Given the likely higher cost of healthy food in a rural supermarket or the added cost of traveling outside one's community to obtain healthier foods, a rural family may opt for less expensive (and less healthy) foods when faced with competing demands for their resources such as for housing and fuel. Chapter Fourteen covers this specific topic in greater depth.

Preventive Care–Seeking Behavior

Health screening behavior is influenced by contextual characteristics (e.g., SES, education, and rurality) and lack of access to health care can result in under-utilization of preventive services in rural areas, even when they are available, affordable, or even free (Lane & Martin, 2005; Zhang, Tao, & Irwin, 2000). When it comes to getting an annual influenza vaccination, older rural and urban residents do so in about equal proportions (64.6 percent versus 63.8 percent). Among older rural residents, however, ethnic differences compound the picture. Although 66 percent of whites are immunized, only 42 percent of blacks are. Rural Asian elders have the highest rates of any racial group, with over three-fourths being immunized (76.6 percent). Conversely, only 61.2 percent of older Asians living in urban areas are immunized (Bennett et al., 2008).

In terms of behaviors affecting women's health, the picture is equally complex. Fewer rural than urban women receive mammograms as recommended by national guidelines (70.7 percent versus 76.6 percent). In rural areas, black women are less likely than white women to be screened (66.0 percent versus 71.3 percent), whereas in urban areas black women were slightly more likely to be screened than white women (78.5 percent versus 76.7 percent; Bennett et al., 2008).

Pap tests are recommended every three years for all women over the age of twenty-one or earlier if sexually active. Though the overall percentages are relatively high for both, rural women report following these guidelines less frequently than their urban peers (86.3 percent versus 91.4 percent). Rural black women report getting screened more regularly than whites in the same areas (89.7 percent versus 86.0 percent). Native American women living in remote rural areas reported a higher screening rate than other rural women, reflecting the results of successful screening and health education campaigns (Bennett et al., 2008).

Summary of Behavioral Patterns

A large and growing body of research has demonstrated the impact of culture and society on human behavior. When it comes to making healthy lifestyle and preventive care–seeking choices, much of a person's resolve is affected by one's cultural experiences and contextual circumstances (e.g., SES, education, and rurality). These disparate influences offer some explanation for the complex differences between rural and urban America. What can be said with confidence, however, is that disparities in health behavior tend to increase along the urban-rural continuum, with the greatest disparities appearing in the most isolated rural regions and among the most vulnerable populations.

Cultural Influences on Health in Rural America

Every society has a system of shared beliefs, values, behaviors, and symbols that create meaning and order. Because each population is unique in the way it defines the meaning of these attributes, **culture** refers to the indigenous and cultural factors that differ from one locale to another and between distinct groups co-located in particular settings. Culture informs perceptions of health risks, attitudes toward health professionals and institutions, and also behaviors and health-related practices among individuals, agencies, and communities (Betancourt & Flynn, 2009; Kline & Huff, 2008; Rosal & Bodenlos, 2009).

Not only is the whole relationship of culture to human health greater than the sum of its parts, but the whole also influences the sum and the parts. Hammond (1978) offered a comprehensive framework for understanding the influence of culture that can be employed to understand the determinants of rural health disparities. He posited that culture originates from two distinct organizing systems: (1) the shared language, symbols, and worldview that are endogenous to each population and (2) the environmental and social structures through which the members interact with one another and create meaning. Kagawa-Singer et al. (2010) suggest that culture represents a "multilevel, multidimensional dynamic, biopsychosocial, and ecological system in which a population exists" (p. 17). Culture reflects a population's unique geopolitical and sociodemographic context. Variety in culture is nearly endless; uniqueness abounds in ethnicity and national origin, regional norms and customs, religious traditions and beliefs, organizational values, and in countless other ways.

The Social Implications of Culture

Culture provides a framework for understanding normative beliefs and practices regarding aspects such as gender roles, the meaning of life and death, and conceptions of health and disease. There is growing recognition of a culture of rurality that contributes to lifestyle practices and beliefs associated with many of the primary risk factors for chronic health conditions, such as diabetes, cardiovascular disease, obesity, and arthritis (Hartley, 2004; Thomas, Fine, & Ibrahim, 2004). Arguably, this system of normative beliefs and cues has a significant impact on the health decision-making processes and models of care in rural settings. For example, there are specific cultural attributes such as perceived lack of anonymity in some communities where care facilities are scarce and mental health conditions are stigmatized (Kagawa-Singer et al., 2010).

Rural Culture and Its Impact on Health Outcomes

Although rural residence does not always indicate a health disparity, rurality is often associated with a constellation of socioeconomic and structural health disadvantages. The impact of unemployment, underemployment, limited access to health services, and lower educational attainment is best seen through the lens of culture-specific health perceptions and behaviors in rural communities. It is the cumulative and synergistic effects of these contextual experiences and impact of each individual's life experience that have important implications to the overall health and health outcomes and health care delivery system in rural settings (Hartley, 2004; Thomas et al., 2004).

Differences in health status are associated with cultural factors such as regional variations in dietary preferences among rural populations. Diets in rural Greece (Crete), Japan, and China, for example, are thought to have a protective effect on health and mortality when compared with the fattier and more westernized diets of the urban regions of these countries (Keys et al., 1986; Segelken, 2001).

Pervasive cultural messages in rural settings are known to reinforce the stigma of mental disorders and mental health treatment. For example, it is widely recognized that the acceptance of treatment for depression by rural residents is hindered by stigma and adherence to a system of core beliefs promoting self-reliance, belief that life experiences cause depression, and use of spirituality or religion to self-manage depression burden and determine treatment decisions (Kemppainen et al., 2009).

There are parts of the country and certain population groups for which a distrust of the health care delivery system has been reported (Institute of Medicine, 2003; Kennedy, Mathis, & Woods, 2007). Such distrust has been suggested especially for minority populations with a negative perception of past and current interactions with the health care and health research systems, and for undocumented alien populations that may be unwilling to seek care for fear of legal repercussions. Although it is difficult to quantify the extent or impact of this distrust, it could potentially affect the willingness of these populations to interact with the health care delivery system and result in lower levels of care-seeking behaviors.

There is also a culture, at least in some parts of the country, of self-reliance and independence (Behringer & Friedell, 2006). Although this aspect of culture is difficult to quantify, when superimposed against a historical background in which health care was simply not available, it may affect the willingness of rural residents to seek health care even when it is needed and available.

Summary of Cultural Influences

Sociocultural interactions and influences on health and disease are important concepts in the determination of health care solutions that are congruent with the system of beliefs and values in rural settings (Thomas et al., 2004). An improved understanding of cultural currency and milieu and its impact on health beliefs and behaviors can inform public health practice and assist policy makers to create targeted and innovative initiatives to reduce rural health disparities.

Determinants of Socioeconomic Origin in Rural America

The **social determinants of health** include circumstances in which people are born, raised, and reside. These circumstances are in turn shaped by a wider set of social forces, such as economics, policies, and politics (WHO, 2011). A growing body of literature argues that social conditions are one of the fundamental causes of health disparities (Link & Phelan, 2005). Poverty, education, and health are inextricably linked in a dynamic reciprocal relationship. This section outlines aspects of social determinants that public health practitioners should consider when planning rural health programs.

Educational Attainment

Rural residents are much less likely to go to or finish college compared to urban residents in the United States (40 percent versus 53 percent, respectively; Mississippi State, 2006). In the most rural US counties, it is common for less than 10 percent of residents to be college graduates (Gibbs, 2005). There is also great disparity in the quality of educational programming available to rural youth, including enrichment activities. Educational attainment and the expectation of it for youth are markedly different for those in rural compared with urban settings.

Rural residents are much less likely to go to or finish college compared to urban residents in the United States

Though rural Americans now have more education than ever before and the increase has been marked in the past generation, they still lag far behind their urban counterparts (26 percent college graduation rate for urban dwellers against 15 percent for rural). Degree attainment notwithstanding, rural residents do about as well in school as their urban counterparts (Gibbs, 2005).

There is strong evidence that healthier students are better learners (Basch, 2010), and there is increasing focus on providing coordinated health activities to children in schools, at least in several states (e.g., Texas, Tennessee, Colorado). The challenge has been and will be in integrating school health activities with family and community activities in resource-poor settings, where parents and youth may be physically distant from schools and other social networks.

At least one state, Tennessee, has enacted a version of the Centers for Disease Control (CDC) model for coordinated school health (CSH) in every county in the state, resourcing the activities through the state Department of Education. Although evaluation activities are ongoing, preliminary results indicate progress in screenings, physical activity, and number of programs for urban and rural youth in Tennessee.

Education, Income, and Health

In a study reported by the Department of Education, high school sophomores were more than ten times as likely to have completed college in ten years if their parents had professional degrees than if their parents were high-school noncompleters (Robert Wood Johnson Foundation, 2009).

Infants born to mothers who have finished less than a high school degree are almost twice as likely to die in the first year of life as those born to mothers who have finished college (Robert Wood Johnson Foundation, 2009). There is a more than sixfold difference between the two groups when considering the percentage of children under seventeen years old who were reported by their parents to be in fair or poor health (0.7 days compared to 4.4 days in the past month). Similarly, there is a five- to seven-year difference in life expectancy at age twenty-five for men and women when comparing the two groups. Although all of the ways in which educational achievement affect health outcomes have not been identified, it is reported that this impact extends beyond the direct relationship between education and income (Robert Wood Johnson Foundation, 2009).

Wealth Distribution and Social Status

There is a great inequity in how wealth is distributed in the United States. Since the 1970s, the greatest income gains have been seen by the wealthiest few percent of Americans, with all but the top 10 percent having inflation-adjusted incomes that are largely static (Sherman & Stone, 2010).

There has been a dramatic widening of the gap between the richest and poorest Americans (see Figure 4.1). Between 1969 and 2009, the income of the lowest quintile of Americans increased about 15.6 percent and the income of the highest quintile increased about 61 percent. As a result, the ratio of income between the top and bottom quintile has grown from 10.6 to 14.8.

As the income gap between the wealthiest and the poorest Americans has widened, it is anticipated that those parts of the country with disproportionately high rates of less wealthy citizens, including many rural areas, will see a widening income gap with other parts of the country.

One of the central tenets of changing the social determinants that lead to inequities in health is changing the economic forces that shape inequities in income. In rural areas, with the noted exceptions of farms and small business, the vast majority of workers are employed in low-wage, skilled, or unskilled

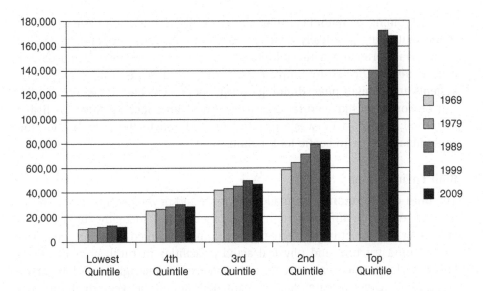

Figure 4.1. Income Change in the United States: 1969–2009
Source: US Census Bureau (2010).

labor positions with relatively few prospects for dynamic income growth or potential change in social status.

Summary of Social Determinants

It is recognized that the three-legged stool of education, wealth, and social status should be considered key social determinants of health in the United States. Rural areas have a lower level in each of these three categories. Intervention programming or studies aimed at understanding rural health should account for these forces and seek to make changes in them to support positive health action.

Environment and Health in Rural America

The physical environment is a key feature in rural health. There are many healthful aspects to living in a clean environment with ample opportunity for relaxation and recreation, and many rural environments can offer these benefits. This section of the chapter focuses, however, on modifiable environmental risk factors found disproportionately in rural areas.

Air, Water, and Soil

Although air, water, and soil are generally cleaner in rural areas, some important exceptions should be noted. First, air quality can be affected by industry, such as mining or manufacturing. For example, Hendryx and Ahern (2008) found that living physically near to a coal mining, finishing, and processing facility was correlated with multiple negative health outcomes. Water quality can be greatly affected by untreated sewage in rural areas from failing septic systems and straight pipes draining sewage into creeks and rivers. Soil quality can be compromised in rural areas because of improper facilities for heavy metal, oil, or industrial waste disposal, in addition to the potential for soil contamination due to septic tank failure.

Built Environment

The **built environment** (manmade structures and developments in communities that enable or hinder certain kinds of activities) in many rural areas is lacking in infrastructure for recreation or human-powered transportation. The lack of infrastructure and physical activity facilities in rural areas has been linked to lower physical activity and increased overweight (Gordon-Larsen et al., 2006). Other research has substantiated the link between the built environment and obesity (e.g., Humpel, Owen, & Leslie, 2002).

Rural walking and cycling promotion campaigns have shown some success in increasing physical activity and use of existing facilities in small cities and towns (e.g., Reger-Nash et al., 2005). The feasibility of promoting such fitness activities in some rural areas can be challenging given the relatively low population density and type and condition of roadways. A walking promotion campaign, for example, in a mountainous mining community with no sidewalks may actually place a person at risk for injury or death.

Social Environment

The social networks that are found in many rural areas are deep and in many ways protective against poor mental health outcomes. As Phillips and McLeroy (2004) have stated, "Rural areas frequently have strengths including dense social networks, social ties of long duration, shared life experiences, high quality of life, and norms of self-help, and reciprocity" (p. 1663). These networks influence the social environment and are key to supportive relationships.

Injury

Occupational and other injuries are more common in rural areas than in urban communities. Farming, mining, and timbering are all very hazardous rural jobs with high injury rates. Also, injuries are common in recreational motor sports, for example, all-terrain vehicles (ATVs) and other motor vehicles (Helmkamp et al., 2008). The impact of an injury in a rural area may be further exacerbated by the distance to emergency health care.

Summary of Environmental Forces

The environment should be carefully considered when evaluating health disparities that may exist in a rural community. Although those living in rural areas may benefit from the health-promoting aspects of rural life, there may also be significant environmental risks that may have strong negative effects on health.

Conclusion

Considering access to care, behavior, culture, social determinants, and the environment is a useful starting place for understanding the depth of rural health disparities in the United States. Although the impact of the ABCDEs will vary in different rural areas, they provide a structure by which public health professionals can systematically and quickly assess the relative health status of any rural community.

Some communities will pose specific challenges not directly covered by an ABCDE assessment, for example, a community recently affected by a natural or human-made disaster. However, for most situations, this systematic assessment will provide the public health professional with a useful tool for quickly evaluating the health status of any rural community.

Access to health care, behavior, genetics, social determinants, and the environment work together to positively or negatively influence health. ABCDE assessment components are all highly interrelated and mutually dependent. By paying attention to the interdependence of these factors and acknowledging their influence, the public health professional is best positioned to improve the health of those living in rural areas. Hence, public health practitioners should take the time to consider their ABCDEs when taking public health action in rural communities.

Summary

- It is necessary for rural health care professionals to systematically evaluate *a*vailability and access to health care in rural America, *b*ehavioral patterns, *c*ultural influences, *d*eterminants of socioeconomic origin, and *e*nvironmental factors affecting health in rural areas to understand and address the unique health challenges of the rural community in which they serve.

- A number of factors limit availability and access to health care in rural communities, such as having a shortage of health care professionals practicing in rural areas, affordability of the health care services, and geographic barriers.

- Cultural and societal norms greatly affect health behavioral patterns in rural communities, including whether to engage in a healthy lifestyle and whether to make preventive care–seeking decisions. An improved understanding of sociocultural influences and their effect on health beliefs and behaviors can inform public health practice and assist policy makers in creating targeted and innovative initiatives to reduce rural health disparities.

- Rural areas have lower levels of education, wealth, and social status compared to their urban counterparts. These three social determinants are key factors to consider when conducting interventions and research to improve the health of rural communities.

- Environmental forces such as air, water, and soil quality; the quality of the built environment; social environment; and rates of injury should be thoroughly assessed when evaluating health disparities that may exist in rural communities.

For Practice and Discussion

1. Working with a colleague or two from class, select a rural community for which health data are available. Discuss and explain how the ABCDEs could inform efforts to address the health challenges of this community and explain how they are interrelated.

2. You have been hired by the local health department to address heart disease. How do the ABCDEs inform your programmatic planning?

3. Robust evidence implicates poverty as a primary cause of poor health outcomes. How might this relationship be similar or different between people living in rural areas compared to those living in urban areas?

Key Terms

access   health behavior

built environment   social determinants of health

culture

References

The Access Project. (2007, September). *Issue brief no. 1: 2007 health insurance survey of farm and ranch operators*. Retrieved from http://www.accessproject.org/adobe/issue_brief_no_1.pdf

Agency for Healthcare Research and Quality, Center for Financing, Access and Cost Trends. (2008). *Medical expenditure panel survey HC-105: 2006 full year consolidated data file.* Retrieved from http://meps.ahrq.gov/mepsweb/data_stats/download_data/pufs/h105/h105doc.pdf

Basch, C. E. (2010). *Healthier students are better learners: A missing link in school reforms to close the achievement gap.* New York: Campaign for Educational Equity, Teachers College, Columbia University.

Behringer, B., & Friedell, G. (2006). Appalachia: Where place matters for health. *Preventing Chronic Disease, 3*(4), A113.

Bennett, K. J., Olatosi, B., & Probst, J. C. (2008). *Health disparities: A rural-urban chartbook.* Columbia: South Carolina Rural Health Research Center.

Berk, M., Feldman, J., Schur, C., & Gupta, J. (2009). *Satisfaction with practice and decision to relocate: An examination of rural physicians.* Final report. Bethesda, MD: NORC Walsh Center for Rural Health Analysis.

Betancourt, H., & Flynn, P. M. (2009). The psychology of health: Physical health and the role of culture and behavior. In F. A. Villarruel, G. Carlo, J. M. Grau, M. Azmitia, N. J. Cabrera, & T. J. Chahin (Eds.), *Handbook of U.S. Latino psychology* (pp. 347–361). Thousand Oaks, CA: Sage.

Bird, D., Dempsey, P., & Hartley, D. (2001). *Addressing mental health workforce needs in underserved rural areas: Accomplishment and challenges.* Portland: Edmund S. Muskie School of Public Service, Maine Rural Health Research Center. Retrieved from http://muskie.usm.maine.edu/Publications/rural/wp23.pdf

Chen, F., Fordyce, M., Andes, S., & Hart, G. L. (2010). Which medical schools produce rural physicians? A 15-year update. *Academic Medicine, 85,* 594–598.

Coburn, A. F., MacKinney, A. C., McBride, T. D., Mueller, K. J., Slifkin, R., & Ziller, E. (2009). *Assuring health coverage for rural people through health reform.* Robert Wood Johnson, Rural Policy Research Institute (RUPRI). Retrieved from http://www.rupri.org/Forms/Health_ReformBrief_Oct09.pdf

Coffman, J., Rosenoff, E., & Grumbach, K. (2002). *Improving recruitment and retention of primary care practitioners in rural California.* Berkeley: California Program on Access to Care, California Policy Research Center. Retrieved from http://www.ucop.edu/cpac/documents/carerural.pdf

Contributing factors to racial and ethnic gaps in health. (1999). *Improving the collection and use of racial and ethnic data in HHS* (ch. 2). Joint report of the HHS Data Council Working Group on Racial and Ethnic Data and The Data Work Group of the HHS Initiative to Eliminate Racial and Ethnic Disparities in Health. Department of Health and Human Services. Retrieved from http://aspe.hhs.gov/datacncl/racerpt/chap2.htm

Council on Graduate Medical Education. (1998). *Tenth report: Physician distribution and health care challenges in rural and inner-city areas.* Washington, DC: Department of Health and Human Services.

Diez Roux, A. V., & Mair, C. (2010). Neighborhoods and health. *Annals of the New York Academy of Sciences, 1186,* 125–145.

Doescher, M. P., Fordyce, M. A., & Skillman, S. M. (2009). *Policy brief: The aging of the primary care physician workforce: Are rural locations vulnerable?* Seattle:

WWAMI Rural Health Research Center, University of Washington. Retrieved from http://depts.washington.edu/uwrhrc/uploads/Aging_MDs_PB.pd

Doescher, M. P., Jackson, J. E., Jerant, A., & Hart, L. G. (2006). Prevalence and trends in smoking: A national rural study. *Journal of Rural Health, 22*(2), 112–118.

Eberhardt, M. S., Ingram, D. D., Makuc, D. M., et al. (2001).*Urban and rural health chartbook. Health, United States, 2001.* Hyattsville, MD: National Center for Health Statistics. Retrieved from http://www.cdc.gov/nchs/data/hus/hus01cht.pdf

Florence, J. A., Goodrow, B., Wachs, J., Grover, S., & Olive, K. E. (2007). Rural health professions education at East Tennessee State University: Survey of graduates from the first decade of the community partnership program. *Journal of Rural Health, 23*(1), 77–83.

Fordyce, M. A., Chen, F. M., Doescher, M. P., & Hart, L. G. (2007). *2005 physician supply and distribution in rural areas of the United States.* Final Report #116. Seattle: WWAMI Rural Health Research Center, University of Washington.

Gamm, L. D., Hutchison, L. L., Dabney, B. J., & Dorsey, A. M. (Eds.). (2003). *Rural healthy people 2010: A companion document to Healthy People 2010* (Vol. 1). College Station: The Texas A&M University System Health Science Center, School of Rural Public Health, Southwest Rural Health Research Center. Retrieved from http://srph.tamhsc.edu/centers/rhp2010/Volume1.pdf

Ganong, L., Coleman, M., Beckmeyer, J., Benson, Jamison, T., McCaulley, G., & Sutton, E. (2007). *Poverty in America: Rural and urban differences* (Research Brief). Columbia: University of Missouri, Human Environmental Sciences Extension. Retrieved from http://missourifamilies.org/cfb/briefs/ruralurban.pdf

Gibbs, R. (2005). Education as a rural development strategy. *Amber Waves, 3*(5), 20–25.

Gordon-Larsen, P., Nelson, M. C., Page, P., & Popkin, B. M. (2006). Inequality in the built environment underlies key health disparities in physical activity and obesity. *Pediatrics, 117*(2), 417–424.

Halaas, G. W. (2005). The rural physician associate program: New directions in education for competency. *Education for Health, 18*(3), 379–386.

Hammond, P. (1978). *An introduction to cultural and social anthropology* (Vol XIV, 2nd ed.). New York: Macmillan.

Hartley, D. (2004). Rural health disparities, population health, and rural culture. *American Journal of Public Health, 94*(10), 1675–1678.

Helmkamp, J., Furbee, P. M., Coben, J. H., & Tadros, A. (2008). All-terrain vehicle-related hospitalizations in the United States, 2000–2004. *American Journal of Preventive Medicine, 34*(1), 39–45.

Hendryx, M., & Ahern, M. M. (2008). Relations between health indicators and residential proximity to coal mining in West Virginia. *American Journal of Public Health, 98*(4), 669–671.

Humpel, N., Owen, N., & Leslie, E. (2002). Environmental factors associated with adult's participation in physical activity: A review. *American Journal of Preventive Medicine, 22*, 188–199.

Institute of Medicine. (2003). *A shared destiny: Community effects of uninsurance.* Washington, DC: The National Academies Press.

Jensen, L. (2006). At the razor's edge: Building hope for America's rural poor. *Rural Realities*, *1*(1). Retrieved from http://web1.ctaa.org/webmodules/webarticles/articlefiles/razor.pdf

Jolliffe, D. (2004). *Rural poverty at a glance*. Rural Development Research Report no. 100. USDA Economic Research Service. Retrieved from http://www.ers.usda.gov/Publications/RDRR100

Kagawa-Singer, M., Dadia, A. V., Yu, M. C., & Surbone, A. (2010). Cancer, culture, and health disparities: Time to chart a new course? *CA: A Cancer Journal for Clinicians*, *60*, 12–39.

Kemppainen, J. K., Taylor, J., Jackson, L. A., & Kim-Godwin, Y. S. (2009). Incidence, sources, and self-management of depression in persons attending a rural health clinic in Southeastern North Carolina. *Journal of Community Health Nursing*, *26*(1), 1–13.

Kennedy, B. R., Mathis, C. C., & Woods, A. K. (2007). African Americans and their distrust of the health care system: Health care for diverse populations. *Journal of Cultural Diversity*, *14*(2), 56–60.

Keys, A., Menotti, A., Karvonen, M. J., Aravanis, C., Blackburn, H., et al. (1986). The diet and 15-year death rate in the seven countries study. *American Journal of Epidemiology*, *124*(6), 903–915.

King, J., Geiger, L., Silberman, P., & Slifkin, R. (2007). *State profiles of Medicaid and SCHIP in rural and urban areas*. Retrieved from http://www.shepscenter.unc.edu/rural/pubs/report/FR91.pdf

Kline, M. V., & Huff, R. M. (2008). Health promotion in the context of culture. In M. V. Kline & R. M. Huff (Eds.), *Health promotion in multicultural populations: A handbook for practitioners and students* (ch. 1, 2nd ed.). Thousand Oaks, CA: Sage.

Lane, A. J., & Martin, M. (2005). Characteristics of rural women who attended a free breast health program. *Online Journal of Rural Nursing and Health Care*, *5*(2), 12–27. Retrieved from http://www.rno.org/journal/index.php/online-journal/article/viewFile/40/50

Lang, F., Ferguson, K. P., Bennard, B., Zahorik, P., & Sliger, C. (2005). The Appalachian preceptorship: Over two decades of an integrated clinical-classroom experience of rural medicine and Appalachian culture. *Academic Medicine*, *80*(8), 717–723.

Lin, B. H., Guthrie, J., & Blaylock, J. R. (1996). *The diets of America's children: Influence of dining out, household characteristics, and nutrition knowledge*. Report no. AER746. Washington, DC: US Department of Agriculture, Economic Research Service.

Link, B. G., & Phelan, J. C. (2005). Fundamental sources of health inequalities. In D. Mechanic (Ed.), *Policy challenges in modern health care*. New Brunswick, NJ: Rutgers University Press.

Liu, J., Bennett, K. J., Harun, N., Zheng, X., Probst, J. C., & Pate, R. R. (2007). *Overweight and physical inactivity among rural children aged 10–17: A national and state portrait*. Columbia: South Carolina Rural Health Research Center. Retrieved from http://rhr.sph.sc.edu/report/(7–1)Obesity%20ChartbookUpdated10.15.07-secured.pdf

Liu, J., Jones, S. J., Sun, H., Probst, J. C., & Cavicchia, P. (2010). *Diet, physical activity, and sedentary behaviors as risk factors for childhood obesity: An urban and rural comparison.* Columbia: South Carolina Rural Health Research Center.

McIntosh, W. A., & Sobal, J. (2004). Rural eating, diet, nutrition, and body weight. In N. Glasgow, L. W. Morton, & N. E. Johnson, (Eds.), *Critical issues in rural health* (ch. 10). Ames, IA: Blackwell.

Mississippi State, Stennis Institute of Government. (2006, August). *Urban vs. rural: Educational attainment for population 25 and older.* Retrieved from http://www.sig.msstate.edu/files/CompEd.pdf

National Highway Traffic Safety Administration. (2008). *Traffic safety facts 2008: Rural-urban comparison.* DOT HS: 811 164. Washington, DC: National Center for Statistical Analysis.

Phillips, C. D., & McLeroy, K. R. (2004). Health in rural America: Remembering the importance of place. Editorial. *American Journal of Public Health, 94*(10), 1661–1663.

Rahilly, C. R., & Farwell, W. R. (2007). Prevalence of smoking in the United Stated: A focus on age, sex, ethnicity, and geographic patterns. *Current Cardiovascular Risk Reports, 1,* 379–383.

Reger-Nash, B., Baumann, A., Booth-Butterfield, S., Cooper, L., Smith, H., Chey, T., & Simon, K. J. (2005). Wheeling walks: Evaluation of a media-based community intervention. *Family & Community Health, 28*(1), 64–78.

Ricketts, T. C. (Ed.). (1999). *Rural health in the United States.* New York: Oxford University Press.

Robert Wood Johnson Foundation, Commission on Health. (2009, September). *Education matters for health.* Issue Brief 6: Education and Health. Retrieved from http://www.commissiononhealth.org/PDF/c270deb3-ba42-4fbd-baeb-2cd65956f00e/Issue%20Brief%206%20Sept%2009%20-%20Education%20and%20Health.pdf

Rogers, C. C. (2005). *Rural children at a glance.* Economic Information Bulletin no. 1. USDA Economic Research Service. Retrieved from http://www.ers.usda.gov/publications/EIB1/eib1.pdf

Rosal, M. C., & Bodenlos, J. S. (2009). Culture and health-related behavior. In S. A. Shumaker, J. K. Ockene, K. A. Riekert (Eds.), *Handbook of health behavior change* (ch. 3, 3rd ed.). New York: Springer.

Rosenblatt, R. A., Andrilla, C. H., Curtin, T., & Hart, L. G. (2006). Shortages of medical personnel at community health centers: Implications for planned expansion. *Journal of the American Medical Association, 295*(9), 1042–1049.

Schoenborn, C. A., Adams, P. F., Barnes, P. M., Vikerie, J. L., & Schiller, J. S. (2004). Health behaviors of adults: United States, 1999–2001. *Vital and Health Statistics, 10*(219), 1–79.

Schroeder, S. A. (2007). We can do better—improving the health of the American people. *New England Journal Medicine, 357,* 1221–1228.

Segelken, R. (2001). China study II: Switch to Western diet may bring Western-type diseases. *Cornell Chronicle, 32*(39). Retrieved from http://www.news.cornell.edu/chronicle/01/6.28.01/China_Study_II.html

Seshamani, M., Van Nostrand, J., Kennedy, J., & Cochran, C. (2009). Hard times in the heartland: Health care in rural America. Rural Health Research Centers. Retrieved from http://www.healthreform.gov/reports/hardtimes/ruralreport.pdf

Sherman, A., & Stone, C. (2010, June 25). *Income gaps between very rich and everyone else more than tripled in last three decades, new data show.* Center on Budget and Policy Priorities. Retrieved from http://www.cbpp.org/cms/index.cfm?fa = view&id = 3220

Skillman, S. M., Palazzo, L., Hart, L. G., & Butterfield, P. (2007). *Registered nurse workforce from 1980 to 2004.* Final Report #115. WWAMI Rural Health Research Center, University of Washington. Retrieved from http://depts.washington.edu/uwrhrc/uploads/RHRC%20FR115%20Skillman.pdf

Skillman, S. M., Palazzo, L., Keepnews, D., & Hart, G. L. (2005). *Characteristics of registered nurses in rural vs. urban areas: Implications for strategies to alleviate nursing shortages in the United States.* Working Paper #91. WWAMI Center for Health Workforce Studies, University of Washington. Retrieved from http://depts.washington.edu/uwrhrc/uploads/CHWSWP91.pdf

Thomas, S. B., Fine, M. J., & Ibrahim, S. A. (2004). Health disparities: The importance of culture and health communication. *American Journal of Public Health, 94*(12), 2050.

US Census Bureau. (2010, September). *Income, poverty, and health insurance care coverage in the United States, 2009.* Retrieved from http://www.census.gov/prod/2010pubsp60–238.pdf

Whaley, A. L. (2003). Ethnicity/race, ethics and epidemiology. *Journal of the National Medical Association, 95*(8), 736–742.

World Health Organization. (2011). *Social determinants of health.* Retrieved from http://www.who.int/social_determinants/en/

Williams, D. R., Mohammed, S. A., Leavell, J., & Collins, C. (2010). Race, socioeconomic status, and health: Complexities, ongoing challenges, and research opportunities. *Annals of the New York Academy of Science, 1186,* 69–101.

Zhang, P., Tao, G., & Irwin, K. (2000). Utilization of preventive medical services in the United States: A comparison between rural and urban populations. *Journal of Rural Health, 16*(4), 349–356.

Ziller, E. C., Coburn, A. F., & Yousefian, A. E. (2006). *Out-of-pocket health spending and the rural underinsured. Health Affairs, 25*(6), 1688–1699.

Part Two

Rural Public Health Systems

Public Health Systems, Health Policy, and Population-Level Prevention in Rural America

Angela L. Carman
F. Douglas Scutchfield

Learning Objectives

- Describe the importance of public health governmental agencies in providing individual- and population-level health services in rural communities.
- Articulate the three core functions of public health: assessment, policy development, and assurance.
- Learn about the diversity in infrastructure, services, partnerships, financing, and workforce issues in local health departments.
- Recognize the importance of technology, education, and funding to changes in rural health policy.
- Understand the value of community needs assessments and community health improvement plans.

•••

Public health governmental agencies and the larger public health systems are major, though overlooked, contributors to the community's health. They provide a substantial portion of the primary preventive services in many communities and are the only community resources for population-based public health services, such as enforcing environmental laws designed to protect the public's health. In many communities, and more often in rural communities, they become the last resort provider of care when patients who require illness care have no place else to turn. Public health represents a significant governmental presence in the health care system and maintains a substantial fiduciary responsibility for the health of a community. This chapter attempts to introduce the governmental and system descriptions of public health and to examine briefly population-based prevention approaches and rural health policy development.

Because this text focuses on rural health, it is necessary to understand the role of public health in rural areas. Public health departments and the public health system represent a major community investment in health and health care, particularly in rural areas of our nation. The care of individual patients is certainly important but the capacity to deal with population-level health problems and risk, as well as focus on health promotion and disease prevention, is probably a more important predictor and influence on the health status of the community. In order to understand how best to focus on rural community health, it is imperative to understand public health and how to use the knowledge and skills of public health professionals to improve the health of communities. This chapter provides introductory knowledge and skills to understand and work with health departments and public health systems in rural communities. It explores the nature of public health, the character of rural public health departments, and major policy issues and activities that affect rural communities. Finally, there is a discussion of issues in rural public health that need attention in further policy development to address shortcomings and concerns about the delivery of public health services in rural areas.

Key Concepts

Public health services, many of which are provided at the local level, are vital to the maintenance and improvement of the public's health. In the past, public health focused on infectious diseases; now the focus is on chronic diseases and the influence of multiple factors on our health, ranging from individual to community-level risk factors. As noted throughout this text, rural communities experience an undue burden of health disparities due to a variety of factors including poor health behaviors, geographic isolation, increased concentrations of minority and medically underserved populations, lack of access to medical care, and lower socioeconomic status. Public health agencies have a significant role in addressing rural health disparities through the application of the three core functions of public health: assessment, policy development, and assurance. However, application of these three core functions is dependent on the diversity found within local health departments. Specifically, rural local health departments vary in governance, service provision, partnerships, infrastructure, financing and revenue sources, and workforce and staffing. Further, there is a need for increased technology resources, education, and funding for rural public health agencies. Finally, it is vital that rural health departments conduct an assessment of community health needs to guide programming, training, collaborative partnerships, and financial expenditures.

A Brief History of Public Health

The early history of public health in the United States focused primarily on epidemic disease and its control in ports, which was driven by a concern for the economic impact of disease on commerce. After the emergence of the germ theory of disease and an understanding of how infectious disease was transmitted and controlled, the role of public health shifted from quarantine and control of broad epidemics to control of those infectious diseases for which the new sciences of microbiology and immunology had provided tools and knowledge to successfully control. A review of the major causes of death at the turn of the twentieth century illustrates the nature of those disease problems. Many of these were amenable to basic environmental sanitation, clean water, and management of sewage; others were controlled by the new vaccines that emerged from the understanding of disease immunology. With the control of these infectious agents, at the mid-twentieth century, public health attention to controlling infectious disease turned to controlling the effects of chronic disease (Fee, 2009). Figure 5.1 shows that chronic diseases are now responsible for the ten leading causes of death.

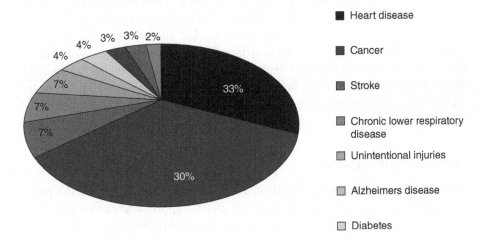

Figure 5.1. Ten Leading Causes of Death: 2007
Source: Data from CDC. http://www.cdc.gov/nchs/fastats/lcod.htm

The new public health paradigm has now shifted to issues of socioecologic factors that influence disease and the presence of disparities in the health status of our diverse population. Issues of poverty, social class, educational achievement, built environment, and social justice are major issues of concern (Scutchfield & Howard, 2011).

Rural Health Problems

Although rural living, defined in this chapter as living in areas with a population of less than fifty thousand, was once synonymous with clean, healthy living (Meit & Knudson, 2009), a look at today's rural population identifies significant health problems. *Rural Healthy People 2010*—modeled after the national *Healthy People 2010* goals and objectives but specific to rural health issues—used a series of roundtables composed of public health faculty members to identify a number of priority health problems. These were heart disease and stroke; diabetes; mental health; oral health; tobacco use; substance abuse; maternal, infant, and child health; nutrition and overweight issues; and cancer (Gamm & Hutchinson, 2005). In addition, others have identified that unintentional injury death rates increase as counties become more rural (Morgan, 2002). The prevalence of these health problems in rural America and the connection of many problems to high-risk health behavior suggest that there is a rural culture health determinant, defined as the impact of living in a rural area, on health (Hartley, 2004).

The *Rural Health Snapshot 2010* produced by the North Carolina Rural Health Research & Policy Analysis Center provides a comparison between rural and metropolitan areas of health insurance coverage, smoking, obesity, infant mortality, diseases of the heart, diabetes, chronic obstructive pulmonary disease (COPD), unintentional injuries, and suicide. In each of these categories rural areas had more people without health insurance coverage and higher levels of each measured health item (North Carolina Rural Health Research & Policy Analysis Center, 2010). Rural residents experience these health issues in addition to persistent poverty (Meit, 2007) and the lack of primary care and emergency medical services (Gamm & Hutchinson, 2005).

Public Health Systems

The advent of contemporary public health was ushered in largely by the publication of the 1988 Institute of Medicine (IOM) report, *The Future of Public Health*. The report described a once-proud system of public health services as being in "disarray." The report was a major turning point, resulting in a public health renaissance in the early 1990s. It also galvanized the public health community and led to many of the innovations and activities subsequently described in this chapter. The report first established a mission for public health, "assuring conditions in which people can be healthy" (IOM, 1988, p. 7). It pointed out that this mission encompassed a variety of actors. Many organizations and agencies, nonprofit, governmental, and private, share this mission; it is not unique to any one sector. These organizations and agencies comprise the **public health system** that is defined as "governmental and non-governmental organizations that contribute to the performance of essential public health services for a defined community or population" (Scutchfield & Keck, 2009, p. 792).

The 1988 IOM report focused specifically on the governmental sector of public health at the federal, state, and local levels. It defined the functions of governmental public health as assessment, policy development, and assurance. **Assessment** is "regular and systematic collection, assembling, analyzing and making available information on the health of the community, including statistics on health status, community health needs, and epidemiologic and other studies of health problems." **Policy development** is best conceived as "public health agencies exercising their responsibility to serve the public interest in the development of comprehensive public health policies by promoting the use of the scientific knowledge base in decision making about public health and by leading in developing public health policy." **Assurance** is "public health agencies assuring their constituents that services necessary to achieve agreed upon goals are provided by encouraging actions by other entities (private or public sector), by requiring such action though regulation, or by providing services directly" (Scutchfield & Keck, 2009, p. 39). The report also had a series of recommendations for various levels of government to discharge the functions described in the document. Many of these recommendations were adopted and many were not (Scutchfield, Beversdorf, et al., 1997; Scutchfield, Hiltabiddle, et al., 1997). These three public health functions—assessment, policy development, and assurance—were further developed and defined in the early 1990s during the debate on the Clinton health reform efforts. Efforts by a working group co-led by the CDC's Public Health Practice Program office and the secretary of the Department of Health and Human Service's Office of Disease Prevention and Health Promotion resulted in the establishment of ten essential public health services that further develop and define assessment, policy development, and assurance. These ten essential public health services and their relations to the functions are illustrated in Figure 5.2.

The 1988 IOM report focused specifically on governmental public health organizations and not the broader public health system. The public health system was addressed in a later IOM report, published in 2002, that dealt specifically with this broader public health system and the potential contributions of some of the sectors in this system to the mission of public health (Institute of Medicine, 2002).

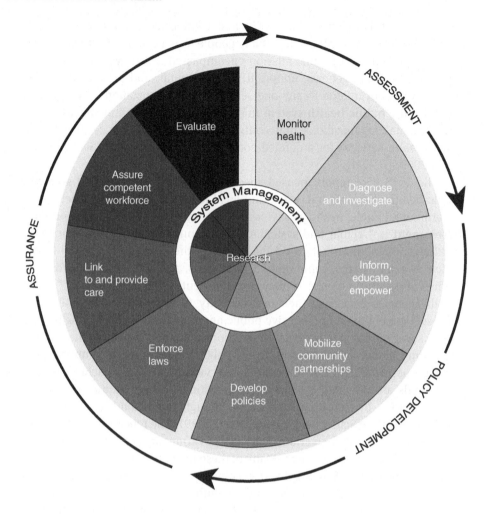

Figure 5.2. Ten Essential Public Health Services

Public Health System Diversity

Of particular interest in governmental public health entities is the great diversity of public health department infrastructure found across the United States. Each state public health system developed independently along with its associated local public health systems and are not necessarily in concert with each other. Such independence of development leads to the much-used statement "if you have seen one local health department, you have seen one local health department" (Meit, 2009, p. S31). This diversity creates difficulty in trying to examine, in any detail, the nature of these health departments. Recently, however, Mays, Bhandari, and Smith (2010) created a typology that attempts to classify local health departments. This typology should allow for more detailed examination of local health departments and provide some measure of comparability for analysis of structure and function.

There are major differences in the governance relations between state and local health departments across the United States. In the majority of states, local health departments are governed by local government (decentralized). However, in other states, local health departments are units of state government (centralized), and still other states have local health departments that are a mix of local and state government units (mixed). Jurisdictions in which local health departments provide public health services are also varied, such as county, city-county, town-township, multicounty, district or region, city, or some other configuration, and are the source for the provision of public health services (NACCHO, 2008). Even with mounting rural public health issues, however, many rural areas still have no local health department at all (Meit, 2007). Traditionally, small rural health departments, where they exist, are without the resources to carry out their defined functions.

Local Health Departments

Local health departments (LHDs) are defined as "an administrative or service unit of local or state government concerned with health and carrying some responsibility for the health of a jurisdiction smaller than the state" (Scutchfield & Keck, 2009, p. 785). The National Association of City and County Health Officials (NACCHO) has conducted surveys of local health departments since the early 1990s. The most recent survey was completed in 2008 and describes local health department infrastructure, practice, and capacity. The 2008 NACCHO survey shows that, of the 2,794 total local health departments in the United States, approximately 64 percent serve rural populations (populations less than fifty thousand). Although the majority of health departments serve rural areas, they actually provide services to less than 12 percent of the nation's population. There are other characteristics of rural health departments that set them aside from their urban counterparts; for example, they are more likely to have a governing board of health compared to larger jurisdictions. In terms of resources, overall, the unadjusted median per capita LHD expenditures was $36, which ranged from a low of $32 per person for LHDs serving jurisdictions of 25,000 to 49,999 people to $42 per person for LHDs serving populations of one million or more. Figure 5.3 shows the distribution of local health departments by size of population served.

The 2008 NACCHO *National Profile of Local Health Departments* indicates that the most frequent services available directly through the local health department include adult and child immunizations, communicable and infectious disease surveillance (including tuberculosis), and food service

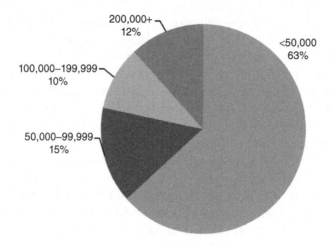

Figure 5.3. Percentage of Distribution of LHDs by Size of Population Served
Source: NACCHO (2008).

establishment inspection. These services were conducted by over 75 percent of all local health departments (NACCHO, 2008). Additional services provided by some health departments include sexually transmitted disease diagnosis and treatment; HIV-AIDS testing; counseling and education; environmental health services such as rabies control; septic tank, swimming pool, and well-water inspection; license and inspection of personal care homes and child care facilities; and the initiation and maintenance of vital records. In addition, most health departments receive federal categorical grants to provide specific public health programs such as Women, Infants and Children (WIC) and other nutritional programs, tobacco use prevention and cessation, maternal and child health services, and emergency preparedness (Wellever, 2006).

The majority of public health department services are population-based services as opposed to individual patient care. The fact these population-based services are provided more often by LHDs is indicative of the transition during the late twentieth century of public health from individual health service delivery to population-based services. This transition away from individual health services, however, has moved much more slowly in rural areas (Meit & Knudson, 2009). Although nearly 25 percent of Americans live in rural areas, only 10 percent of physicians practice there (National Rural Health Association, 2010). With limited access to health care services, rural residents rely on health departments to provide well-baby visits, Pap smears, breast exams, pregnancy testing, perinatal care, and other individual health services (Wellever, 2006). In addition, when compared to urban health departments, very small rural health departments, those serving fewer than twenty-five thousand people, offer home health services more often than those LHDs serving large populations of five hundred thousand or more and offer school-based clinics in equal numbers to urban counterparts (NACCHO, 2008). Rural health departments often resist transitioning away from such individual health services due to dependence on the revenue that such services bring (Meit & Knudson, 2009).

Partnerships

Partnerships between the local health department and other members of the public health system are crucial to delivering the ten essential public health services in rural areas. Literature and practice reveal a variety of collaborations around specific health concerns that involve members of the public health system such as faith-based organizations (Zahner & Corrado, 2004), correctional facilities (Lobato et al., 2004), universities (Goldhagen & Chiu, 1998), nonprofit community organizations, businesses, cities, and other governmental organizations (Public Health Institute, 2010). However, such partnerships vary greatly in the amount of formality with only 13 percent, primarily those offering laboratory services, involving contracts, and the vast majority of relationships involving information exchange only (NACCHO, 2008). Each partner's expertise, resources, and desire to improve the health of communities are critical to the impact of partnerships on public health. Given the nature of rural communities, it is likely that partnerships are more frequent because there are fewer health actors in rural communities and they are more likely to be familiar with each other and to have a track record of working together.

Infrastructure Issues of Rural Health Departments

The ability of rural local health departments to provide public health services is affected by federal- and state-level infrastructure and financing mechanisms available for such services. In some cases, federal funding for specific programs from sources such as the CDC are distributed to states, but in quantities that cannot support service delivery in all of the state's local health departments. In these cases, states often resort to minigrants or contracts awarded on the basis of competitive grant requests by the local health department or allocations to those departments deemed "best able to utilize the funding" (Meit et al., 2009, p. 213). Rural health departments, without infrastructure for grant writing or program management, may fall behind urban counterparts in their ability to access these funds and thus deliver specific services.

The ability of rural local health departments to provide public health services is affected by federal- and state-level infrastructure and financing mechanisms available for such services.

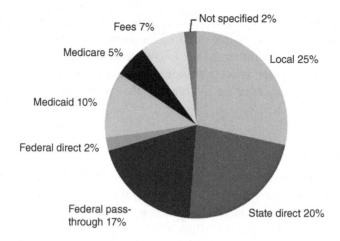

Figure 5.4. Percentage Distribution of Total Annual LHD Revenues by Revenue
Source
Source: NACCHO (2008).

Financial Issues

Local health departments receive revenues from a variety of sources. Although
the majority of revenue (2 percent) comes from city or township and county
sources labeled as *local*, revenues are also received from state direct sources,
federal pass-through sources, private foundations, private health insurance,
patient personal fees, regulatory fees, tribal sources, and others. Figure 5.4
shows the percentage distribution of total annual LHD revenues by revenue
source (NACCHO, 2008).

Revenue sources do vary by the size of population served by the local
health department. Rural health departments, particularly those serving fewer
than twenty-five thousand people, have greater proportions of revenue from
Medicaid and Medicare. In rural areas the limited availability of medical care
prompts local health departments to provide more individual services, such as
clinical preventive services and sickness care. That being the case, it is not
unexpected that a greater amount of their funding comes from medical care
payment sources. Figure 5.5 shows the mean percentage of total LHD revenues
from selected sources by size of population served (NACCHO, 2008).

Per capita expenditures by LHDs also vary by size of population served.
To adjust for the larger receipt of Medicare and Medicare funds and patient
fees by smaller health departments, per capita expenditures shown in Table
5.1 have subtracted these funds from all population size categories. The
smallest LHDs, those serving fewer than twenty-five thousand people, spend

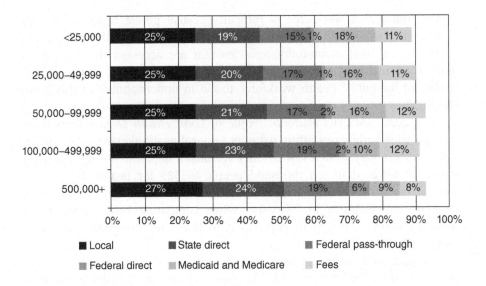

Figure 5.5. Mean Percentage of Total LHD Revenues from Selected Sources by Size of Population Served
Source: NACCHO (2008).

Table 5.1. Adjusted Per Capita Expenditures by Size of Population Served

LHD Characteristics	Adjusted Median
Size of Population Served	
<25,000	$29
25,000 to 49,999	$24
50,000 to 99,999	$27
100,000 to 249,999	$31
250,000 to 499,999	$32
500,000 to 999,999	$36
1,000,000+	$39

Source: NACCHO (2008).

approximately $10 less per person than the largest health departments after this adjustment (NACCHO, 2008).

Workforce Issues

The ability to deliver quality public health services to meet community needs is dependent on a well-prepared public health workforce. However, understanding this workforce is difficult because public health is a compilation of a variety of professions employed by public health agencies and a number of other community agencies that are accessed through collaborations (Scutchfield & Keck, 2009). There have been very few empirical studies of the public health workforce to aid in understanding of this group (Beck, 2010).

The 2008 NACCHO *National Profile of Local Health Departments* documents a wide variety of staffing patterns for local health departments. Median staff numbers vary from a low of three for health departments serving populations of fewer than ten thousand people to 585 for health departments serving one million or more. The median number of employees nearly doubles from eighteen to thirty-five when comparing health departments serving 25,000 to 49,999 in population to those serving 50,000 to 99,999 (NACCHO, 2008).

Occupational categories employed by local health departments also vary by size of the population served. The vast majority of all LHDs reporting in the NACCHO 2008 survey indicate that they employ clerical staff, nurse(s), and a manager or director. However, numbers of other public health occupational categories decline with the size of the health department. For example, health educators are employed by 57 percent of those health departments serving populations of 25,000 to 49,999 and 97 percent of the largest health departments (one million or more population) employ health educators. In addition, over 90 percent of large health departments (five hundred thousand or more population served) employ an epidemiologist and only 7 percent or fewer of smaller health departments (fewer than fifty thousand people served) have these services (NACCHO, 2008). Because of the lower numbers of actual staff to provide public health services in rural areas, rural public health employees, especially nurses, must perform a wide variety of duties for which they are sometimes unprepared. Moreover, due to the limited number of trained epidemiologists, small communities may be less able to quickly identify and respond to disease outbreaks. Only a small percentage of public health workers, more often in rural LHDs, are formally educated in public health, with most relying on short courses or on-the-job training, which cannot keep up with the increasing demands of the public health landscape (Meit, 2009). Improved training methods will be needed, particularly in rural areas, as local health departments seek accreditation, changes in demographics make cultural competencies more relevant, and emergency preparedness (e.g., agroterrorism) and environmental issues (e.g., cleanup of toxic methamphetamine laboratory sites) become a part of rural public health demands (Meit & Knudson, 2009).

Only a small percentage of public health workers, more often in rural LHDs, are formally educated in public health, with most relying on short courses or on-the-job training, which cannot keep up with the increasing demands of the public health landscape.

Of concern for the public health establishment is the issue of employees, especially nurses, who are retiring from public health at greater rates than are entering the field (Gamm & Hutchinson, 2005). Recruitment and retention of new public health workers is especially difficult due to financial constraints that limit the ability to pay competitive salaries, more remote geographic locations for work, lack of educational opportunities, and the expansion of programs and services expected of the rural staff (Hajat, Stewart, & Hayes, 2003). In addition, effects of the economic recession of 2008–2010 resulted in a cumulative loss of twenty-three thousand public health jobs due to layoffs or attrition (NACCHO, 2010) and reductions in federal programmatic funds, such as bioterrorism dollars, which have supported epidemiology and emergency preparedness personnel, may place additional public health workers at risk (Beck, 2010).

Rural Health Policy

The combination of growing health problems in rural populations, financing issues of public health agencies, and the lack of an educated public health workforce may have created a window of opportunity for public health. A **window of opportunity** is a time period in which events converge to make conditions favorable for specific policy implementation (Ricketts, 2009). The Patient Protection and Affordable Care Act of 2010 includes strategies and goals to address "service locations" and eliminating disparities of care including those resulting from geographic disparities (MacKinney & Lundblad, 2010). High-level changes to the direction of rural public health are likely to take the form of uniform expectations of local health departments and governmental incentives for public health infrastructure development (Wellever, 2006) to enhance the efficiency of current public health expenditures, regardless of the population size served.

High-level rural health policy must include attention to three specific areas: technology, education, and funding. Investment in technology, specifically in data systems, can provide needed information for better decision making and resource allocation, thus buffering the impacts of understaffing in rural areas. In addition, policies such as those implemented at the CDC's leadership and management development programs help to subsidize training and tuition reimbursement for rural public health professionals and raise the level of expertise in the leadership and management of scarce resources. Finally, funding sources provided through nongovernmental sources, such as the Robert Wood Johnson Foundation, provide potential rural public health infrastructure development opportunities, such as data information systems, workforce competencies, and health improvement plans (Gamm & Hutchinson, 2005).

Local health departments are trying to affect policy development by supporting community efforts to change the causes of health disparities, using data to describe health disparities in particular jurisdictions, training the **public health workforce** (the population employed in public health professions) (Scutchfield & Keck, 2009, p. 403) on health disparities and their causes, prioritizing resources and programs, specifically for the reduction of health disparities, and taking public policy positions on health disparities through testimony, in written statements, or in the media (NACCHO, 2008). For each type of effort intended to affect the reduction of health disparities through policy, rural health departments are less likely to participate than those health departments representing larger populations. According to the NACCHO 2008 survey, 40 percent of rural health departments reported supporting community efforts to change causes of health disparities, trained their workforce, or used data to describe health problems. In addition, rural health departments are less likely than larger health departments to communicate with legislators, participate on boards or advisory panels, prepare issue briefs, or testify regarding specific health issues (NACCHO, 2008).

Population-Level Prevention in Rural America

Public health programs and interventions should result from an assessment of community health needs. Yet, often public health decisions are generated without input from the citizens such assessments are meant to help (Downey & Scutchfield, 2009). Particularly in rural areas there is often a lack of resources, technical expertise, and information technology capacity to monitor the health of a community (Gamm & Hutchinson, 2005). However, to be most effective, public health initiatives must be rooted in the values, knowledge, expertise, and interests of the individual community and its citizens (Citrin, 2001). Although many models exist for a **community needs assessment,** all share common attributes of bringing together empowered citizens to examine the community's health: collecting and analyzing statistics that measure community health and reviewing the data that identify problems that need to be addressed (Downey & Scutchfield, 2009). The following sections describe some of the more frequently used models for community needs assessment.

Planned Approach to Community Health (PATCH)

Developed by the CDC, PATCH follows the format of community needs assessment by including community mobilization, data collection, development of health priorities, and intervention design. Of note with the PATCH model is the partnership required between the CDC and state and local health departments (US Department of Health and Human Services, 1993).

Assessment Protocol for Excellence in Public Health (APEXPH)

Created by NACCHO in collaboration with the CDC, APEXPH includes an assessment of local health department capacity to address community health needs, organization of a community group to examine community data indicators, and a connection of local health department capacity to a focus on specific community problems (US Department of Health and Human Services et al., 1993).

Mobilizing for Action Through Planning and Partnership (MAPP)

Developed by NACCHO and the CDC, MAPP involves the local health department and other groups and agencies that make up the public health system of the area. MAPP begins with community organization and a visioning process followed by four separate assessments: community themes and strengths assessment, local public health system assessment, community health status assessment, and forces of change assessment (NACCHO, 2000).

Of these three models for community needs assessment, MAPP is currently the most frequently used. The others are of historic importance because they represent the early development of an approach to working with the community to define its needs and what public health programs were appropriate for that community.

Notably, the 2008 NACCHO profile indicates that participation in community health needs assessments varies by size of population served, ranging from a low of 53 percent for jurisdictions of less than 25,000 population, 66 percent for jurisdictions 25,000 to 49,999, to 80 percent for large jurisdictions of 500,000 or more (NACCHO, 2008). Bridging the gap from assessment of community needs to implementing public health programs is the **community health improvement plan** (CHIP). A CHIP follows the assessment of community needs, is used by members of the public health system, and enables priority setting, coordination, and targeting of resources as well as developing health polices and defining the actions to promote health (Public Health Accreditation Board, 2009). Participation in CHIPs, possibly due to the complexity of working with a wide variety of public health system partners, is lower than participation in community needs assessments. The 2008 NACCHO profiles report CHIP participation at a low of 43 percent for health departments serving jurisdictions of less than twenty-five thousand population up to 60 percent for jurisdictions of five hundred thousand or more (NACCHO, 2008).

After completing a community needs assessment and a community health improvement plan, health departments must find a way to use this information to generate useful community interventions. A source of information for local health departments is the *Community Guide to Preventive Services*. This guide was developed by the Community Preventive Services Task Force, an independent, nonfederal group of voluntary public health and prevention experts whose members are appointed by the CDC director. The guide is a credible resource that provides evidence-based information on the effectiveness of interventions, the populations and settings in which the interventions were used, cost of interventions, and when, necessary, the caveat that a specific intervention needs more research before its effectiveness is known (Community Preventive Services Task Force, 2010). Although the goal of the *Community Guide to Preventive Services* is to make evidence-based information accessible to community decision makers, the information provides very little, if any, information on implementation or the effects of differing population settings on the intervention (Briss et al., 2004).

Conclusion

As health problems in rural areas continue to grow, the importance of the work done in governmental public health agencies will also continue to grow. However, due to widely diverse infrastructures, these public health entities encounter difficulty in the examination and comparison of structure and methods of work. Keys to the continuation and growth of public health services in rural areas include the creation of partnerships with other entities of similar mission, effective management of the financing mechanisms available to public health, and the increased education of the public health workforce.

Summary

- Health problems in rural populations are growing.
- The infrastructure found in governmental public health entities is widely diverse, which creates difficulty in examination and comparison of their individual needs.
- Partnerships between rural health departments and other community organizations are critical to the ability to provide services.
- The financing mechanisms available to rural health departments affect the capacity to deliver needed services.
- Only a small percentage of the rural public health workforce is formally educated in public health, necessitating improved training methods to meet increasing demands.
- The root of public health programs and interventions should be in the assessment of community needs.

Key Terms

assessment	partnerships
assurance	policy development
community health improvement plan	public health system
community needs assessment	public health workforce
local health departments	window of opportunity

For Practice and Discussion

1. Working with a colleague from class, identify specific partnerships that a rural local health department should seek out and then discuss the importance of such partnerships to the ability to deliver services.

2. Discuss the impact of physician shortages in rural areas on the ability of rural local health departments to provide population-based services.

3. Identify the rural public health workforce issue that you believe has the biggest impact on the provision of services and justify your answer.

Acknowledgments

Partial funding for this chapter was provided by the Robert Wood Johnson Foundation.

References

Beck, A. (2010). *A systematic review of public health workforce literature: 1985–2010* (pp. 1–39). Ann Arbor: University of Michigan School of Public Health.

Briss, P., Brownson, R., Fielding, J., & Zaza, S. (2004). Developing and using the guide to community preventive services: Lessons learned about evidenced-based public health. *Annual Review of Public Health, 25,* 281–302.

Citrin, T. (2001). Enhancing public health research and learning through community-academic partnerships: The Michigan experience. *Public Health Reports, 116,* 74–78.

Community Preventive Services Task Force. (2010, March). *What is the community guide?* Podcast. Retrieved from http://www.thecommunityguide.org

Downey, L., & Scutchfield, F. D. (2009). *Community health planning and programming principles of public health practice* (pp. 289–306). Clifton Park, NY: Delmar.

Fee, E. (2009). *History and development of public health principles of public health practice* (pp. 12–35). Clifton Park, NY: Delmar.

Gamm, L. D., & Hutchinson, L. L. (Eds.). (2005). *Rural healthy people 2010: A companion document for Healthy People 2010* (Vol. 3). College Station: The Texas A&M University System Health Science Center, School of Rural Public Health, Southwest Rural Health Research Center. Retrieved from www.srph.tamhsc.edu/centers/rhp2010/Volume_3/Vol3rhp2010.pdf

Goldhagen, J., & Chiu, T. (1998). The view from the horizon: Strategic partnership of public health and academic medical centers, and managed care. *Journal of Public Health Management and Practice, 4*(1), 29–35.

Hajat, A., Stewart, K., & Hayes, K. (2003). The local public health workforce in rural communities. *Journal of Public Health Management and Practice, 9*(6), 481–488.

Hartley, D. (2004, October). Rural health disparities, population health, and rural culture. *American Journal of Public Health, 94*(10), 1675–1677.

Institute of Medicine. (1988). *The future of public health.* Washington, DC: National Academies Press.

Institute of Medicine. (2002). *The future of the public's health in the 21st century.* Washington, DC: Author.

Lobato, M., Roberts, C., Bazerman, L., & Hammett, T. (2004). Public health and correctional collaboration in tuberculosis control. *American Journal of Preventive Medicine, 27*(2), 112–117.

MacKinney, A. C., & Lundblad, J. P. (2010). *Securing high quality health care in rural America.* Columbia, SC: Rural Policy Research Institute.

Mays, G. P., Bhandari, M. W., & Smith, S. A. (2010). Understanding the organization of public health delivery systems: An empirical typology. *Milbank Quarterly, 88*(1), 81–111.

Meit, M. (2007). Public health in rural America. *Journal of Public Health Management and Practice, 13*(3), 235–236.

Meit, M. (2009). The emergence of local governmental public health: Practice standards and workforce implication. *Journal of Public Health Management and Practice, 15*(6 Suppl.), 531–532.

Meit, M., Ettaro, L., Hamlin, B., & Piya, B. (2009). Rural public health financing: Implications for community health promotion initiatives. *Journal of Public Health Management and Practice, 15*(3), 210–215.

Meit, M., & Knudson, A. (2009, May/June). Why is rural public health important? A look to the future. *Journal of Public Health Management and Practice, 15*(3), 185–190.

Morgan, A. (2002). A national call to action: CDC's 2001 Urban and Rural Health Chartbook. *The Journal of Rural Health, 18,* 382–383.

NACCHO. (2000). *Mobilizing for action through planning and partnership (MAPP).* Washington, DC: Author.

NACCHO. (2008). *National profile of local health departments.* Washington, DC: Author.

NACCHO. (2010). *Local health department job losses an program cuts: Findings from January/February 2010 survey.* Washington, DC: Author.

National Rural Health Association. (2010). *What's different about rural health care?* Podcast. Retrieved from http://www.ruralhealthweb.org/go/left/about-rural-health/what-s-different-about-rural-health-care

North Carolina Rural Health Research & Policy Analysis Center. (2010). *Rural health snapshot*. Retrieved from http://www.shepscenter.unc.edu/rural/snapshot.html

Public Health Accreditation Board. (2009). *Public Health Accreditation Board standards and measures*. Retrieved from http://www.phaboard.org/accreditation-process/public-health-department-standards-and-measures/

Public Health Institute. (2010). *Health reform and local health departments: Opportunities for the Centers for Disease Control and Prevention*. Oakland, CA: Author.

Ricketts, T. (2009). *Public health policy and the policy-making process principles of public health practice* (pp. 86–115). Clifton Park, NY: Delmar.

Scutchfield, F. D., Beversdorf, C., Hiltabiddle, S., & Violants, T. (1997). A survey of state health department compliance with the recommendations of the Institute of Medicine report, *The Future of Public Health*. *Journal of Health Policy*, 13–29.

Scutchfield, F. D., Hiltabiddle, S., Rawding, N., & Violants, T. (1997). Compliance with the recommendations of the Institute of Medicine report, *The Future of Public Health;* a survey of local health departments. *Journal of Public Health Policy, 18*(2), 155–166.

Scutchfield, F. D., & Keck, C. W. (2009). *Principles of public health practice*. Clifton Park, NY: Delmar.

Scutchfield, F. D., & Howard, A. F. (2011). Moving on upstream: The role of health departments in addressing socioecologic determinants of disease. *American Journal of Preventive Medicine, 40*(1S1), S80–S83.

US Department of Health and Human Services. (1993). *Planned approach to community health (PATCH) program descriptions*. Washington, DC: Author.

US Department of Health and Human Services, Public Health Service, Centers for Disease Control, Public Health Practice Program Office, National Association of County Health Officials. (1993). *Assessment protocol for excellence in public health (APEXPH)*. Washington, DC: National Association of City and County Health Officials.

Wellever, A. (2006). *Local public health at the crossroads: The structure of health departments in rural areas*. Topeka: Kansas Health Institute.

Zahner, S., & Corrado, S. (2004). Local health department partnerships with faith-organizations. *Journal of Public Health Management and Practice, 10*(3), 258–265.

Chapter 6

Rural Public Health Systems
A View from Colorado

Julie A. Marshall
Lisa N. VanRaemdonck

Learning Objectives

- Understand how Colorado has dealt with rural issues related to public and environmental health.
- Understand how the distant and recent history of a rural state may influence current public health practice.
- Identify examples of how funding limitations may have a negative impact on rural public health practice.
- Describe differing needs in workforce capacity in rural public health.
- Describe the advantages of partnerships and collaborations to the promotion of rural public health.

•••

Many forces have shaped the diverse public health landscape in rural Colorado including topography and weather, natural resources (wildlife, minerals, oil, and gas), and a history of mining, agriculture, ranching, and tourism. Traveling over the state by air, one appreciates the expansive and sparsely populated land mass—mountains and plains that were home to Native Americans, early Spanish conquistadors, Hispanic settlers, fur trappers, miners, and with time, farmers and ranchers. Today ski areas and surface mines are carved into the mountain tapestry. Traveling by land, the collection of roads still leaves some areas inaccessible. Most rural towns reflect Colorado's unique history. For example, earlier Spanish and Hispanic settlers built churches and water ditches, mining towns built saloons, cattle towns built wide streets, towns were built along the railroad lines, homes of migrant workers were first built in agricultural areas, and now areas near ski resorts attract seasonal workers. So how do the geography and this history define the public health landscape in rural Colorado today?

Geopolitical Determinants of Health

Land area in rural counties makes up more than 60 percent of Colorado (sixty-nine thousand square miles), and it is populated by about 687,293 residents or 14 percent of the state's total population (Figure 6.1). In Colorado, geography and access to roads play a role in the health of the community (Figure 6.2). A flat map does not fully convey the concept of distance. Travel time and access vary by location and season depending on conditions of mountain roads and passes and inclement weather or rock slides that can slow or even close roads for hours or days. Some areas are isolated for much of the winter by seasonal roads and closed mountain passes.

Colorado has sixty-four governmental counties including twenty-four designated as rural (communities with fewer than twenty-five thousand residents and that are not part of an urbanized area) and twenty-three as frontier (fewer than six people per square mile). Many of the remaining seventeen counties with urban areas also contain large rural areas, and only two counties in Colorado (both located in the Denver metro area) do not contain any rural areas.

Most rural counties are governed by three elected county commissioners who manage county-level activities including county finances and revenues from local taxes, county property and facilities, land use, county transportation infrastructure, environmental and human health programs, and social services. This decentralized governance, with a philosophical focus on local control, creates assets and challenges. For example, local control may make it easier to tailor priorities to local needs and to redirect resources and introduce change as new issues emerge in the community. However, state or federal revenues to counties are often saddled with requirements that make it difficult to address larger problems with relevance to multiple funders. Sharing of resources in a region may be limited by lack of common priorities and governance across neighboring counties.

Whereas public health jurisdictions have county boundaries, public health issues are often not limited to these same **geopolitical** boundaries (boundaries defined by geographical features or governing authority). As health care has

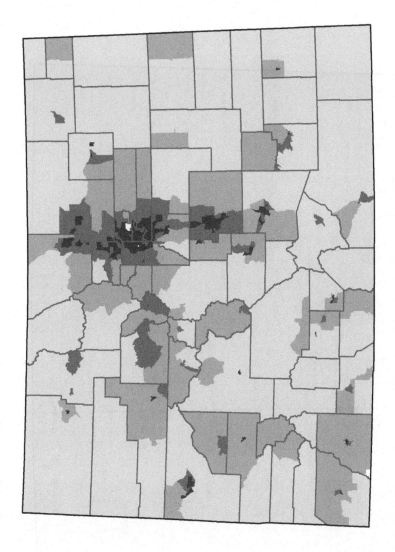

Figure 6.1. Population Density of Colorado, 2010

Source: Devon Williford, Colorado Department of Public Health and Environment.

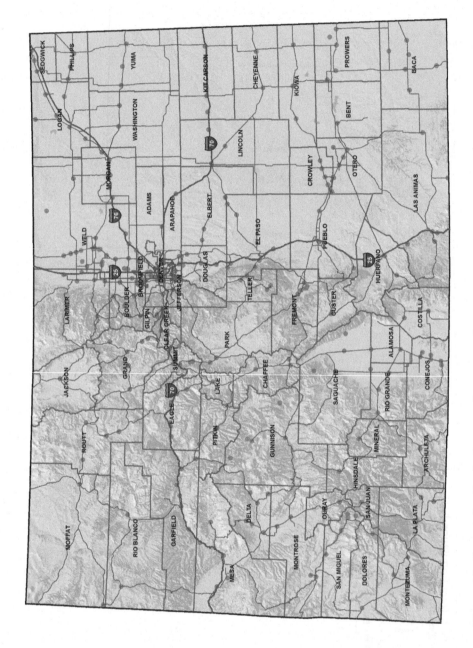

Figure 6.2. Topography, Roads, Towns and Counties of Colorado
Source: Devon Williford, Colorado Department of Public Health and Environment.

transitioned from small, independent, primary care practices to regional medical centers and federally qualified health centers, health care service organizations in rural areas now are likely to have a regional hub that serves a larger catchment area (Figure 6.3). Clients may choose providers based on location, health insurance coverage, or other factors that transcend geopolitical boundaries.

Environmental Determinants of Health

Environmental determinants are natural and human made. Although the types of pollution common to urban environments with high traffic density and concentrated industrial sites may be less of a problem in rural areas, there are other important environmental concerns. The Colorado Rocky Mountains are rich with natural resources that are tapped through oil and gas extraction and surface and underground mining. The history of mining in Colorado has left areas of the land scarred and contaminated with mine tailings and runoff. Similar to other areas in the Southwest, there are aquifers used for drinking water throughout Colorado that contain naturally occurring arsenic, uranium, and radon at concentrations above EPA limits. Many people in rural areas are served by untested well water systems and onsite wastewater systems (septic systems) that are in need of updating and repair. In rural Colorado, air pollution can result from confined animal feeding operations, windblown dust, wood-burning stoves, and oil and gas mining operations. Although environmental health is a concern in rural Colorado, the human health and environmental health professionals in communities can be fragmented due to county structure. In most rural counties, environmental health specialists work within building or planning departments and the public health agency covering human health is a separate department. It takes extra time and effort to collaborate across county-level agencies to manage environmental health issues through a human health lens.

Measures of the built environment and understanding of its relationship to physical activity, food resources, and other resources in rural Colorado are beginning to be explored. In some areas, parks and trails may promote activity but in many rural areas, destination exercise, walking, or biking as a mode of transportation is challenging. State and local foundations have provided strategic funding for rural communities in Colorado to support coalition-focused community change to affect obesity by increasing healthy eating and active living. Rural communities have invested in playground equipment, biking and hiking trails, health coaches, transportation assessments, and community awareness and education campaigns. They are also engaging with community members to build new opportunities for further developing healthy communities.

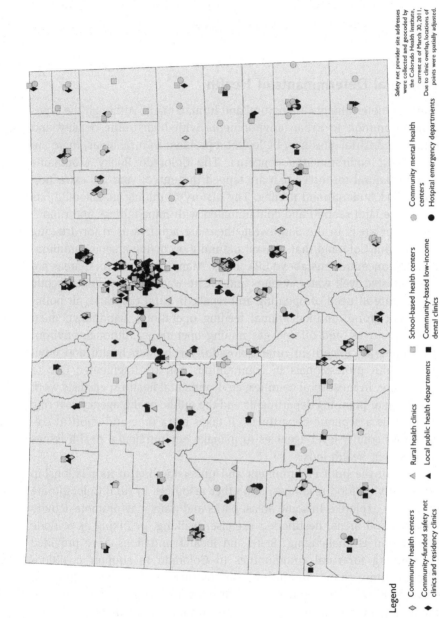

Legend

◇ Community health centers
◆ Community-funded safety net
　 clinics and residency clinics

△ Rural health clinics
▲ Local public health departments

▦ School-based health centers
■ Community-based low-income
　 dental clinics

◉ Community mental health
　 centers
● Hospital emergency departments

Safety net provider site addresses
were collected and geocoded by
the Colorado Health Institute,
current as of March 30, 2011.
Due to clinic overlap, locations of
points were spatially adjusted.

Figure 6.3. Public Health and Safety Net Clinics by County, Colorado 2011

Source: The Colorado Health Institute.

Social Determinants of Health

On average, rural communities in Colorado tend to have lower median incomes, more children living in poverty, fewer educational and economic opportunities, and limited health care access when compared to urban areas. Although these statistics are similar to other rural areas in the United States, it is important to recognize that there is a large degree of variation from one rural community to the next. For example, the proportion of children living in poverty ranges from 6.4 percent in Pitkin County to 44.9 percent in Saguache County (US Census Bureau, 2009).

Rural communities in Colorado tend to have lower median incomes, more children living in poverty, fewer educational and economic opportunities, and limited health care access when compared to urban areas.

Ethnic disparities are also common in rural Colorado. For example, Hispanic ethnicity is associated with higher rates of obesity and type 2 diabetes and the percent of residents who are Hispanic varies from 2.8 percent in Hinsdale County to 66.0 percent in Costilla County.

Although Colorado is considered a healthy state by many accounts, health trends and disparities data show that Colorado residents are experiencing poor health outcomes at an increasing rate. For example, although Colorado is known as the leanest state based on prevalence estimates of obesity in adults, increasing temporal trends parallel other states (United Health Foundation, 2010). Moreover, Colorado is ranked tenth for childhood obesity (Trust for America's Health, 2009) with variation by school ranging from 5 percent to 46 percent of children being overweight or obese (Marshall et al., 2008) and forty-third for geographic disparities in mortality (United Health Foundation, 2010). The state Office of Health Disparities, housed at the state public health department, has chosen to focus primarily on racial and ethnic disparities concluding that little progress has been in made in reducing these critical health inequalities (Palacio et al., 2009). Although important, this focus on racial and ethnic disparities has resulted in limited reporting and focus on health disparities in rural or frontier areas.

The Public Health System in Rural Colorado

The public health system in rural Colorado is different from the urban areas of the state in terms of its history, the impact of funding and funding changes, the recruitment and retention of a public health workforce, and the depth of partnerships required to provide health and public health services. These core infrastructure components provide a backbone to understanding public health service provision.

Rural Public Health History

The history of public health in Colorado is a fascinating one with traveling nurses, disease outbreaks on the trail, rumors of tuberculosis cure in the mountain air, rampant mining without regard to the environment, and a steady influx of new residents. This evolution is filled with fits and starts as Colorado became a state and attempted to manage the transient groups and sparse populations across vast land areas. Public health in the rural areas began with a small group of traveling nurses affiliated with the Denver Flower Mission who attended to the residents in mining and trapping camps. In 1944, Dr. Florence Sabin, a renowned scientist and the first woman member of the Academy of Sciences, came out of retirement when she was appointed by the Colorado governor to chair a subcommittee on health (Colorado Department of Health, Public Information Office, 1969). This began a campaign that would provide great inspiration and momentum to public health in Colorado. Dr. Sabin was able to get laws passed that developed public health services in every Colorado county. Rural counties were served by nursing services and the urban areas were served by organized health departments. The diverse agencies had different authority and requirements, resulting in the current variation in the breadth and depth of public health services provided in rural communities.

Public Health Act of 2008

Great strides were made in the 1940s and during the 1980s there were calls for updating the public health laws to remove reference to outdated activities including managing cholera and contaminated rags and to add a set of core public health services that should be provided to every resident. In the large majority of rural areas, public health was still served by nursing services. Only those services falling within the scope of the practice of nursing and deemed necessary by the local board of health were required. This requirement meant there was not direct provision for environmental health services and the services provided were often a result of history rather than current needs (Colorado Department of Public Health and Environment, the State Board of Health, and the Public Health Act Advisory Group, 2009). However, it was not until 2007 that the possibility of updating the public health laws became a reality. Updating the Public Health Act of Colorado involved a complete review and editing process for the entire public health law. The act, passed in 2008, removed the multiple structures of public health agency and made all local governmental public health entities into "local public health agencies." The act is in the implementation phase and former nursing services in rural areas are working to understand the changes in service mix that will be required by the development of core public health services. The public health act also requires that the state health department and local public health agencies undertake a community health assessment and a community health improvement plan (prerequisites for the public health accreditation process). It is anticipated that the implementation of the act will result in more uniform public health services being provided across the state with a standard level of quality.

Public Health Funding

As with many other states, funding for governmental public health in Colorado has ebbed and flowed over time. Limited funds are mandated for public health services so there are many service areas, such as chronic disease prevention, that rely on competitive grants to distribute federal, state, and private funds. These grants come from a variety of sources, are relatively short term, often address funder priorities first, and often come with complicated administrative overhead with differing rules and reporting requirements for each grant. This funding system makes it difficult to coordinate and provide services that respond to local priorities and that can be sustained over time. Availability of funding has changed with the state's political ideology, programs, and philosophy at the state health department, federal-level programs, new taxes and fees, the growth and contraction of industry, and the local, state, and national economies. With this inconsistency in funding comes the building of programs and infrastructure followed by the destruction and dissolution of those same programs and the loss of staff, expertise, and infrastructure.

Two recent examples highlight the funding instability: the loss and reinstatement of state-level per capita funds and the passing of a tobacco tax and subsequent transfer of those funds away from local public health and community-based organizations. In 2002, a governor's decision resulted in the total loss of state-level funding that was provided through the state health department. These funds had been unrestricted and distributed according to a per capita formula to all public health agencies across the state. Public health directors who led agencies during the subsequent years consider it a gloomy time in local public health. Agencies lost well-qualified and experienced staff, programs, and services to community members were drastically reduced. In 2006, funds were reinstated by a new governor but not before the damage was done to local public health agencies. With the national economic decline that followed, the state legislature had to consider whether the general per capita funding for local public health should be used to fill holes in the state budget.

In 2004, the citizens of Colorado passed a tobacco tax with legislative restrictions on how the funds could be used. The collected dollars were required to fund specified public health and community health care programs. Millions of dollars flowed from the state health department to local public health agencies and community-based organizations to build tobacco prevention and cessation programs, tackle health disparities in communities, and perform and support local screening and treatment programs for cancer, cardiovascular disease, and pulmonary disease.

Colorado built a tobacco prevention and cessation program across the state that funded local communities and supported experts providing technical assistance at the state level, which provided momentum to pass the Colorado Clean Indoor Air Act in 2006. By 2007 a wide range of public health programming was funded in every Colorado county. One provision in the tobacco tax legislation allowed the funds to be revoked from the stated programs when two-thirds of state legislators voted that the state was in a fiscal emergency. In summer 2009, a fiscal emergency was declared and the funds were taken away from local public health agencies and community-based organizations. Staff were lost to these funding cuts, networks of professionals were disintegrated, and agencies terminated prevention and screening services.

Public Health Workforce

Although Colorado was host to various public health education programs, it wasn't until 2008 that Colorado and the Rocky Mountain region opened its first formal school of public health (accredited in 2010). This collaborative school offers degrees at the University of Colorado, Colorado State University, and University of Northern Colorado. It has provided broader access to public health professional education and professional development. Two new undergraduate public health programs in Denver and in rural Durango will help in training entry-level public health professionals. Prior to 2008, there were few opportunities for working professionals in rural areas to obtain an advanced degree in public health.

Colorado's public health history has created a public health workforce in rural Colorado of primarily public health nurses. Most rural public health directors are registered nurses and several have master's degrees. Approximately 16 percent of the local public health workforce serves in a jurisdiction of fewer than twenty-five thousand people.

Rural public health directors report a challenge in recruitment and retention of qualified staff. Teller County public health director, Christina Rubin, has a unique approach to hiring and managing staff to increase retention and job satisfaction. Teller County is similar to several counties in Colorado—within driving distance from a metro area but far enough away to experience the traditional rural challenges in recruiting and retaining qualified health professionals. Chris concentrates on high standards, employee involvement, and finding the right fit for employees and the organization.

Rural public health work requires employees to be true generalists and have the ability to perform a wide variety of public health activities, including providing immunizations and health care, facilitating a community coalition meeting, collecting and analyzing community health data, creating community health plans, and working with partners to plan for public health emergencies. It takes a particular type of person to fit well into this broad role. In Teller, Chris requires all staff to hold at least a bachelor's in nursing, and ensures they have had some education in community health. This high standard allowed her to increase the base salary for staff positions, which is used with a more flexible schedule and ample holidays and sick time as a recruiting tool. Staff members are involved in strategic planning for the agency and are asked to offer ideas for improvement and programs. They are also encouraged to get involved in the community so they can gain leadership skills and see community issues from outside the walls of the public health agency.

As happens in most rural public health agencies, Chris spends part of her time working as a nurse practitioner in the public health clinic. This keeps her close to the clinic processes and community members so she can make more informed decisions toward quality improvement and program development. She works closely with nursing, medicine, and other students to help give them a glimpse into the rigors and benefits of working in rural public health.

Partnerships and Collaboration

Partnerships are critical in rural public health because single organizations rarely have the resources and capacity to manage comprehensive services. In rural Colorado, local public health agencies also take on significant responsibility for providing and ensuring access to care. The network of community health centers, rural hospitals, and rural health centers provides a foundation of access, but local public health also fills gaps in clinical care. In rural public health agencies this often means that a public health director also serves as a nurse or nurse practitioner who provides clinical services. In some communities, the local public health director is the school nurse or the jail nurse as well. Also, due to the limited number of organizations in rural communities and the limited potential for stable funding, some public health agencies provide home care services whose revenues may support public health infrastructure.

In some communities, the local public health director is the school nurse or the jail nurse as well.

Partnerships at the state level provide support for public health professionals across the state through the Public Health Alliance of Colorado (the Alliance). In 2006, public health leaders and foundations came together to create a unique way to support many of the nationally affiliated professional associations and provide a united voice for public health. The Alliance is an umbrella organization for ten major public health professional associations in the state. This collaboration has allowed the statewide, professional organizations to retain their individuality while providing high-quality administrative support in an efficient manner. The Alliance serves as a unified voice for public health in questions of policy and philosophy and provides a neutral place for public health professionals to connect, collaborate, gain leadership skills, and work toward improving public health at the system level.

The role of the Alliance office is primarily one of a convener, coordinator, and administrative hub. It was in the Alliance office that public health leaders crafted the Public Health Act of 2008. Participation in Alliance organizations builds and connects rural public health leaders across the state. Board members and leaders in all of the organizations come from all areas of Colorado, and rural areas are well represented. The professional networks provide support and opportunities to learn from colleagues and develop partnerships.

Rural Public Health Innovations

The following sections of this chapter feature three rural communities, each with a story that provides insights into how their public health agencies addressed challenges.

Weld County: Maximizing Opportunities for Collaboration

Communities house resources in a variety of public and private agencies, each with their own mission and funding sources. These resources can be mobilized to effectively address community health when a culture of collaboration is built and nurtured. Partners in Weld County in northeast Colorado have created an organization of organizations, the North Colorado Health Alliance, committed to integrated and seamless provision of broadly defined health services.

Weld County covers 3,999 square miles at an altitude of 4,400 to 5,000 feet with rolling prairies and low hills in the western part of the county. Fertile fields and rain have helped make Weld County a leading producer of cattle, grain, and sugar beets and it is the second leading oil- and gas-producing region in the state (Weld County Colorado, n.d.). The county borders Wyoming on the north, rural communities on the east, and urban areas on the west and south. With 253,000 residents (US Census Bureau, 2010), Weld County includes one principal city, Greeley, and rural areas that include thirty-one municipalities, seventeen school districts, and twenty-four fire districts resulting in a large number of entities to work with in order to ensure provision of public health services to all residents. It is legislatively designated as a home rule county. The estimated median household income, $57,578, is just above the state average of $55,735 (US Census Bureau, 2009), yet 19.5 percent of residents are uninsured (US Census Bureau, 2007) and 18.5 percent of children live in poverty (US Census Bureau, 2009). The majority of health disparities occur among Hispanic residents living in poverty.

Alignment of the organizations that later became the North Colorado Health Alliance began in 2001 when, in spite of working so hard to decrease the teen birth rate, increase the percent of pregnant women receiving prenatal care, and decrease low birth weight, the county continued to rank low in these areas. It finally "made us mad," said public health director, Dr. Mark Wallace. It was at this juncture that public health "reached across the table" to the Community Health Center, who could best reach the population at risk, in a new way, saying "we need you," "we trust you." Transcending current interagency issues, the agencies committed 100 percent to work together. Coordinating when and where services were provided, free pregnancy testing was made available every day. Family planning was linked with prenatal care. Even though multiple agencies were providing services, every effort was made to make this seamless to the women seeking care. Partners began to see the health indicators turn around.

Since this precipitating event, the North Colorado Health Alliance has developed organically on a foundation of collaboration—a way of seeing the world and modeled by leaders every day. Employees are recognized for successes resulting from partnerships. This foundation is supported by four pillars:

- Access to physical, mental, oral, and public health services
- A workforce with a capacity to design and support systems that are **collaborative** (working together to achieve community goals) and integrated, culturally competent, and will address needs of the future
- Services and activities that are integrative in nature and resulting in a seamless interface for the person using the service
- Accountability to the community

Exemplifying the vision, mission, and pillars of the Alliance, integrative priorities have resulted in a shared community electronic health record. As a result, a child identified by her physician with high blood lead levels was seamlessly referred to environmental health. The family was contacted and an environmental assessment was conducted by the county's water chemist, a shared community resource, trained in environmental assessment. After determining that the source of exposure was leaded pipe dope brought home from work on the father's clothing, the Occupational, Safety, and Health Administration, and the work site successfully joined forces to remove the worksite exposure without litigation. Training was put in place for workers and physicians to promote practices that avoided human lead exposure. This example demonstrates the power of collaboration not only in addressing an individual child's lead exposure but also in addressing an environmental issue that may have affected many children and adults.

The culture of collaboration and engagement in Weld County runs deep. They have brought the process of community health assessment to life by the inclusion of community partners. A detailed community assets inventory helps clarify what resources can be realigned or leveraged to address health priorities. The process creates tangible success, which demonstrates the benefits of a collaborative approach.

The San Luis Valley: Shared Infrastructure for Research and Practice

Universities house faculty members and resources that can be mobilized to support not only rural workforce development (e.g., area health education centers, a variety of public health training centers) but also shared services and infrastructure that serve the local public health system (e.g., cooperative extensions, community-based research). The rural San Luis Valley (SLV) in south central Colorado is a six-county area of forty-six thousand people who have decades of experience collaborating among local health providers, public health officials, educators, community members, and academic partners. Here we feature links between community-based research and public health infrastructure and services.

The SLV is a rural intermountain valley surrounded by the Rocky Mountains, adjacent to the New Mexico border, and covering a land area the size of Connecticut. The valley economy relies on agriculture, tourism, and its role as a regional government center. Three of the six counties are designated as frontier counties, with fewer than six people per square mile. The estimated median household income in the SLV is $33,660 compared to the Colorado median of $55,735 (US Census Bureau, 2009). The percent of children living in poverty is extremely high, ranging from 29 to 45 percent in five of the six counties (US Census Bureau 2009). Approximately 22 percent of residents are uninsured (US Census Bureau, 2007) and many rely on Medicaid for access to health care. The SLV is identified as a Health Professional Shortage Area and a Medically Underserved Area, two key federal designations that identify areas with severe health care provider access issues and areas in need of assistance with health care delivery. Despite these lower socioeconomic conditions, the people of the SLV have a strong history of working together to improve health and the environment.

Researchers from the University of Colorado, School of Medicine, and now, the recently established Colorado School of Public Health, have conducted studies of type 2 diabetes and related conditions in the SLV since 1983. The SLV has had a relatively stable population for decades. About half of residents are Hispanic and half are non-Hispanic white. These two ethnic groups have lived side by side for generations with little intermarriage. In part because of the relative geographic isolation of the valley, first-line medical care is usually sought locally. These conditions provided a unique opportunity to study the etiology and natural history of type 2 diabetes in two ethnic groups known to have different disease rates.

Early observational studies in Alamosa and Conejos counties extended the reach of medical care providers with blood glucose, lipid, and blood pressure testing reported back to participants and their providers. In 1,351 participants without a history of diabetes, about 5 percent were determined to have previously undiagnosed diabetes and 12.5 percent had impaired glucose tolerance. Detailed studies conducted to understand the microvascular and macrovascular complications of diabetes brought otherwise unavailable clinical technology to the SLV. For example, there was not a retinal camera in the SLV and about 80 percent of identified adults with diabetes in the two-county area received photographs read by an ophthalmologist. The first dual-energy X-ray absorptiometry machine in the SLV was leased by the university to conduct studies of body composition and shared with local providers for bone density assessments. In a later study, a similar machine was purchased by a study, housed in the regional medical center, and became their property when the study ended. A recent study analyzed water samples from well and public water supplies, mapped water arsenic concentrations throughout the valley, and related this to development of heart disease and diabetes. A project studying the translation of a cooking-based nutrition curriculum focused on healthy eating to be implemented in low-income rural schools (Belansky et al., 2006) has led to dissemination and sustainability of the curriculum in twelve of fourteen elementary schools in the SLV. Partnerships between researchers and community partners deepened as school and family intervention projects grew out of community-identified needs and as partners began to ask researchers for program evaluation support. With this experience came recognition that research and practice partners often have related needs that could be supported by common infrastructure.

In 2009, Green et al. comprehensively reviewed theories on diffusion and knowledge dissemination, use, and integration in public health and then put the composite application of these theories to a test. The resulting use-focused surveillance framework provides a unifying system for integrating research and practice in the SLV where the small population size characteristic of rural communities makes it difficult to obtain locally relevant data regarding emerging health issues.

Grand County: Public Health and Community Partnerships

Grand County is a land filled with mountains and meadows north of the I-70 corridor and is home to two ski resorts and the western side of Rocky Mountain National Park, which sees fewer visitors than the main entrance to the park. The county lies in northern part of the "rural resort" area in the central mountains of Colorado. The economy relies on tourism and vacation homes to support its construction, retail and food service, and real estate industries.

Grand County is designated as rural, with approximately eight people per square mile. The estimated median household income is $58,209 compared to the Colorado median of $55,735 (US Census Bureau, 2009). The percent of children living in poverty is 12 percent compared to 16 percent across Colorado (US Census Bureau, 2009). Approximately, 25 percent of residents are uninsured (US Census Bureau, 2007) and those who are eligible rely on Medicaid for access to health care. Grand is in close-enough proximity (sixty-seven miles) from Denver, however, far enough away that many residents struggle with access to primary and specialty health care.

Partnerships across the health and public health communities have led to increased access to health care in this county. Here, partnership is more than just sitting at a table together or attending meetings. True partnership begins with a deep-seated belief in the value of community connections. Health leaders, such as Brene Belew-LaDue, director of Grand County Public Health, and Jen Fanning, director of the Grand County Rural Health Network, work to consistently create and maintain functional partnerships.

The Grand County Rural Health Network was created in 2000 through a HRSA-funded rural development grant. The network is an independent 501(c)3 with a mission to "work in partnership to improve and direct the future of healthcare in Grand County." In the competitive and often turf-based environment of health care, and in a conservative community where the role of government is constantly questioned, it is beneficial to have a nongovernmental, neutral convener. The Grand County Rural Health Network provides a **nonpoliticized** (not directly influenced by politics or political decisions) venue for community members and health professionals to make strategic decisions based on data, community need, and existing community capacity.

Assessments in 2005 indicated that most residents received health care services outside of the county. Grand County had one critical-access hospital and several physicians but most residents had to drive to Denver or other

counties to receive care. The network determined that there were two important reasons to tackle this issue of access to care. First, all residents deserve
to be able to get care close to their home. Second, because most of the health
care dollars spent by Grand County residents were spent outside of the county,
a significant economic opportunity was not being realized.

The partnership has led to the development of two health care voucher
programs developed to increase access within the county. Vouchers are accepted
by local providers for acute medical, pharmacy, dental, and mental health
care needs for children and medical and pharmacy needs for adults. In addition to the gap-filling voucher programs, the partnership has created a greater
vision for an integrated medical center co-locating the range of health organizations and including an outpatient center connected with the local critical
access hospital. The economy and other issues got in the way of the development but leaders in the community still envisioned a robust health care
community site.

The Grand County Rural Health Network took on the role of connecting
rural health care providers through providing administrative support to the
Grand County Healthcare Professionals Society. This group has existed as a
volunteer organization for years but has achieved a new level of activity
with formal staff support. An initial project created by the members was to
achieve a goal of 100 percent of county primary care physicians using the
assuring better childhood development (ABCD) tool. This change in practice
across all providers built their capacity to engage in quality improvement
activities.

Community partnership and involvement exists beyond the traditional
community leaders. Not only do the public health and rural health network
directors participate on advisory and community boards within the county, but
they also encourage staff to participate as well. This builds leadership and
connections among staff members and prevents typical burnout of the same
leaders who participate in many committees within a rural area.

Conclusion

Colorado is an example of a largely rural state that has experienced a host of
challenges to public health. Some of these challenges are inherent while others
are a product of financial cutbacks. Fortunately, orchestrated efforts have
resulted in the formation of health partnerships, alliances, and coalitions
which, in turn, have catalyzed efforts to improve rural public health infrastructures. Recent success stories of three distinctly different rural counties serve
as strong evidence that creative collaborations in rural America can have a
tremendously powerful influence on the health and well-being of the public.

Summary

- Colorado is an example of a largely rural state that has experienced a host of challenges to public health.

- Rural public health workers in Colorado are oftentimes generalists in the field, performing a multitude of tasks such as providing health care, collaborating with the community, and organizing for emergency preparedness.

- Orchestrated efforts have resulted in the formation of health partnerships, alliances, and coalitions that in turn have catalyzed efforts to improve rural public health infrastructures.

- Success stories of three distinctly different rural counties serve as strong evidence that creative collaborations in rural America can have a tremendously powerful influence on the health and well-being of the public.

- On average, rural communities in Colorado tend to have lower median incomes, more children living in poverty, fewer educational and economic opportunities, and limited health care access when compared to urban areas.

- Geopolitical determinants of health such as geography, climate, road access, and decentralized governance are characteristic of a predominantly rural Colorado.

- Environmental determinants in Colorado are results of nature and human-made events, including water sources with naturally occurring arsenic, uranium, and radon; contamination from the mining industry; and pollution from animal operations.

- Partnerships and collaboration between and among state and local governments and resources are imperative in addressing the increasing health disparities in rural Colorado.

Key Terms

collaborative   nonpoliticized

geopolitical

For Practice and Discussion

1. Use the Internet to investigate rural health coalitions in your own state. Find one best example of a rural health coalition and compare that to each of three examples presented in this chapter.

2. Working with a colleague identify all of the advantages (stated in this chapter) that stem from partnerships in public health. Then, for each advantage mutually decide if it (1) is unique to rural counties, (2) is more likely to occur in nonrural counties, or (3) has an equal probability of occurring in rural and nonrural counties.

Acknowledgments

This publication was supported by cooperative agreement number 1U48DP001932–01 from the Centers for Disease Control and Prevention. The findings and conclusions in this article are those of the author(s) and do not necessarily represent the official position of the Centers for Disease Control and Prevention. We would also like to thank Devon Williford, Colorado Department of Public Health and Environment; the Colorado Health Institute; Dr. Mark Wallace, Weld County Department of Public Health and Environment; E. Brene Belew-LaDue, Grand County Public Health and Grand County Nursing Services director; Jen Fanning, executive director, Grand County Rural Health Network; and Christina G. Rubin, director, Teller County Public Health Department.

References

Belansky, E. S., Romaniello, C., Morin, C., Uyeki, T., Sawyer, R. L., Scarbro, S., Crane, L., Auld, G. W., Hamman, R. F., & Marshall, J. A. (2006). Dissemination of a school-based nutrition and physical activity program in a low income, rural community. *Journal of Nutrition Education and Behavior, 38*, 106–113.

Colorado Department of Health, Public Information Office. (1969). *Health in Colorado: The first one hundred years.* Denver: Author.

Colorado Department of Public Health and Environment, the State Board of Health, and the Public Health Act Advisory Group. (2009). *Colorado's public health improvement plan.* Denver: Author. Retrieved from http://www.cdphe.state.co.us/opp/resources/FINALDRAFT_COPHIP.pdf

Green, L.W., Ottoson, J. M., Garcia, C., & Hiatt, R. A. (2009). Diffusion theory and knowledge dissemination, utilization, and integration in public health. *Annual Review of Public Health, 30*, 151–174. doi:10.1146/annurev.publhealth.031308.100049.

Marshall, J. A., Poniers, A., Drisko, J., White, C., & Tenney, M. (2008). *Obesity surveillance in Colorado children.* Presented at the Colorado Public Health Association annual meeting, Breckenridge, CO. Retrieved from http://ucdenver.edu/academics/colleges/PublicHealth/research/centers/RMPRC/resources/Pages/Presentations.aspx

Palacio, M., Reynolds, R., Drisko, J., Lucero, C., Hunt, C., & Phi, K. (2009). Racial and ethnic disparities in Colorado 2009. Denver: Colorado Department of Public

Health and Environment, Office of Health Disparities. Retrieved from http://www.cdphe.state.co.us/ohd/ethnicdisparitiesreport/HD%202009%20LowRes.pdf

Trust for America's Health. (2009). *F as in fat: How obesity policies are failing America*. Retrieved from http://healthyamericans.org/reports/obesity2009/

United Health Foundation. (2010). *America's health rankings*, 2010 Edition. Retrieved from http://www.americashealthrankings.org/

US Census Bureau. (2007). *Model-based small area health insurance estimates (SAHIE) for counties and states*. Retrieved from http://www.census.gov/hhes/www/sahie/index.html

US Census Bureau. (2009). *Model-based small area income & poverty estimates (SAIPE) for school districts, counties, and states*. Retrieved from http://www.census.gov/hhes/www/saipe/

US Census Bureau. (2010). *2010 census data for Colorado*. Retrieved from http://dola.colorado.gov/dlg/demog/census2010/census_2010.html

Weld County Colorado. (n.d.). *About Weld*. Retrieved from http://www.co.weld.co.us/AboutWeld/

Chapter 7

Rural Public Health Systems
A View from Kentucky

Baretta R. Casey

Learning Objectives

- Understand Kentucky's health status ranking.
- Gain knowledge of the health disparities affecting Kentucky citizens.
- Understand the barriers to assess of tertiary and subspecialty health care.
- Understand the critical role county assessments play in planning to meet the needs of a community.
- Gain knowledge of unique models to alleviate barriers to assessing health care for rural Kentucky.

• • •

The Commonwealth of Kentucky is geographically made up of three distinct areas: the Appalachian highlands of eastern Kentucky, the Bluegrass region of central Kentucky, and the Upper Mississippi Delta region of western Kentucky. Kentucky has an abundance of lakes for recreational activities, mostly human-made to prevent flooding of the regions. There are many species of wildlife (e.g., white tail deer, wild turkey, and elk) and the commonwealth has a fair number of avid hunters. Kentucky is also known for its thoroughbred horses, cattle and crop farms, and bourbon distilleries. Vineyards and wineries are quickly becoming a new source of economic growth in the commonwealth.

The air pollution in Kentucky is low compared to some states in the United States with less industry and large amounts of forest throughout the Kentucky landmass.

The Appalachian highlands are defined by the Appalachian Regional Commission (ARC) as those counties that are within the Appalachian Mountain chain. ARC's definition encompasses fifty-four counties in Kentucky (Appalachian Regional Commission, 2010). All these counties within Appalachian Kentucky are rural counties. The topography of this mountain chain is made up of beautiful vistas with high mountain peaks intertwined by valleys and mountain streams boasting scenic waterfalls. However, this same mountain chain has labored under the burden of sustaining the economic engine through coal mining, timbering, and farming. Even though the region has sustained some with employment, the economy has caused many detrimental effects on the population making their homes in the mountains. Some of the health-related diseases tied to employment in Appalachia include coal worker's pneumoconiosis (black lung), musculoskeletal degenerative disease, and injuries resulting in disability. An example of coal mining in Kentucky is seen in Figure 7.1.

Some of the health-related diseases tied to employment in Appalachia include coal worker's pneumoconiosis (black lung), musculoskeletal degenerative disease, and injuries resulting in disability.

The Bluegrass region in central Kentucky holds the majority of the metropolitan areas in the commonwealth including Lexington, Louisville, and northern Kentucky (Ona & Davis, 2011). The landscape includes beautiful horse farms just miles from the cities with swaying fields of bluegrass for which

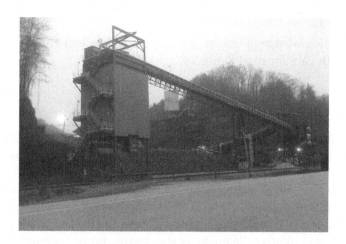

Figure 7.1. A Kentucky Coal Mine

it is named. This region also sustains the largest tertiary care hospitals in the commonwealth. Rural residents must travel to the hospitals located in the Bluegrass region when needing subspecialty care. The three metropolitan areas are located on major interstate highways, thus allowing for interstate commerce and large factories providing better job markets.

The Upper Mississippi Delta region begins at the far western part of the commonwealth along the Mississippi River. Two of the largest lakes, Barkley and Kentucky, are found in the Delta region. The majority of the counties in this region are rural.

Key Concepts

The demographics of Kentucky include topography, rurality, socioeconomic, and the uninsured creating a climate for numerous health disparities. The health care delivery systems strive to meet the needs of the people but the current delivery system remains in silos and coordination for the care of the patient is lacking.

Kentucky Demographics

Kentucky's land mass is divided into 120 counties. The smallest of these counties (Gallatin County) has ninety-nine square miles and a total population of 7,870. Gallatin County is bordered by the Ohio River and is one of the most northern Bluegrass region counties. The most eastern county (Pike County) is the largest county with 788 square miles and a total population of sixty-eight thousand. Pike County lies within the Cumberlands of eastern Kentucky and produces 25 percent of the entire state's coal production at thirty-five million tons per year. This county also has the third largest banking center in Kentucky.

Of these 120 counties, 85 are noted to be rural by the Kentucky Institute of Medicine (2007). These rural counties are home to almost 50 percent of the commonwealth's population. The total population of Kentucky is 4,262,400. Of this, 946,900 (22 percent) are living in **poverty** (ratio of income to poverty) and the median annual income is $41,489. There is an unemployment rate of 10.2 percent. Of its residents, the commonwealth has 688,000 (16 percent) uninsured. Of those with medical insurance, 49 percent are covered by their employers, with the remainder being covered by Medicaid (17 percent), Medicare (16 percent), individual (4 percent), and other public sources (1 percent) (Kaiser Family Foundation, 2010). Kentucky is predominately white (90 percent) with smaller populations of African Americans (8 percent) and Hispanics (2 percent).

Kentucky Health Disparities

Kentucky is one of the **unhealthiest** states in the United States. The United States ranks states according to disease-related health statistics with the number one state being the healthiest and the number fiftieth being the unhealthiest. Kentucky's rankings include the following:

- Total mortality—fiftieth
- Cancer deaths—fiftieth
- Percentage of smokers—forty-ninth
- Poor physical health—forty-eighth
- Cardiovascular deaths—forty-sixth
- Percentage adults obese—forty-fifth
- Premature deaths—forty-second (Kentucky Institute of Medicine, 2007)

Kentucky has a disproportionately high rate of disease-related **health disparities** including the following:

- An infant mortality rate of 7.0 per thousand live births
- Heart disease death rate of 288.9 per one hundred thousand
- A 29.8 percent rate of high blood pressure
- A 27.5 percent rate of adult obesity
- A 24.8 percent prevalence of disability
- A total of $49.00 per capita of state expenditures spent for mental health (Kaiser Family Foundation, 2010)

Other health disparities in Kentucky include the following:

- High cholesterol rate of 38.5 percent (CDC, 2008)
- Diabetes death rate of 30.0 per one hundred thousand
- A current smoker rate of 28.2 percent (CDC, 2008)
- Highest age-adjusted death rate for cancer out of all fifty states, with 187.2 deaths per one hundred thousand (CDC, 2007).

County-level statistics are needed to develop an effective health plan for the Commonwealth of Kentucky. To address this need, the Kentucky Institute of Medicine published *The Health of Kentucky: A County Assessment* in 2007. The publication centered on behavioral risk factors, health access, demographics, cancer mortality rates, and health outcomes for each county. The findings showed smoking to be the number one preventable behavior directly related to a number of Kentucky's highest health disparities including chronic

Table 7.1. Most and Least Healthy Counties in Kentucky

Most Healthy Counties		Least Healthy Counties	
Oldham	1 (most healthy county)	Owsley	111
Boone	2	Powell	112
Jessamine	3	Hart	113
Anderson	4	Knott	114
Woodford	5	Lee	115
Fayette	6	McCreary	116
Spencer	7	Perry	117
Daviess	8	Harlan	118
Calloway	9	Clay	119
Clark	10	Wolfe	120 (least healthy county)

Source: Kentucky Institute of Medicine (2007).

obstructive lung disease, lung cancer, and cardiovascular disease to name a few. Other modifiable behaviors include sedentary lifestyle with little or no exercise and obesity mostly related to poor dietary choices high in saturated fats and carbohydrates. As quoted from the report, "Only 10 of Kentucky's counties are above the national average for physical activity and 78 are above the national average for obesity" (Kentucky Institute of Medicine, 2007, p. 7) Kentucky's challenges were not just poor behavioral choices but poor economic status, a growing population of older residents, and lower-than-average high school graduation rates. The **county assessment** also looks at health access from the prospective of residents having a primary care physician, having immunization coverage, the lack of health insurance, and having adequate prenatal care. These four factors heavily determine whether residents receive many preventive services. The county assessment report is aimed to be a resource for others to focus on the critic needs of the rural counties. Using twenty-five measures of the county's health status as compared to the other Kentucky's counties, the county assessment ranked each county from the most healthy to the least healthy (Kentucky Institute of Medicine, 2007). Table 7.1 lists the top ten most healthy counties and the bottom ten least healthy counties. The county assessment points out that more of the metropolitan counties are in the top healthiest counties whereas the most rural counties are in the bottom as far as health status.

Rural Health Care Delivery Systems

There are many health care **delivery systems** (the population enters to obtain health care) to address the multitude of disease related health disparities in

Kentucky. At best these health care delivery systems are loosely affiliated but lack the synergies necessary to provide adequate patient care, and at worst they are designed in such a way that many priorities compete with patient care. The health care delivery systems are categorized as follows:

- Small critical access hospitals
- Small regional hospitals
- Federally qualified health care centers (community health centers)
- Primary care centers and rural health clinics
- County and regional health departments
- Independent provider practices
- Mental health comprehensive care centers

The following sections describe each of these rural health delivery systems.

Small Critical Access Hospitals

Because of a number of small rural hospital closures across the United States since the 1990s, mainly as a result of economic distress, the US Department of Health and Human Services (DHHS) HRSA created the Medicare Rural Hospital Flexibility Grant Program (RHFGP) in 1997. This program is administered through their Office of Rural Health Policy. The design of the program gave hospitals in rural America the opportunity to convert to critical access certification. The certification gave increased cost-based reimbursement for Medicare inpatient and outpatient services. Receiving payment for the true cost of caring for the patient increased the financial viability of the rural hospitals. This program greatly reduced the closure of small rural hospitals. These rural hospitals must meet certain criteria to be eligible to become a critical access hospital (CAH). These criteria include the following:

- Located in a rural area
- Thirty-five miles from another hospital or shorter distance if poor road structure
- Classified as a necessary provider
- Maximum of twenty-five beds
- Must provide twenty-four-hour emergency services
- Must have at least one physician onsite or on call
- Must have at least one registered nurse onsite twenty-four hours a day
- Must be an agreement with an acute care hospital for patient referral and transfer options

Kentucky had thirty CAHs as of 2008. The goal of these CAHs is to provide quality health care to local residents. Without these hospitals in their local community, residents would need to travel long distances for care or elect not to seek care at all (Ona & Davis, 2011). To an impoverished family, having to travel long distances adds to the cost of care and may not be acceptable. Thus, many poor rural Kentuckians do not seek care until they are critically ill or in the late stages of a chronic disease.

CAHs in Kentucky are also an economic bond to local communities. These hospitals provide jobs to highly skilled health care professionals and in turn stimulate the local economy by purchases made though local businesses by the hospital and its employees. Having local health systems spurs the attraction of professionals into the community as well as retirees wishing to return home. The hospital brings in outside dollars (payments for Medicare and Medicaid) to the local community (Ona & Davis, 2011). A 2000 economic impact study of CAHs in Kentucky showed around 4,682 local jobs were created, $140 million of labor income was generated within the hospital local community, and $285 million was added to the local community reserve (Scorsone, 2004). Figure 7.2 shows the county distribution of CAHs. This illustrates the large areas of the rural population in Kentucky without timely access to hospital services.

Small Regional Hospitals

There are small regional hospitals that did not seek the CAH designation. These hospitals have been able to sustain their economic viability on their own. They provide much the same level of services as the CAHs. They also contribute to the economic base of their communities and care for the population.

Federally Qualified Health Care Centers

Federally qualified health care centers (FQHCs), also known as community health centers (CHCs), are funded by grants from the Bureau of Primary Health Care, HRSA, and DHHS. FQHCs receiving these funds are mandated to report data about the patients served through a uniform data system. This health system was placed in the highest areas of need for US health care. The criteria included a high rate of poverty, infant mortality, and a physician shortage area. Further, the FQHC must be open to all patients regardless of their ability to pay for the services or their insurance status. The services must be tailored to the needs of the population in the community in a culturally competent and linguistic manner. The care must be comprehensive in providing primary care as well as assisting the patients in navigating the health delivery system, including transportation, pharmacy, lab, radiology, and case management. As an FQHC, the program is eligible to apply for a 340B pharmacy status. The

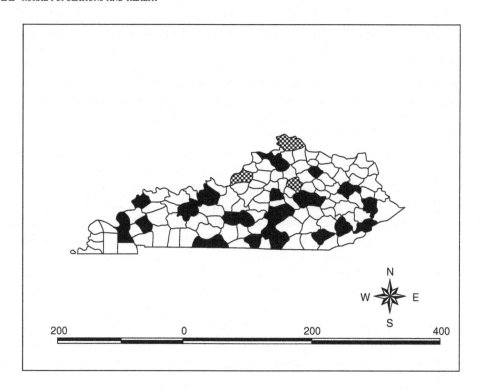

Figure 7.2. Critical Access Hospitals (CAH) Counties in Kentucky
Note: Kentucky CAH counties are shaded; counties with major cities are shown with dots.

pharmacy status allows the FQHC to purchase medications at the federal drug price and to pass this savings on to the patients to decrease the cost of necessary drug treatments. The mission of FQHCs is to provide quality care by improving patient outcomes and reducing health disparities. A reduction in the number of emergency room visits, hospital stays, and specialty care by FQHCs results in a cost savings to the medical system. This health delivery system places uninsured patients on a sliding fee scale related to the poverty level. Many patients do not pay anything for their care at the FQHC.

A reduction in the number of emergency room visits, hospital stays, and specialty care by FQHCs results in a cost savings to the medical system.

In 2006, Kentucky had fifteen FQHCs with sixty-nine delivery sites for a total of 216,635 patients. Of the patients, 2,813 were migrant farm workers and 10,968 were homeless patients. Of Kentucky's vulnerable population in 2005, those served by FQHCs included 21 percent low-income uninsured, 12 percent at or below the **poverty** level (ratio of income to poverty) and in 2007, 10 percent of total Medicaid beneficiaries (National Association of Community Health Centers, 2010) (see Figure 7.3).

Primary Care Centers and Rural Health Clinics

Primary care centers (PCCs) are state designated through the Medicaid program to provide rural primary care to the state population. To qualify for the designation, a PCC must adhere to a set of regulations by the Commonwealth of Kentucky (Kentucky Cabinet for Health and Family Services, 2004). Rural health clinics (RHCs) are federally designated through Medicare to provide primary care to rural residents. RHCs must also adhere to the regulations set forth by the federal government (US Department of Health and Human Services, Centers for Medicare and Medicaid Services, 2010). Both of these designations afford the clinics a prospective payment system reimbursement to help cover the cost of the uninsured seen in the clinics. The clinic must perform a yearly cost report to the respective agency, state or federal.

County and Regional Health Departments

The Institute of Medicine's 1988 report, *The Future of Public Health,* identified three core functions for public health that are widely accepted by the public health policy and academic communities: assessment, policy development, and assurance. In 1994, several revised versions appeared from different groups in the public health arena. To coordinate a single language for the public health community to use, Philip Lee, assistant secretary for health, developed the Core Public Health Functions Project. The local health department's responsibility is to prevent disease and injury and protect and promote health. Services that are provided by public health are population based and focus on the improvement of the population's health.

The essential public health services supply the foundation for the National Public Health Performance Standards Program (NPHPSP) instruments. This foundation describes the public health activities that every public health department should undertake in its community.

The CDC's ten essential public health services provide a common definition of public health responsibilities and a guide for local public health systems:

- Monitor health status to identify and solve community health problems
- Diagnose and investigate health problems and health hazards in the community
- Inform, educate, and empower people about health issues

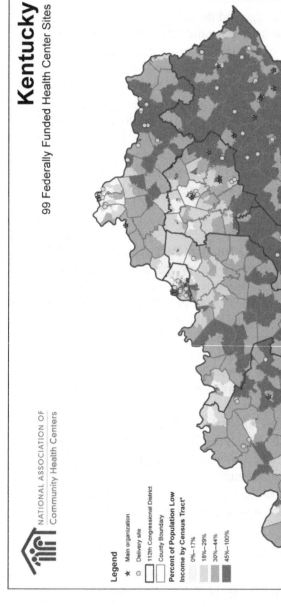

Figure 7.3. Kentucky's Ninety-Nine Federally Funded Health Center Sites

Notes: *Congressional district boundaries are as of the 110th Congress. **Low income represents under 200 percent of FPL. Health center and look-alike organizations: Health Services and Resources Administration (HRSA) data warehouse, June 2, 2011; low-income and population data: US Census Bureau's American community five-year (2005–2009) estimates; geographic boundaries: 2000 and 2010 census and ArcGIS.com; federally funded health center sites count: HRSA data warehouse, June 27, 2011.

Source: National Association of Community Health Centers (2008).

- Mobilize community partnerships and action to identify and solve health problems
- Develop policies and plans that support individual and community health efforts
- Enforce laws and regulations that protect health and ensure safety
- Link people to needed personal health services and ensure the provision of health care when otherwise unavailable
- Ensure a competent public and personal health care workforce
- Evaluate effectiveness, accessibility, and quality of personal and population-based health services
- Identify new insights and innovative solutions to health problems (CDC, 2010)

Each local health department is expected to perform public health planning. Through partnerships, an LHD and a community health board assess not only their internal capacity but also the health of the community. This public health planning is used to identify top priority public health issues and decide on appropriate interventions. Local, state, and federal funding agencies access planning performed by LHDs to ensure accountability. This is an essential part of the process to ensure effective targeting of public services (CDC, 2010). Figure 7.4 shows the location of district health departments with several counties in each district and the independent health departments that represent a single county.

Independent Provider Practices

Throughout Kentucky there are small independent health systems. These clinical operations usually have one or more physicians and many have other health professionals, nurse practitioners, or physician assistants. Most of these privately owned and operated practices are on a fee-for-service reimbursement rate for all health insurers. Many of the providers have worked in their rural communities since completing medical training. However, those same physicians are facing retirement and are having great difficulty recruiting young physicians to take their place. In some rural areas, physicians in their seventies and eighties are still seeing patients for fear no one will be there to care for the rural community.

Mental Health Care Centers

Kentucky provides community services for mental health, intellectual disability, or other developmental disability, and substance abuse through fourteen publicly funded mental health and mental retardation boards located in rural

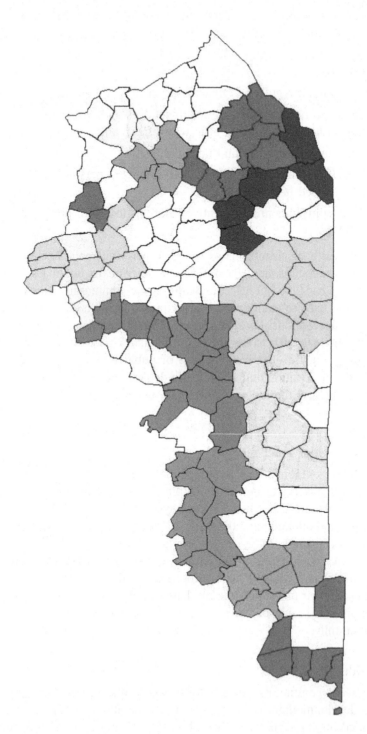

Figure 7.4. Kentucky Public Health Local Departments, Districts, and Independent Counties
Source: Kentucky Cabinet for Health and Family Services (2011).

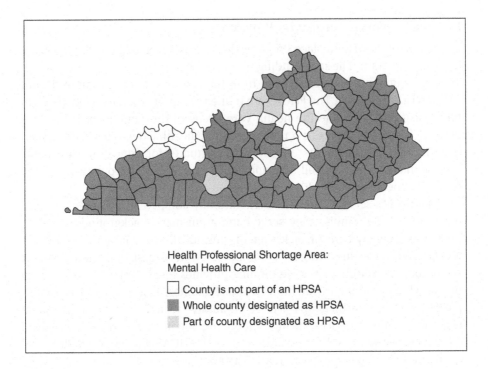

Figure 7.5. Kentucky Counties in Health Professional Shortage Areas: Mental Health Care, 2007
Source: Bureau of Health Professions, Health and Human Services (2007).

multicounty-designated regions of the state. The regional boards were established by state statute and are private, nonprofit groups.

Kentucky's Department for Behavioral Health, Developmental, and Intellectual Disabilities (DBHDID) is administered by the Kentucky Cabinet for Health and Family Services. DBHDID operates several inpatient hospitals across the state for mental health and substance abuse. The provided services include psychiatric and rehabilitative services to its clients (Kentucky Cabinet for Health and Family Services, 2011). Figure 7.5 illustrates the severe shortage of mental health professionals.

Models That Are Improving Systems of Care in Kentucky

Since about 2000, innovative models have been developed to improve the systems of care by filling some of the health care gaps in Kentucky. The next section of the chapter will cover a few of these innovative models.

Lay Health Worker Navigation Program

In 1994, Kentucky Homeplace Program (KHP) was developed thorough a state-legislated program. The state funding supports the infrastructure of the program. This program employs local people from the community called family health care advisors (FHCAs). The FHCAs are trained paraprofessionals. They perform home visits to determine the health care needs of the families in their community. The FHCA serves as a navigator of the health care system and human services. These home visits afford the opportunity for education of chronic disease management as well as empowering families to improve their quality of life (Schoenberg et al., 2001).

The FHCAs serve as first contact, culturally competent, accepted community leaders. The families they serve come from many backgrounds as far as their faith, employment or lack thereof, and location in the community but the families have one thing in common: they need assistance due to their socioeconomic status. KHP state funding provides for the infrastructure of the program but does not provide funds to assist families. This assistance is accomplished through partnerships with community, regional, state, and federal resources. These services include providing medications, durable medical equipment, eyeglasses, hearing aids, and food. FHCAS also help schedule free or discounted medical services (Schoenberg et al., 2001).

Health Care Professional Workforce Shortage

There has remained a shortage of a professional health care workforce since the time of Mary Breckinridge, who founded the Frontier Nursing Service in Hyden, Kentucky, in 1925. Mary was a nurse who lost her husband and two children while still a young woman. Afterward, Mary dedicated her life and nursing career to the women of eastern Kentucky. She was affectionately dubbed the *angel on horseback.* Mary was determined to bring health care and to decrease mother and infant mortality to an area with poor roads usually accessible only by horseback (Goan, 2008).

Although Mary Breckinridge's successes were emulated across the United States in many rural areas, the shortage of physicians remains a reality for rural Kentucky. ARC addressed this issue by using the Conrad State 30 J-1 Visa Waiver program, a national program that allows an international medical graduate (IMG) to enter the United States for residency training on completion of medical school. The IMG is required to return to his or her home country for at least two years after residency training. If the IMG agrees to work in a designed medically underserved area, the IMG can remain in the United States and the requirement to return to the home country can be waived. The J-1 program mandates that the IMG must work a minimum of three years in an HPSA. The HPSA areas are designated by the US Bureau of Primary Health

Care using the median household income and the physician-to-population ratio (Appalachian Regional Commission, 2010).

To help address the rural physician shortage, a new medical school was established in Pikeville, Kentucky. In September 1997, the Pikeville College School of Osteopathic Medicine (PCSOM) enrolled the first class of sixty students. The first dean for the college, John Strosnider, announced that the school was established to address the chronic underlying problem of rural Kentucky's health access issue: the extreme shortage of physicians, especially primary care physicians (Castro, 2001).

PCSOM was the dream of Paintsville resident and attorney Chad Perry III, who had dedicated much of his professional career representing disabled coal miners as a result of occupational health issues. Perry wished to make a lasting contribution to addressing the health needs of eastern Kentuckians. To make his dream of an area medical school a reality, Perry generated local support from community leaders, foundations, corporations, and government agencies. An application was submitted to the ARC for grant funds to build the additional buildings and provide the equipment needed for teaching (Baldwin, 1999). "When the idea of a medical school in Pikeville was first proposed," says Strosnider, "many people felt it was foolish and impossible. We've proven them wrong. We have residency programs established. We have post-doctoral programs established. So we pick students from the mountains and train them in the mountains. They can do their residencies in the mountains, and we believe most of them will stay and practice in the mountains" (Castro, 2001, p. 2).

Medical Care for the Indigent

Health Kentucky–Kentucky Physicians Care (KPC) is a group of health professionals that includes physicians, pharmacists, and dentists as well as pharmaceutical manufacturers. These health professionals donate their time and expertise to care for patients in Kentucky who are uninsured. The program is designed to treat acute care and minor health issues. The pharmaceutical manufacturers provide free medications for the indigent patients. By using the KPC program, indigent patients may apply and once approved they are then paired with a participating provider nearest where they live. The eligibility criteria include the following:

- US citizen and a Kentucky resident
- Between the ages of eighteen and sixty-four
- Uninsured for medical care
- Household income at or below the federal poverty guideline (Health Kentucky, 2005)

Telehealth

The availability of access to quality health care in rural areas of Kentucky is limited. Telemedicine (telehealth) is a relatively new and unique way to provide health care in rural areas. Through the use of specialty cameras and diagnostic tools by using videoconferencing, the patient can be connected to medical specialists at the University of Kentucky (UK). The equipment uses electronic stethoscopes and other tools for this telelink visit, reduces the need for patient travel over long distances, and provides a decreased cost to patients and their families. The subspecialty physician can provide a full assessment and recommendations to the local primary care provider.

Kentucky TeleCare Network, at the UK Chandler Medical Center, was established in 1994. This program helped initiate a statewide telehealth linkage: the Kentucky TeleHealth Network (KTHN). KHTN is legislatively mandated by a statewide telehealth initiative and is comanaged by UK and the University of Louisville since 2000, providing administrative, clinical, and educational services throughout rural Kentucky. KHTN provides medical care videoconferencing at seventy health care facilities across Kentucky (Capalbo, Kruzich & Heggem, 2002).

Conclusion

The Commonwealth of Kentucky has many advantages that could help improve the health of its people. Low levels of factory pollution compared to other states, miles and miles of waterways, large areas of forest, and native wildlife all provide favorable environments in which to live. This state also has numerous health delivery systems all working to improve the health of those in the local communities. In addition, there are a vast number of organizations developing unique models to further improve the health of the state population through research, altruistic efforts, and partnerships with others.

The glaring omission in all the systems of care shows they are not designed in such a way to give total care for the patient. The patient should be the recipient of these efforts. Appropriate, caring, cost-effective care can only be achieved through coordination of all the potential services the patient needs. By placing the patient in the center of each visit, the health delivery system can function as a wheel moving in all directions from the center (the patient) to ensure the patient's needs are met at each visit. Only then can the systems of care in Kentucky overcome the current silos in which patients now find themselves.

Summary

- Kentucky is one of the unhealthiest states in the United States, ranking in the lowest ten out of the fifty states in total mortality, cancer deaths, percentage of smokers, poor physical health, cardiovascular deaths, percentage of obese adults, and premature deaths.

- Kentucky has a disproportionately high rate of health disparities in infant mortality, heart disease, high blood pressure, adult obesity, prevalence of diabetes, and extremely low rates per capita of state expenditures spent for mental health.

- Kentucky's Bluegrass region holds the majority of the metropolitan areas and the largest tertiary care hospitals in the state, in which rural residents must commute to when seeking subspecialty care.

- Rural Kentucky communities in Appalachia experience a multitude of health disparities, mostly from working in the coal mining, timbering, and farming industries, which lead to health-related diseases such as coal worker's pneumoconiosis, muscoskeletal degenerative disease, and work injuries.

- Measures have been taken to address Kentucky's drastic health disparities by conducting a county assessment on behavioral risk factors, health access, demographics, and cancer mortality rates and health outcomes. These steps are intended so that the assessment would become a resource for others to use to evaluate the critical needs of rural counties.

- Rural Kentucky health delivery systems fall short in providing adequate patient care to residents due to a shortage in the health care professional workforce, limited access to quality health care, and other factors.

Key Terms

county assessment	poverty
delivery systems	unhealthy(iest)
health disparities	

For Practice and Discussion

1. Working with a colleague, compare and contrast the rural health care systems of Kentucky to those described in Chapter Six for Colorado.

2. In addition to the health care systems described in this chapter, please identify at least three opportunities to protect people against premature morbidity and mortality for a rural state such as Kentucky

(think about primary prevention services rather than those aimed at secondary or tertiary prevention).

References

Appalachian Regional Commission. (2010). Counties in Appalachia. Retrieved from http://www.arc.gov/counties.

Baldwin, F. D. (1999). Access to care: Overcoming the rural physician shortage. *Appalachia, 32*(2), 8–15.

Bureau of Health Professions, Health and Human Services. (2007). *RUPRI state demographic and economic profiles.* Retrieved from http://www.rupri.org/Profiles/Kentucky2.pdf

Capalbo, S. M., Kruzich, T. J., & Heggem, C. N. (2002). Strengthening a fragile rural health care system: Critical access hospitals and telemedicine. *Choices, 17*(4), 26–29.

Castro, J. E. (2001). *A medical school for the mountains: Training doctors for rural care.* Appalachian Regional Commission. Retrieved from http://www.arc.gov/magazine/articles.asp?ARTICLE_ID = 48&F_ISSUE_ID = 6&F_CATEGORY_ID =

Center for Disease Control and Prevention (CDC). (2007). *National Program of Cancer Registries (NPCR). United States Cancer Statistics (USCS).* Retrieved from http://apps.nccd.cdc.gov/uscs/state.aspx?state = Kentucky.

CDC. (2008). Kentucky: Burden of Chronic Diseases. Retrieved from http://www.cdc.gov/chronicdisease/states/pdf/kentucky.pdf

CDC. (2010). National Public Health Performance Standards Program (NPHPSP). Retrieved from http://cdc.gov/nphpsp

Goan, M. B. (2008). *Mary Breckinridge: The frontier nursing service and rural health in Appalachia.* Chapel Hill: University of North Carolina Press.

Health Kentucky, Inc. (2005). Health Kentucky, a network of caring. Retrieved from http://www.healthkentucky.org

Institute of Medicine. (1988). *The future of public health.* Washington, DC: National Academies Press.

Kaiser Family Foundation. (2010). *Kentucky—Kaiser state health facts.* Retrieved from http://www.statehealthfacts.org/profileglance.jsp?rgn = 19

Kentucky Cabinet for Health and Family Services. (2004). *Legislative Research Commission. 902 Kentucky administrative regulations (KAR)20:058.* Retrieved from http://lrc.ky.gov/kar/902/020/058.htm

Kentucky Cabinet for Health and Family Services, Department for Behavioral Health. (2011). Developmental and intellectual disabilities. Retrieved from http://dbhdid.ky.gov/

Kentucky Institute of Medicine. (2007). *The health of Kentucky: A county assessment.* Retrieved from: http://kyiom.org/assessment.html

National Association of Community Health Centers. (2010). *Kentucky health center fact sheet, 2009.* Retrieved from www.nachc.com/client/documents/KY10.pdf

National Association of Community Health Centers. (2008). *Kentucky: 81 health center sites; 231,033 patients served.* Retrieved from http://www.nachc.com/client/documents/research/2007-state-maps/KY-map-11202008.pdf

Ona, L., & Davis, A. (2011). Economic impact of the critical access hospital program on Kentucky's communities. *The Journal of Rural Health, 27,* 21–28.

Schoenberg, N. E., Campbell, K. A., Garrity, J. F., Snider, L. B., & Main, K. (2001). The Kentucky Homeplace Project: Family health care advisors in underserved rural communities. *The Journal of Rural Health, 17*(5), 179–186.

Scorsone, E. (2004). *The economic impact of critical access hospitals on 20 rural Kentucky counties.* Lexington: Kentucky Rural Health Works Program.

US Department of Health and Human Services, Centers for Medicare and Medicaid Services. (2010). *Rural health clinic.* Retrieved from http://www.cms.gov/MLNProducts/downloads/RuralHlthClinfctsht.pdf

Chapter 8

Rural Public Health Systems
A View from Alabama

Theresa A. Wynn
Mona N. Fouad

Learning Objectives

- Understand the role history has played in the health of residents in the Black Belt counties of Alabama.
- Describe the intersection of limited primary care services, sociodemographic characteristics of rural communities, and increased breast cancer burden among African American women.
- Recognize the role of community-based participatory research in the REACH 2010 project.
- Learn how community health advisors can serve as a bridge between the health care systems and medically underserved rural populations to affect breast cancer screening rates.

•••

The purpose of this chapter is to highlight the work of volunteers in Alabama's Racial and Ethnic Approaches to Community Health by 2010 (REACH 2010) project. If the problem is in the community, then the answer is also in the community (Nguyen et al., 2003). This phrase emphasizes the importance of active community participation in affairs that affect the lives of community members. Communities are more than geographical boundaries defined by census tracks and zip codes. They are composed of natural helpers (Jackson & Parks, 1997) who genuinely care about the vitality of their community. Often these natural helpers do not wear badges and uniforms, yet their acts of kindness, bravery, and sacrifice are worthy of recognition. Thus, we call them *angels in the field,* and this chapter features their successful work in the Alabama REACH 2010 project. Specifically, 143 community volunteers were trained to address breast cancer issues among rural African American women residing in some of the most underserved Alabama counties (Fouad et al., 2006).

Communities are more than geographical boundaries defined by census tracks and zip codes. They are composed of natural helpers who genuinely care about the vitality of their community.

Ranked the thirtieth largest state in the United States, Alabama spans 52,423 square miles (see Figure 8.1). To geographers, Alabama is a state with a diverse natural landscape that includes fertile land, historic plantations, wooded regions, winding rivers, and expansive lakes (Alabama, 2011). Alabama is home to an estimated 4.7 million people. Nearly 30 percent of Alabamians live in rural areas. Whites comprise 61 percent of the population, followed by African Americans at 26 percent and Hispanics and Latinos at 3 percent (US Census Bureau, 2010). According to the US Census Bureau (2010), nearly 16 percent of Alabamians live in poverty, compared to a US average of 13 percent.

From the US Civil War until World War II, agriculture was a significant part of Alabama's economy. Similar to many southern states, Alabama experienced economic challenges because of its dependence on agriculture (Agriculture in Alabama, 2010). After World War II, Alabama shifted from a predominantly rural, agrarian state to an area dependent on nonagricultural jobs, such as heavy manufacturing, mineral extraction, education, and technology. Considered home to the largest industrial growth because of the automotive industry, Alabama has generated nearly sixty-eight thousand new jobs since 1993 (Active USA Center, n.d.). Although some areas have been successful in attracting well-paying jobs, others have not. Mostly rural, high-minority counties continue to experience population declines as a result of decreased economic opportunity (Center for Business and Economic Research, 2006).

Alabama has sixty-seven counties (US Census Bureau, 2010); fifty-five counties are classified as rural and twelve are considered urban (Alabama Rural Health Association, n.d.). Traditionally, twelve to eighteen rural counties extending east to west across central Alabama are known as the **Black Belt** (University of Alabama Institute for Rural Health Research, 2002) (See darker gray area of Figure 8.1). Once named for its dark, rich, and fertile soil, the Alabama Black Belt currently represents a poverty-stricken area where more than 60 percent of the population is African American. Furthermore, eight Black Belt counties are among the one hundred poorest counties in the United States (University of Alabama Institute for Rural Health Research, 2002).

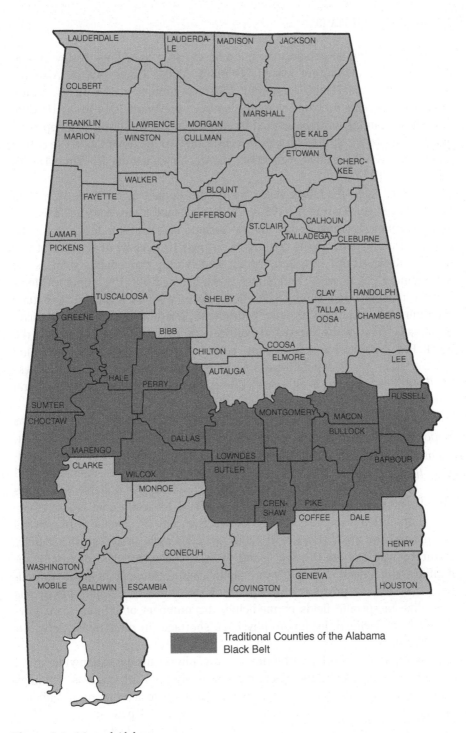

Figure 8.1. Map of Alabama

Note: Traditional Black Belt counties are shaded. Counties in dark gray are historically considered part of the Black Belt region and counties in light gray are sometimes considered part of the geographic region.

From a historical perspective, this region has connections to slavery and the plantation agriculture system (Phillips, 2004; University of Alabama Institute for Rural Health Research, 2002). Beginning in the 1830s, cotton plantations became Alabama's greatest source of revenue. Prior to the US Civil War, these plantations were worked by African American slaves. Soil depletion and the infestation of the boll weevil contributed to the downfall of the cotton plantations (Phillips, 2004: University of Alabama Institute for Rural Health Research, 2002).

Decades later, the Black Belt became the hotbed of the American Civil Rights Movement. During the 1950s and 1960s, small towns such as Tuskegee, Marion, Selma, Hayneville, and Eutaw became the front line for some of the most critical moments in the civil rights struggle (University of Alabama Institute for Rural Health Research, 2002). Noteworthy movements such as the Montgomery bus boycott (Agriculture in Alabama, 2010), the Selma to Montgomery marches, and voter registration reform were orchestrated to outlaw discriminatory practices and the widespread disenfranchisement of African Americans. Despite the success of political and social protest campaigns, the Black Belt continues to suffer from severe economic stagnation, declining populations, high unemployment rates, and poor access to health care (University of Alabama Institute for Rural Health Research, 2002).

The Black Belt continues to suffer from severe economic stagnation, declining populations, high unemployment rates, and poor access to health care.

Health care access is a major problem for rural areas (Gamm & Hutchinson, 2005) such as the Black Belt, where the population is more likely to be African American, older, and uninsured, with lower education and income, and living in medically underserved areas (Rural Assistance Center, 2011). Although access to health care is a complex and multifaceted issue, it is widely known that only 10 percent of physicians practice in rural areas (Hyer et al., 2007). Factors associated with the scarcity of rural physicians are the social and professional remoteness of rural communities, the limited availability of hospitals and technology in nonmetropolitan areas, and the prospect of urban affluence. However, as more physicians specialize in specific fields of medicine, the numbers of primary care physicians have declined, leading to physician shortages in rural areas (Colwill & Cultrice, 2003).

Although the shortage of primary care physicians is nationwide, rural communities are feeling its effects more severely than urban areas. Findings from the Alabama Rural Health Association (2004) revealed that rural Alabama primary care physicians have twice as many potential patients (2,125.9) as their urban counterparts (1,027.5). Consequently, rural doctors may have to work longer hours and provide a wider array of services (Debellis, 2008).

A paper published by the American College of Physicians (2008) indicated that the number of US medical graduates entering residencies in family medicine plummeted by 50 percent from 1997 to 2005. Further, a 2007 study of the career decision making of fourth-year medical students revealed that only 2 percent intended to pursue careers in general internal medicine (Hauer et al., 2008). As the number of primary care physicians in rural areas dwindles, the burden of providing care falls on those who remain, which can have serious implications for providers and patients.

Although the number of primary care physicians is decreasing, the number of older Americans is increasing. In 2006, Americans ages sixty-five and older comprised 2 percent of the population. By 2030, it is projected that almost 20 percent of the population, an estimated 71.5 million people, will be sixty-five and older (Federal Interagency Forum on Aging-Related Statistics, 2008). Rural areas are aging as a result of aging-in-place, out-migration of young adults, and in-migration of older persons from metro areas (Rogers, 2002).

Older Americans in rural areas face an array of challenges that negatively affect their health and quality of life (Gerrior & Crocoll, 2008). Factors such as traveling long distances to access services, limited financial resources, lower literacy, and lack of access to medical treatment present serious barriers to long-term care for rural elders (Buckwalter et al., 2002). More than 75 percent of adults aged sixty-five and older suffer from at least one chronic medical condition that requires ongoing care and management. Currently, 20 percent of Medicare beneficiaries have five or more chronic health conditions (Tanner & Mechanic, 2007).

According to *Rural Healthy People 2010*, chronic diseases such as cancer are more prevalent in rural areas (Gamm & Hutchinson, 2005). It has been documented that compared to urban women, rural women are less likely to engage in preventive behaviors such as breast examinations (Bushy, 2011) and less likely to comply with mammography screening guidelines (Bennett, Olatosi, & Probst, 2008). A study conducted by Brustrom and Hunter (2001) documented that women would defer having a mammogram if the travel distance was greater than twenty miles. Compounded by limited finances and lack of health insurance, rural women have an increased risk of being diagnosed with breast cancer in later stages of the disease than urban women (Rural Assistance Center, 2010).

In addition to urban-rural regional differences, cancer incidence and mortality rates vary considerably among racial and ethnic groups (American Cancer Society, 2009). Although in recent years we have seen an improvement in overall breast cancer mortality rates, a disparity between African American and white women still exists. National and state-level data show that African American women experience higher breast cancer mortality rates despite having lower incidence rates (Jemal et al., 2010). Based on these findings, it is necessary to examine the contributing factors associated with health disparities between African Americans and the general population (US Department of Health and Human Services, n.d.).

Examining the factors that contribute to cancer health disparities is a challenging task because multiple issues for which there are no easy solutions contribute to poor outcomes. Given the complex interplay between cancer health disparities and individual, community, and societal factors, alternative methods of scientific inquiry need to be employed—methods that ask research questions within the social context of the disease (Minkler, 2000; Wallerstein & Bernstein, 1994). **Community-based participatory research** (CBPR) is defined as scientific inquiry conducted in partnership with communities and researchers (Israel et al., 2001). Described as an iterative process incorporating research, reflection, and action in a cyclical manner, CBPR allows all research participants to gain a deeper understanding of the disease within the social context of human life circumstances (Minkler & Wallerstein, 2003). This collaborative partnership produces a level of trust that improves the quality and impact of the research (Viswanathan et al., 2004).

Recognizing the importance of community involvement in efforts to eliminate cancer health disparities, a number of endeavors—from federally funded projects to government initiatives to university-sponsored programs to state health plans to local grassroots efforts—are under way in Alabama. The dilemma of rural Alabama has not gone unnoticed; leaders from different walks of life have emerged to work together with the citizens of the Black Belt to create measurable and sustainable change (Sumners & Lee, 2003). **Racial and Ethnic Approaches to Community Health by 2010** (REACH 2010), a demonstration project funded by the CDC, serves as an example of a rural health initiative designed to lessen racial and ethnic cancer health disparities in the Alabama Black Belt region by implementing CBPR principles (CDC, 2007).

In response to *Healthy People 2010s* national goal of eliminating health disparities (US Department of Health and Human Services, n.d.), in 1999 the CDC established cooperative agreements with more than forty communities across the United States to reduce disparities in six health areas, including breast and cervical cancer (CDC, 2007). The Alabama REACH 2010 Breast and Cervical Cancer Coalition, known as Alabama REACH 2010, was one of the projects funded to eliminate breast and cervical cancer disparities among African American women by enlisting the expertise of community volunteers trained as community health advisors (CHAs) (Fouad et al., 2004). Although the project was a multilevel intervention, the next section focuses specifically on how CHAs were identified and trained and shares outcomes of the CHA-led intervention.

Key Concepts

Community health advisors are known by many other titles, such as *community health workers, community advocates, peer educators,* and *lay health* *educators* (CDC, 1994). Academicians, researchers, and clinicians often use their expertise to implement and translate services, provide culturally appropriate education and information, advocate for individual and community health needs, and give informal guidance on health behaviors. Eng and Young (1992) noted that CHAs can serve as a bridge between health care institutions and groups that have traditionally lacked adequate access to health care services. CHAs are able to address the needs of underserved or hard-to-reach populations in a culturally sensitive manner because they usually share ethnicity, language, socioeconomic status, and life experiences with the community members they are serving (Earp & Flax, 1999). Interventions using CHAs to promote behavior change build on the strengths of the community and create behavioral and social changes through natural social ties (Eng & Young 1992). Furthermore, breast and cervical cancer interventions promoted by CHAs have resulted in an increase in mammography and Pap smear use among disadvantaged community women (Duan et al., 2000; Margolis et al., 1998).

Trust is a critical factor to consider when engaging underserved African Americans in research, given the history of distrust by this population in the health care system (Corbie-Smith, Thomas, & St. George, 2002). Because the Alabama REACH 2010 project was working in some of the poorest counties in the nation, it was crucial for the staff and coalition members to establish a relationship of trust with local community leaders prior to implementing the project. To create such opportunities, a series of meetings were held with community leaders to give them an overview of the project and to request their assistance in identifying ten to twelve well-respected African Americans, twenty-one years and older, to participate as REACH 2010 CHAs (Wynn et al., 2006).

To complement the efforts and recommendations of community leaders, the project staff hosted one-hour informational meetings throughout the county to further highlight the REACH 2010 project. During these meetings, an overview of the cancer burden in the African American community was presented along with a synopsis of the project and description of the roles and responsibilities of CHAs. Consent forms were available for those who wanted to participate in the project and attend the six-week CHA training session (Fouad et al., 2006).

The six-week, twelve-hour CHA training curriculum provided volunteers with cancer education and skill-building opportunities. Role-playing and return demonstrations were included in each of the six lessons, along with homework assignments. During lesson one, volunteers consented and received an introduction to cancer, including a review of common terminology, followed by a discussion on cancer facts and myths. Lessons two and three focused on breast and cervical cancer and included information on risk factors, signs and symptoms, screening recommendations, treatment options, and how to perform breast self-examination.

Lesson four was a discussion on the importance of ethical issues in research and incorporated topics such as respect for persons, beneficence, and justice from the *Belmont Report* (National Institutes of Health, 1979), along with a review of the roles, responsibilities, expectations, and limitations of CHAs. Lesson five was an activity-based session that demonstrated how to communicate effectively and how to collect data. A graduation ceremony was held during lesson six. All CHAs received a signed certificate of completion and a $50 gift card for attending the training sessions (Fouad et al., 2006; Hardy et al., 2005).

Over the course of three months, 143 CHAs graduated from the REACH 2010 training across eight counties, an average of fifteen to twenty CHAs per county. Seventy-six percent of the CHAs were between the ages of forty and sixty-nine years, 96 percent were African Americans, 32 percent had a high school degree, and 28 percent were community college graduates.

Each CHA was responsible for assessing the breast and cervical cancer screening practices of ten to twelve African American women aged forty and older in their county; following up with each woman for two years to ensure receipt of a mammogram and Pap smear; and conducting outreach activities to promote awareness of breast and cervical cancer, such as health fairs, town-hall meetings, paint-the-town-pink events, and so on (Fouad et al., 2006; Wynn et al., 2011). Some CHAs even volunteered to drive women without transportation to their screening appointments (Fouad, Wynn, et al., 2010). The detailed CHA assessment and follow-up protocol are described elsewhere (Fouad, Partridge, et al., 2010). Figure 8.2 depicts REACH CHAs in action.

To retain CHAs in the project and maintain their skills, one-hour monthly maintenance meetings were instituted following the graduation ceremony. During these meetings, CHAs received additional leadership and skill-building training (Fouad et al., 2006; Hardy et al., 2005).

The 143 CHAs were able to assess the breast and cervical cancer screening needs of 1,513 African American women. This caseload was triaged into three groups and stages based on the women's responses to cancer screening questions. For example, women were categorized as stage one if they did not have a prior mammogram. Stage two represented women with a previous mammogram but not in the past year. Stage three comprised women who had a mammogram during the past year (Fouad, Partridge, et al., 2010).

Based on the woman's stage, CHAs provided tailored messages to support, encourage, or reinforce participation in screening. Tailored messages for women in stage one centered on reducing fear and increasing awareness that early detection of breast cancer can save lives. Tailored messages for stage two were designed to reduce fear but also motivate, remind, and support women in scheduling and keeping their mammography screening appointments. Tailored messages for stage three commended women for keeping their mammography screening appointments (Fouad, Partridge, et al., 2010).

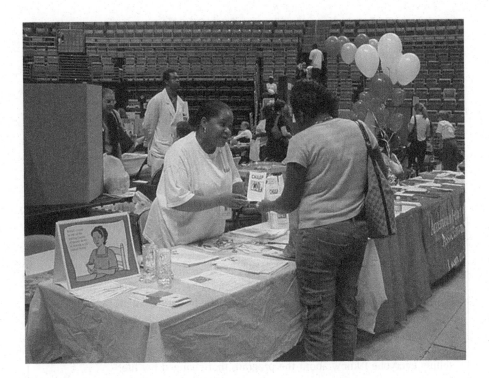

Figure 8.2. REACH CHAs

Results from the self-reported mammography survey revealed that more women received mammography screenings after participating in the intervention. For example, the number of women who reported never having a mammogram (stage one) decreased, whereas the number of women who were infrequently (stage two) and regularly (stage three) screened increased. At baseline, 14 percent ($n = 211$) of the women were in stage one, 16 percent ($n = 247$) in stage two, and 70 percent ($n = 1,055$) in stage three. After the two-year intervention, 4 percent ($n = 61$) were in stage one, 20 percent ($n = 306$) in stage two, and 76 percent ($n = 1,146$) in stage three (see Table 8.1) (Fouad, Partridge, et al., 2010).

Conclusion

The Alabama REACH 2010 project was well received by the CHAs and the community (see Box 8.1). The results from Alabama REACH 2010 indicate that, consistent with CBPR, there are tremendous benefits of broad stakeholder involvement. By enlisting the expertise of natural helpers trained as CHAs, we were able to understand the barriers associated with participation in

Table 8.1. Screening Stages of REACH 2010 Participants at Baseline and at Two-Year Follow-up: African American Women, Alabama, January 2001–November 2005

	Baseline	Follow-up
Stage one	14%	4%
Stage two	16%	20%
Stage three	70%	76%

Box 8.1. Quotes from a REACH CHA and Community Participant

"Before the Alabama REACH 2010 project came to my community, I was afraid to even say the word *cancer.* Perhaps I was afraid because, as a child, I had seen so many relatives die of cancer. When I was asked to attend the REACH training program, I saw a chance to learn more about the *c* word. Now that I've been a community health advisor for the past four years, I can boldly say that cancer is not a death sentence because there are resources and help available. Now, I'm telling everyone I know about the program that changed my life!"

—REACH community health advisor

"REACH 2010 was a blessing to me and my community. It is nice to know that people care about my health. My CHA calls me often to see how I was doing and to ask if I need help to my appointment. That is so thoughtful."

—Community participant

---

mammography screening from the community's perspective and devise viable action plans to overcome them, which resulted in increased rates of mammography use. CBPR principles are a necessary ingredient to sustainable and lasting change.

Summary

- Local community members are interested in partnering with universities and researchers in an equitable manner to address cancer health disparities.
- With the proper guidance and support, community volunteers can be trained as CHAs.

- In addition to the initial six-week training, it was important for CHAs to attend monthly continuing-education classes to reinforce their knowledge and newly acquired skills.
- Based on each woman's screening stage, CHAs offered tailored health messages designed to support, encourage, remind, or reinforce screening practices.
- In addition to sharing tailored messages, CHAs conducted numerous community outreach efforts and even volunteered to transport women to their doctor's appointments.
- As a result of the CHA-led intervention more women participated in mammography screenings.
- Interventions partnering with CHAs to promote behavior change build on the strengths of a community and create behavioral and social changes through natural social ties.

Key Terms

Black Belt

community-based participatory research

community health advisors

Racial and Ethnic Approaches to Community Health by 2010

For Practice and Discussion

1. Identify the various titles used for CHAs and describe how CHAs are able to promote behavior change in rural communities.
2. Working with one or two colleagues from class, discuss why it was important to have monthly skill-building meetings following the initial six-week CHA training.
3. In your opinion, what are the benefits and challenges associated with community-based participatory research?

Acknowledgments

The authors thank all the community health advisors for their labor of love and untiring dedication to assisting women in need. Special thanks to all members of the Alabama REACH 2010 Breast and Cervical Cancer Control Coalition, staff, investigators, and partners. We are grateful to the CDC for funding this project and to Shannon White, our supportive project officer.

This work is supported in part by the Centers for Disease Control and Prevention (cooperative agreement number U50/CCU417409) and the University of

Alabama at Birmingham. The contents of this work are solely the responsibility of the authors and do not necessarily reflect the official views of the Centers for Disease Control and Prevention.

References

Agriculture in Alabama. (2010). *Encyclopedia of Alabama*. Retrieved from http://www.encyclopediaofalabama.org

Active USA Center. (n.d.). *Alabama state economy*. Retrieved from http://www.theusaonline.com/states/alabama/economy.htm

Alabama. (2011). *Encyclopedia Britannica*. Retrieved from http://www.britannica.com/EBchecked/topic/11958/Alabama

Alabama Rural Health Association. (n.d.). *What is rural?* Retrieved from http://www.arhaonline.org/what_is_rural.htm

Alabama Rural Health Association. (2004). *Rural/urban comparisons*. Retrieved from http://www.arhaonline.org/rururbcomp.htm

American Cancer Society. (2009). *Cancer facts & figures for African Americans*. Atlanta, GA: American Cancer Society.

American College of Physicians. (2008). *How is a shortage of primary care physicians affecting the quality and cost of medical care?* Philadelphia: American College of Physicians.

Bennett, K. J., Olatosi, B., & Probst, J. C. (2008). *Health disparities: A rural-urban chartbook*. Columbia: South Carolina Rural Health Research Center. Retrieved from http://rhr.sph.sc.edu/report/SCRHRC_RuralUrbanChartbook_Exec_Sum.pdf

Brustrom, J. E., & Hunter, D. C. (2001). Going the distance: How far will women travel to undergo free mammography. *Military Medicine, 166*(4), 347–349.

Buckwalter, K. C., Davis, L. L., Wakefield, B. J., Kienzle, M. G., & Murray, M. A. (2002). Telehealth for elders and their caregivers in rural communities. *Family and Community Health, 25*(3), 31–40.

Bushy, A. (2011). Populations centered nursing in rural and urban communities. In M. Tanhope & J. Lancaster (Eds.), *Public health nursing: Population-centered health care in the community* (7th ed.). St. Louis: Mosby-Elsevier.

CDC. (1994). *Community health advisors: Programs in the United States, health promotion and disease prevention* (Vol. II). Atlanta, GA: Author.

CDC. (2007). *REACHing across the divide: Finding solutions to health disparities*. Atlanta, GA: Author.

Center for Business and Economic Research. (2006). *Alabama population trends*. Retrieved from http://cber.cba.ua.edu/rbriefs/ab2007q2_poptrends.pdf

Colwill, J. M., & Cultrice, J. M. (2003). The future supply of family physicians: Implications for rural America. *Health Affairs,22*(1), 190–198.

Corbie-Smith, G., Thomas, S. B., & St. George, D.M.M. (2002). Distrust, race, and research. *Archives of Internal Medicine, 162*, 2458–2463.

Debellis, A. (2008). A physician shortage—the rural crisis. *Birmingham Medical News*, p. 6. Retrieved from http://www.birminghammedicalnews.com/news.php?viewStory = 1149

Duan, N., Fox, S. A., Derose, K. P., & Carson, S. (2000). Maintaining mammography adherence through telephone counseling in a church-based trial. *American Journal of Public Health, 90,* 1468–1471.

Earp, J. A., & Flax, V. L. (1999). What lay health advisors do: An evaluation of advisors' activities. *Cancer Practice, 7*(1), 16–21.

Eng, E., & Young, R. (1992). Lay health advisors as community change agents. *Family and Community Health, 15,* 24–40.

Federal Interagency Forum on Aging-Related Statistics. (2008). *Older Americans 2008: Key indicators of well-being.* Washington, DC: US Government Printing Office.

Fouad, M. N., Nagy, M. C., Johnson, R. E., Wynn, T. A., Partridge, E. E., & Dignan, M. (2004). The development of a community action plan to reduce breast and cervical cancer disparities between African-American and white women. *Ethnicity & Disease, 14,* 54–61.

Fouad, M., Partridge, E., Dignan, M., Holt, C., Johnson, R., Nagy, C., Parham, G., Person, S., Scarinci, I., & Wynn, T. (2006). A community-driven action plan to eliminate breast and cervical cancer disparity: Successes and limitations. *Journal of Cancer Education, 21*(Suppl.), S91–S100.

Fouad, M., Partridge, E., Dignan, M., Holt, C., Johnson, R., Nagy, C., Parham, G., Person, S., Wynn, T. A., & Scarinci, I. (2010). Targeted intervention strategies to increase and maintain mammography utilization among African American women. *American Journal of Public Health, 100*(12), 2526–2531.

Fouad, M., Wynn, T., Martin, M., & Partridge, E. (2010). Patient navigation pilot project: Results from the community health advisors in action program (CHAAP). *Ethnicity & Disease, 20*(2), 155–161.

Gamm, L. D., & Hutchison, L. L. (Eds.). (2005). *Rural healthy people 2010: A companion document to Healthy People 2010* (Vol. 3). College Station: The Texas A&M University System Health Science Center, School of Rural Public Health, Southwest Rural Health Research Center.

Gerrior, S. A., &. Crocoll, C. E. (2008). USDA CSREES' role in broadening support for an aging nation. *Journal of Extension.* Retrieved from www.joe.org/joe/2008february/comm2.php

Hardy, C., Wynn, T. A., Lisovicz, N., Huckaby, F., & White-Johnson, F. (2005). African American community health advisors as research partners: Recruitment and training. *Family & Community Health, 28*(1), 28–40.

Hauer, K. E., Durning, S. J., Kernan, W. N., Fagan, M. J., Mintz, M., O'Sullivan, P. S., DeFer, T., Elnicki, M., Harrell, H., Reddy, S., Boscardin, C. K., & Schwartz, M. D. (2008). Factors associated with medical students' career choices regarding internal medicine. *Journal of the American Medical Association, 300*(10), 1154–1164. doi:10.1001/jama.300.10.1154.

Hyer, J. L., Bazemore, A. W., Bowman, R. C., Zhang, X., Petterson, S., & Phillips, R. L. (2007). Rural origins and choosing family medicine predict future rural practice. *American Family Physician, 76*(2), 207.

Israel, B. A., Schulz, A. J., Parker, E., & Becker, A. B. (2001). Community-based participatory research: Policy recommendations for promoting a partnership approach in health research. *Education for Health, 14*(2), 182–197.

Jackson, E. J., & Parks, C. P. (1997). Recruitment and training issues from selected lay health advisor programs among African Americans: A 20-year perspective. *Health Education Behavior, 24*(4), 418–431.

Jemal, A., Siegel, R., Xu, J., & Ward, E. (2010). Cancer statistics, 2010. *CA: A Cancer Journal for Clinicians, 60,* 277–300.

Margolis, K. L., Lurie, N., McGovern, P. G., Tyrrell, M., & Slater, J. S. (1998). Increasing breast and cervical cancer screening in low-income women. *Journal of General Internal Medicine, 13,* 515–521.

Minkler, M. (2000). Using participatory action research to build healthy communities. *Public Health Reports, 115*(23), 191–197.

Minkler, M., & Wallerstein, N. (Eds.). (2003). *Community-based participatory research for health.* San Francisco: Jossey-Bass.

National Institutes of Health. (1979). *The Belmont report: Ethical principles and guidelines for the protection of human subjects of research.* National Commission for the Protection of Human Subjects of Biomedical and Behavioral Research. Retrieved from http://ohsr.od.nih.gov/guidelines/belmont.html

Nguyen, T. N., Kagawa-Singer, M., Kar, S., Chai, J., Hayes, S., & Penniman, T. (2003). *Multicultural health evaluation: Literature review and critique.* The California Endowment. Retrieved from www.calendow.org/uploadedFiles/Publications/Evaluation/multicultural_health_evaluation.pdf

Phillips, D. (2004). Alabama black belt. *Discovering Alabama: Teacher's guide.* Retrieved from http://discoveringalabama.org/wp-content/uploads/2010/05/alabama_black_belt.pdf

Rogers, C. C. (2002). The older population in 21st century rural America. *Rural America, 17*(3), 1–10.

Rural Assistance Center. (2010). *Women's health.* Retrieved from http://www.raconline.org/topics/public_health/womenshealth.php

Rural Assistance Center. (2011). *Minority health.* Retrieved from http://www.raconline.org/info_guides/minority_health

Sumners, J. A., & Lee, L. (2003). *Beyond the interstate: The crisis in rural Alabama.* Auburn, AL: Auburn University.

Tanner, J., & Mechanic, D. (2007). Vulnerable people, groups, and populations: Societal view. *Health Affairs, 26*(5), 1220–1230.

University of Alabama Institute for Rural Health. *Black Belt fact book.* (2002). Retrieved from http://cchs.ua.edu/rhi/

US Census Bureau. (2010). *Alabama quick facts.* Retrieved from http://quickfacts.census.gov/qfd/states/01000.html

US Department of Health and Human Services. (n.d.). Healthy people 2010: What is Healthy People? Retrieved from http://healthypeople.gov/2020/default.aspx

Viswanathan, M., Ammerman, A., Eng, E., Gartlehner, G., Lohr, K. N., Griffith, D., Rhodes, S., Samuel-Hodge, C., Maty, S., Lux, L., Webb, L., Sutton, S. F., Swinson, T., Jackman, A., & Whitener, L. (2004). *Community-based participatory research: Assessing the evidence.* Rockville, MD: Agency for Healthcare Research and Quality.

Wallerstein, N., & Bernstein, E. (1994). Introduction to community empowerment, participatory education, and health. *Health Education Quarterly, 21*(2), 141–148.

Wynn, T. A., Johnson, R. E., Fouad, M., Holt, C., Scarinci, I., Nagy, C., Partridge, E., Dignan, M., Person, S., & Parham, G. (2006). Addressing disparities through coalition building: Alabama REACH 2010 lessons learned. *Journal of Health Care for the Poor and Underserved, 17*(2 suppl.), S55–S77.

Wynn, T. A., Taylor-Jones, M., Johnson, R. E., Bostick, P. B., & Fouad, M. (2011). Using community-based participatory approaches to mobilize communities for policy change. *Family & Community Health, 34*, S102–S114.

Chapter 9

Rural Public Health Systems
A View from Iowa

Faryle Nothwehr
Lauren Erickson
Ulrike Schultz

Learning Objectives

- Describe the sociodemographics of Iowa, a primarily rural state that has experienced an out-migration of young, educated people from many of the farming communities.
- Learn about the CDC-funded Prevention Research Center for Rural Health at the University of Iowa and its community-research partnerships.
- Understand how restaurant table signs can affect healthy food choices.
- Articulate the influence of local newspapers and public libraries in providing nutrition information to rural communities.

• • •

Although the rural Midwest region of the United States offers a high quality of life and many opportunities for businesses and individuals, there remain a number of challenges to promoting optimal health in this population. An aging citizenry, an increasing cultural diversity, and environmental barriers to healthy behavior all require innovative and dynamic approaches to addressing health disparities in this region.

A fair amount of research has been conducted addressing the problem of health care access in rural areas of the United States. Much less work has been devoted to understanding unique challenges of providing health promotion and disease prevention programs and policies in these populations. Although the rural Midwest region of the United States, including the state of Iowa, is often seen as a relatively healthy area of the country, health disparities exist here as well. The area is quite understudied in terms of effective health promotion strategies that are feasible and effective in the many small towns scattered across the state and region. Programs and policies that are successful in urban areas, and even in other rural areas of the United States, do not necessarily translate well to this part of the country because of differences in culture, geography, or available resources. This chapter first provides the reader with an overview of demographic, social, cultural, and environmental factors relevant to health care and health promotion in Iowa. Some commonly held stereotypes about the state and region may be confirmed and others challenged in this review. This is followed by a series of examples of efforts to promote healthy lifestyles through interventions involving small town restaurants, libraries, and newspapers, highlighting the work of the University of Iowa Prevention Research Center for Rural Health (PRC-RH) and affiliated researchers and community partners. Each example is designed to illuminate particular strategies that have been found effective as well as unique challenges to success.

Key Concepts

Planning effective health promotion programs and policies requires an understanding of the demographic, social, cultural, and environmental characteristics of a community. Following is an overview of these characteristics in rural Iowa.

A Demographic Overview of the State of Iowa

In order to have an accurate picture of the rural health disparities in Iowa, one must first gain an overall perspective on the health status of all Iowans. Iowa is a mainly rural state with ninety-nine counties. Fifty-seven percent of the population live in one of the twenty counties considered to be metropolitan statistical areas and the other 43 percent live in counties designated as rural areas (State of Iowa, 2010; University of Iowa and Iowa Department of Public Health, 2011). In comparison, only 25 percent of the US population lives in rural areas (Kaiser Family Foundation, 2010). Iowa has a very strong history and association with a rural lifestyle, with these populations typically experiencing higher poverty rates, decreased access to hospitals and physicians, and higher rates of chronic disease (State of Iowa, 2010). Rural populations, in general, tend to have an overall poorer health status when compared to their urban counterparts (Iowa Center on Health Disparities, 2003d; State of Iowa, 2010).

Depending on the measures used, Iowans can appear to be better or worse off than others. From 2007 to 2009 the median annual household income was ranked thirtieth in the country at $50,422 annually compared with an average annual income of $49,945 nationwide. From 2008 to 2009, 13 percent of the Iowa population lived below the national poverty level compared with 20 percent of the US population (Kaiser Family Foundation, 2010). The average per capita income in Iowa's rural counties is 23 percent lower than in Iowa's urban counties (Iowa Center on Health Disparities, 2003d). Health care spending per capita in 2004 was $5,380 compared with the national average of $5,283, and only 10 percent of the population was uninsured from 2008 to 2009 versus a national average of 17 percent for 2009. The unemployment rate as of November 2010 was 6.6 percent compared with 9.8 percent nationally (Kaiser Family Foundation, 2010). The state also has a high rate of high school graduation, with 86.5 percent of incoming ninth-graders graduating in four years or less (United Health Foundation, 2010).

Iowa's population of 3,002,555 (in 2008) has seen many changes since 2000. Whereas the US population has grown at a rate of 13 percent over this period of time, Iowa's population growth has been much slower, increasing at only 5 percent (Kaiser Family Foundation, 2010; University of Iowa, 2009). Between 1980 and 2000, the number of people living on farms in Iowa dropped from four hundred thousand to two hundred thousand (Iowa State University Extension, 2010). Iowa's population distribution has also changed as well. The state median age rose from 36.6 in April 2000 to 38.1 in 2008, and the proportion of people over the age of sixty-five continues to grow while the proportion of young people in the state has been decreasing (Iowa State University Extension, 2010; State of Iowa, 2010). Many young, educated people have left Iowa's rural areas in recent years, leaving a disproportionate number of older adults and a changing economic climate. In one poll, 95 percent of farmers either agreed or strongly agreed that "young people have left their communities because larger communities offer higher paying jobs," and 94 percent agreed or strongly agreed that "a lack of good jobs in their communities has contributed to young people leaving." The majority of farmers also agreed with two other statements: "There is really nothing here to retain young families" (60 percent) and "Young people are no longer interested in farming and rural living" (51 percent) (Iowa State University Extension, 2010).

Many young, educated people have left Iowa's rural areas in recent years, leaving a disproportionate number of older adults and a changing economic climate.

The population distribution has also changed with regards to racial and ethnic minorities. The majority of the rural population in Iowa is Caucasian. White rural Iowans, most often descendants of northern European countries, tend to have a strong sense of independence and self-reliance, which make them less likely to seek out health care when they need it, and they may view assistance with their health care issues as a sign of weakness (Iowa Center on Health Disparities, 2003d). This may be especially prevalent among older adults and those with less education (Rossman, 2003).

From 2000 to 2006 the population of Hispanics in Iowa, predominantly originating from Mexico, increased approximately 24 percent, making them the largest and fastest growing racial and ethnic minority group in Iowa (Iowa Center on Health Disparities, 2003c). This population is somewhat concentrated in small manufacturing towns. Hispanics typically face many barriers when it comes to accessing health care, a significant one being the lack of Spanish-speaking interpreters across the state. Reports have estimated that 50 percent or more of Hispanics do not have health insurance and many are unable to pay for services out of pocket because roughly 20.2 percent of Hispanics live below the poverty level. Hispanics may also lack transportation to reach health care services, and many have work schedules that make it difficult for them to access the typical office hours of hospitals and clinics (Iowa Center on Health Disparities, 2003c).

From 2000 to 2006 the population of African Americans in Iowa has increased by 15 percent across the state, and the majority (89 percent) live in urban areas (Iowa Center on Health Disparities, 2003a). African Americans in Iowa tend to have lower education levels than whites, which can be one of the strongest predictors of poverty and negative health status. African Americans earn 40 percent less per capita than Caucasians in Iowa and are four times as likely as Caucasians to live below the poverty level. African Americans in Iowa also have nearly two times the rate of fetal and infant deaths, low-birth-rate babies, and death from heart disease as Caucasians (Iowa Center on Health Disparities, 2003a).

The **Amish** are descendants of immigrants that came to the United States from Switzerland several hundred years ago. They continue to embrace a traditional lifestyle that has changed very little since their arrival in this country. The Amish follow a very strict interpretation of the Bible and typically shun many forms of modern technology, including western medicine, unless it is absolutely necessary. They typically speak an old form of High German and may need interpreters in a health care setting. They tend to live in rural areas, and Iowa is one of the few states that has a thriving population of Amish people (Iowa Center on Health Disparities, 2003b).

Rural Health Care Issues in Iowa

Of the 121 hospitals in Iowa, 99 are considered rural hospitals and 22 are considered urban. Six of Iowa's counties do not have a hospital at all (Iowa Department of Public Health, 2009a). In addition to these hospitals, Iowa has twelve federally qualified health centers and one incubator health center. These thirteen sites administer a total of eighty-three sites and satellite clinics across the state and served more than 125,000 individuals through more than 423,000 clinic visits in 2008 (Iowa Department of Public Health, 2009a). An estimated 41 percent of the patients served at these health centers were uninsured. These clinics are administered on a sliding fee scale based on the patient's income, and patients cannot be turned away because of their lack of ability to pay for services (Gale & Coburn, 2003). In addition, there are thirty-seven clinics in Iowa that offer no-cost medical services. These clinics are run mainly by volunteer staff. In 2009, there were 142 rural health centers (RHCs) distributed throughout fifty-nine counties in the state where patient services are furnished by a physician's assistant or nurse practitioner at least 50 percent of the time the clinic operates (Iowa Department of Public Health, 2009a).

The population decrease in rural areas coupled with the increasing proportions of elderly persons and immigrants present challenges to Iowa's health care systems as they attempt to improve statewide access to primary care, especially in rural areas. Fifty-four counties in Iowa are currently either partially or fully designated as Health Professional Shortage Areas (HPSAs), meaning that the ratio of patients to primary health care providers is greater than three thousand to one. Sixty-two counties are designated as dental HPSAs with a ratio of patients to dentists of more than five thousand to one. Even more serious, eighty-nine of the state's ninety-nine counties are designated as mental health HPSAs with a ratio of patients to mental health care providers of greater than thirty thousand to one. The ten counties that do not fit into this category are all metropolitan statistical areas. Iowa also ranks forty-seventh among states with psychiatrists per capita and forty-sixth among states with psychologists per capita (Iowa Department of Public Health, 2009a).

The number of primary care physicians practicing in Iowa has increased in recent years but the proportion of providers willing to practice in rural areas has decreased. This can be attributed to younger physicians tending to practice in urban areas and the coincident retirement of elderly physicians. A recent study found that 54 percent of primary care physicians practiced in the eight metropolitan counties, leaving slightly less than half of them to provide access in the remaining ninety-one counties (University of Iowa, 2009). The rural elderly population is also less likely to receive medical checkups, which contributes to a worsening health status. This, along with fewer health care providers available to provide treatment, may cause the health status of rural populations to decline further in the near future (State of Iowa, 2010).

Health Behaviors and Related Outcomes

Iowans have several positive social and health-related behaviors, one being a high percentage of childhood immunization coverage with 93.3 percent of children nineteen to thirty-five months old receiving immunizations (United Health Foundation, 2010). However, Iowa also faces several behavioral health concerns such as a high prevalence of binge drinking at 19.4 percent statewide and a high rate of the population reporting being a current smoker (20.4 percent in 2007). Iowa also has a high prevalence rate of obesity (66.2 percent) among the adult population (University of Iowa and Iowa Department of Public Health, 2011). These factors all contribute to high rates of chronic disease, with four of the top five causes of death from 1997 to 2007 being chronic diseases (diseases of the heart, malignant neoplasms, cerebrovascular disease, and chronic lower respiratory disease). Approximately 68 percent of all deaths in Iowa in 2009 were due to chronic disease, with 28 percent of all deaths attributed to diseases of the heart and 23 percent attributed to cancer (Iowa Department of Public Health, 2009b).

Similar to many other states, the Iowa Department of Public Health has targeted unhealthy eating habits and lack of adequate physical activity as very high priorities for intervention. These behaviors are underlying contributors to the obesity epidemic and many chronic diseases. This focus is also consistent with national public health priorities set by the Centers for Disease Control (CDC). Various collaborative efforts have been developed in the public and private sectors to find solutions to increase healthy behaviors among individuals and within communities, workplaces, schools, and health care systems across the state.

Like many other states, the Iowa Department of Public Health has targeted unhealthy eating habits and lack of adequate physical activity as very high priorities for intervention.

Community-Based Intervention Research in Rural Iowa

When conducting health promotion research in partnership with a community, it is crucial to learn as much as possible about that community: their challenges and their strengths. This learning never stops because communities and their leaders are constantly changing over time, as are the research teams. When first started in 2002, the CDC-funded PRC-RH at the University of Iowa began working with a small town in the southeastern part of the state. This town of just over two thousand people already had some experience interacting with the university and welcomed the PRC-RH as a partner in this new venture. The town also seemed appropriate as a partner because it was, on many levels, very typical of small towns across the state; therefore, research and other lessons learned would translate well to other small towns and the broader region. Although the PRC-RH eventually developed partnerships with many other towns, agencies, and organizations, much of what was learned in those first few years informed future research projects throughout the state.

One early task of the partnership was to bring together community leaders and others interested in the health of the community. An obvious partner was the local health department but others emerged from many sectors of the community and brought their ideas and enthusiasm to the table. The membership of this working group naturally changed somewhat over the years as priority issues emerged and others were discarded. Through these interactions, the various resources and strengths of the community became apparent as well as the challenges and limitations common to many small towns. There were clearly some community capacity issues to consider. Previous efforts with health promoting activities and programs were limited because of lack of local funding, limited grant writing skills to obtain external funding, and a dearth of personnel with time dedicated to these activities. Good intentions and concern for the community were strong but were challenged by such factors. The limited financial and personal resources available also made it difficult to work on multiple issues at one time. Considerable effort was expended trying to focus and prioritize the efforts of the group.

In addition to the level of financial and human resources, the **social environment** of a community can also greatly influence the issues chosen and the strategies that are used in health promotion efforts. For example, religious or civic organizations can provide various forms of support to community members and serve as networks for reaching them with programs and services. In this small community, most people knew one another at least somewhat and had worked with each other on other nonhealth-related issues in the past. Even the most powerful decision makers in town were known as friends and neighbors and not faceless corporate or government entities, as might be the case in larger urban areas. This social cohesion was seen as a clear strength. Residents saw cooperation and civility as essential to the progress and health of the community. Not surprisingly, the partnership chose nonconfrontational and collaborative strategies to organize the community around issues, as opposed to a conflict approach, and tended to avoid very sensitive issues. This isn't necessarily the most effective model of change for every community or every issue (Minkler, Wallerstein, & Wilson, 2008) but it seemed to be the approach this community was most comfortable with. The community eventually developed small work groups that engaged in health promotion activities, with varying degrees of success.

Effective health promotion activities and research can involve almost any entity in a community. It is important to look beyond the seemingly obvious partners when developing community-based health promotion research. In rural Iowa, many county health departments have little or no budget for health promotion and often are consumed with required and reimbursed activities, such as providing home nursing care, with little time or initiative left for health promotion activities. There are exceptional counties that do manage to consistently engage in such activities, primarily because they have learned to effectively partner with other groups and organizations such as schools, churches, local media, and businesses of all types. As a research team, the PRC-RH has often worked directly with these other organizations to develop project ideas with only secondary or no involvement with the county health department or other health-related agencies. The motivation to participate in a given project may vary from one organization to the next but positive results may still be attainable with a strong partnership and commitment to a mutual goal.

The PRC-RH strives to identify entities that are commonly found in even relatively small rural towns and works with them to design simple but effective health-promoting programs and policies, with an eye toward their future dissemination through the state and region. Good candidate partners for this work include, but are not limited to, owner-operated restaurants, libraries, schools, churches, service clubs, grocery stores, and county health departments. The following sections provide examples of specific research projects conducted in partnership with rural communities in Iowa.

The Rural Restaurant Healthy Options Program

From the earliest discussions with community partners, the obesity epidemic, and nutrition in particular as an underlying health factor, became an area of focus. Social and environmental factors that support or hinder healthy eating were emphasized. One concern expressed by residents was that it was difficult to find healthy food choices in local restaurants. Restaurant owners countered that they were reluctant to make major menu changes for fear of losing regular customers. They discussed the difficulty of having fresh fruits and vegetables or other healthy options available when they could not be certain that customers would order such foods. Labeling menus with nutrition information was also ruled out because of the expense involved in this process and the lack of standardized menu items. In time, an idea emerged for a rather simple intervention that was tested in a local restaurant. In collaboration with the restaurant owner, table signs were designed that listed options customers could request that would improve the healthfulness of their order, for example, asking for meat or fish to be broiled instead of fried, requesting low-fat salad dressing, and choosing smaller portions for some menu items. These were all options that the owner was willing to provide even prior to the program but they were just not advertised. Customer surveys conducted before and after placement of the signs showed that customers were noticing the signs and many of them were using the information to adjust their order. Customers also indicated that they were pleased with the program and the owner stated she had received only positive comments about the program. She also expressed

a strong interest having her restaurant become known as a place where customers could find healthy options if they wanted them. Participation in the
study caused her to consider other ways of providing healthy options to customers without having to dramatically change her menu.

These preliminary findings were used to support a grant proposal to the
National Institutes of Health, and funding was subsequently received to test
the program in four other restaurants in similar rural towns. This larger study
was guided by the RE-AIM framework (*reach*, *effectiveness*, *adoption*, *implementation*, *maintenance*) put forward by the United States National Institutes
of Health and intended to guide the design, implementation, evaluation, and
dissemination of health-promotion programs (US National Institutes of Health,
National Cancer Institute, 2012). The research team met personally with each
restaurant owner about the proposed program and secured his or her commitment to participate in the study. A baseline customer survey was conducted
in each restaurant that assessed the demographic characteristics of customers,
whether they were currently trying to change their diet in any way, and asked
about their interest in a variety of healthy options. This survey had been
pretested in the preliminary study and was found to be well understood by
customers. Customers were approached by a research assistant after they
placed their order but before food arrived and asked to complete the anony-
mous, self-administered survey. Most customers indicated they were interested
in the options and over half said they were trying to change their diet in some
way (e.g., to lose weight, cut down on fat or salt) (Nothwehr et al., 2010).
These findings helped encourage the owners that their customers would appre-
ciate the proposed program.

Following the baseline survey, **table signs** (see Figure 9.1) were placed
that were very similar to those placed in the preliminary study but tailored
slightly to the owner's preferences. Customer surveys were again conducted
and included questions about whether people noticed the sign, and if so,
whether it affected their order. If they indicated that it affected their order,
they were asked to write how it did so. Other items about demographics and
interest in changing their diet were also included. These follow-up surveys
were repeated three times in different seasons of the year, with the final survey
occurring one year from the baseline survey. As an incentive for the owner to
participate in the program, a press release describing the study was given
to the local newspaper in each town. All newspapers were interested in the
program, interviewed the owners, and published stories. This free publicity
was greatly appreciated by the owners.

The findings from these surveys were very similar across restaurants and
over time. On average, about 70 percent of customers indicated that they
noticed the signs (reach) and 34 percent of these said it affected their
order in some way (effectiveness). Examples of comments about how the

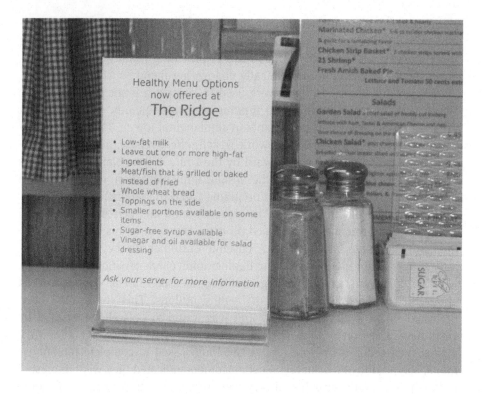

Figure 9.1. Healthy Menu Options at The Ridge Restaurant

orders were affected included: they liked or appreciated the signs and the signs were a "good reminder" to eat healthy; they chose grilled food over fried; chose a smaller portion; chose more fruits and vegetables or something lower in fat or calories; and chose whole wheat bread over white. Customers who had indicated they were currently trying to make dietary changes were no more likely to indicate that they noticed the signs than people who were not trying to make such changes, but they were more likely to indicate that the signs affected their order (Nothwehr et al., in press).

Regular interviews with the owners and waitstaff indicated that the study procedures and the program itself were not a problem for them and that they received many positive comments from customers about the program. All of the signs remained in place for the duration of the program, indicating that implementation of this simple intervention occurred as planned (Nothwehr et al., in press). A statewide dissemination study involving this program is underway to further understand issues related to program adoption, implementation, and maintenance on a larger scale.

This study demonstrated the importance of working closely with community partners in designing and evaluating a program. A program that required significant changes in a restaurant's menu, for example, would not have been acceptable to restaurant owners. However, the owners want to please customers who are looking for healthy options and this program was a relatively painless way to meet that need. There are often challenges to collecting good evaluation data in community settings and this study was no exception. The owners were willing to tolerate the administration of customer surveys as long as the flow of business was not disrupted. This meant the survey needed to be short and customers were not bothered once their food arrived. There were no sales data available that might have been useful to show changes in ordering behavior. An analysis of the order slips was undertaken but it was clear that these were not good measures of the many small adjustments customers reported they made to their order. Given the consistency of the self-reported data across restaurants and over time, the findings do suggest that the program led to small changes in ordering behavior in a segment of the population. Similar to other nutrition environment interventions, the program by itself is not expected to bring about changes in body weight, but when combined with other programs and policies, it could help create an environment more supportive of healthy choices. It is important to note that the findings may not be the same in a nonrural environment or in different restaurants across the country.

Nutrition Information in Public Libraries Study

Many small towns in rural Iowa have **public libraries.** Besides providing traditional library services, the libraries are frequently involved in activities in their communities, and their buildings often serve as meeting places for a variety of community functions. Past studies found that libraries are successful in providing consumer health information and are excellent partners for promoting health (Linnan et al., 2004; Pifalo et al., 1997). A recent Internet-based survey of 119 directors or managers of Iowa public libraries, guided by the constructs of self-efficacy, outcome expectations, and behavioral capability within social cognitive theory (Bandura, 2004), found that the libraries are open, on average, about forty-three hours per week and most serve populations between five hundred and nine thousand (data not published). The majority of directors stated that providing accurate nutrition information to the public was important, that their community was in need of more of this information, and that it would be of value to increase nutrition information in their library. Although the majority stated that they were confident in their ability to provide nutrition information to patrons of their library, about 70 percent also indicated that they would be interested in receiving training to enhance their abilities.

When asked about barriers to providing nutrition information, the most frequent responses had to do with providing space for materials and finding funds for new materials or programming. Additional qualitative research is under way to discuss a possible pilot intervention with several rural libraries that would take into account their challenges and interests. This research involves individual interviews with rural public librarians in their own libraries so that the research team can gain a better understanding of the physical and social environment of the library: for example, the physical layout of the space, availability and use of computers and other media, the nature of interactions between patrons and library workers, as well as feasible ideas to promote nutrition information within libraries. Interviews or surveys with library patrons are also planned to better understand the types of nutrition information that is of most interest and the best means for delivering it (e.g., online, paper format, video or other media, personal presentations). As with the restaurant study described previously, it will be crucial to work closely with these community partners in order to develop an intervention study that will be acceptable for rural public libraries, feasible, effective, and will have potential for long-term maintenance and eventual dissemination to other sites.

The Rural Newspaper Study

Various forms of media may contribute to an environment that makes it difficult to eat healthfully. One of the critical channels for receiving nutrition information in rural communities is local daily and weekly newspapers (Flora, Flora, & Fey, 2007). Even though more people go to the Internet and other news media channels to get important information, including health and nutritional information (Beckjord et al., 2007; Fox, 2006), several recent reports have demonstrated that **local newspapers** are still among the most important means for local residents in the United States to get food and nutritional information in their everyday lives (Academy of Nutrition and Dietetics, 2008; Borra, Earl, & Hogan, 1998). Although newspapers have suffered in recent years because of competition with the Internet (Franklin, 2008), newspapers in US rural areas are still strongly embedded in their local communities as a key source of community information for residents (Viswanath, Randolph Steele, & Finnegan, 2006). A 2010 survey found that 86 percent of rural Iowans read a newspaper each week (Iowa Newspaper Association, 2010). Therefore, rural newspapers will likely remain as one of the major sources of food and nutrition information for their local residents. In addition, older adults are disproportionately represented in the rural Midwest, and some research suggests they prefer to receive health information in written form (McKay et al., 2006).

Few studies have examined the prevalence of various forms of nutrition-related content in newspapers serving rural communities. Therefore, establishing an analysis framework and reliable methods for characterizing a newspaper's nutrition-related content are essential first steps toward measuring the effects of interventions designed to improve such content.

The content of local newspapers is determined by many factors, with reporters and editors serving as key decision makers or gatekeepers in this regard (Schudson, 1989). In order to influence rural newspapers to include more stories about healthy eating, it is essential to understand a number of issues from the perspective of reporters and editors. To meet the second aim of this study, we will conduct telephone interviews with editors at local daily and weekly newspapers in rural Iowa to determine their knowledge of reliable and accurate sources of nutrition information, their interest in improving nutrition-related content, and their perspective on barriers to doing so. Interviews will be guided by elements of social cognitive theory (Bandura, 2004), specifically, the triadic determinants of "person" (e.g., knowledge and attitudes, including self-efficacy and outcome expectations), "behavior" (e.g., decision making and information seeking), and "environment" (e.g., institutional and social factors affecting behavior). Improving the quality and quantity of nutrition-related content in newspapers in rural communities could serve as an effective strategy toward improving dietary knowledge and ultimately behaviors among the residents in those areas. The findings of the current study will be used to develop a future intervention study designed to assist local newspapers to deliver evidence-based nutrition information in their news stories and to be advocates for improving the nutrition environment in their local communities.

Conclusion

The State of Iowa has a variety of strengths and challenges when it comes to addressing health disparities. An aging and increasingly diverse population is requiring public health professionals in practice settings and in research to devise novel approaches to health care delivery and community-based health promotion. Drawing on the power of community partnerships, progress is being made and valuable lessons learned about how to most effectively reach this geographically dispersed population.

Summary

- All rural communities have unique strengths and challenges that must be taken into account when planning health promotion programs and research. Simply transplanting programs and policies tested only in urban areas, or even other rural areas, is not likely to be successful.

- Community partners have local knowledge and experience that is essential to designing and evaluating interventions that may be feasible and have the best potential for sustainability and dissemination. Such partners may include traditional health-related organizations, such as hospitals, clinics, and public health departments, but should not be limited to these.

- No single program or policy is likely to solve the complex health problems faced by communities but this should not deter communities and researchers from taking action where they can to improve the health of their communities. Small changes, added together, have the potential to contribute to larger changes in social norms and an environment better supportive of a healthy life.

Key Terms

Amish   social environment

local newspapers   table signs

public libraries

For Practice and Discussion

1. What are the most critical factors that should be considered when attempting to bring together a rural community to plan a health promotion intervention?

2. In this chapter we described what have been some of the unique strengths and challenges faced when designing and implementing health promotion interventions in rural Iowa. How are these strengths and challenges similar to or different from the strengths and challenges of rural communities in your state?

3. Working with a colleague or two from your class, discuss which different community groups or organizations you would involve (and why) when planning a health promotion program of your choice in a rural community.

Acknowledgments

This publication was supported by cooperative agreement number 1-U48DP001902-01 from the Centers for Disease Control and Prevention. The findings and conclusions in this document are those of the authors and do not necessarily represent the official position of the Centers for Disease Control and Prevention.

We also acknowledge the sincere cooperation and encouragement of our various community partners as we conduct our research projects and work together to improve the health of rural Iowans.

References

Academy of Nutrition and Dietetics. (2008). *Nutrition and you: Trends 2008.* Retrieved from www.eatright.org/Media/content.aspx?id = 6442465073

Bandura, A. (2004). Health promotion by social cognitive means. *Health Education & Behavior, 31*(2), 143–164.

Beckjord, E., Finney-Rutten, L., Squirers, L., Arora, N., Volckmann, L., Moser, R., et al. (2007). Us of the Internet to communicate with health care providers in the US. Estimates from the 2003 and 2005 Health Information National Trends Surveys (HINTS). *Journal of Medical Internet Research, 9*(3), 20.

Borra, S. T., Earl, R., & Hogan, E. H. (1998). Paucity of nutrition and food safety "news you can use" reveals opportunity for dietetics practitioners. *Journal of the American Dietetic Association, 98*(2), 190–193.

Flora, C., Flora, J., & Fey, S. G. (2007). *Rural communities: Legacy and change* (3rd ed.). Boulder, CO: Westview Press.

Fox, S. (2006). *Online health search 2006.* Pew Internet. Retrieved from http://www.pewinternet.org/Reports/2006/Online-Health-Search-2006.aspx

Franklin, B. (2008). The future of newspapers. *Journalism Studies, 9*(5), 630–641.

Gale, J., & Coburn, A. (2003). *The characteristics and roles of rural health clinics in the United States: A chartbook.* Retrieved from http://muskie.usm.maine.edu/Publications/rural/RHChartbook03.pdf

Iowa Center on Health Disparities. (2003a). *African Americans in Iowa: A snapshot of health disparity issues.* Retrieved from http://www.iowahealthdisparities.org/documents/africa_2003.pdf

Iowa Center on Health Disparities. (2003b). *The Amish.* Retrieved from http://www.iowahealthdisparities.org/documents/amish.pdf

Iowa Center on Health Disparities. (2003c). *Hispanics in Iowa: A snapshot of health disparity issues.* Retrieved from http://www.iowahealthdisparities.org/documents/HispanicsFact2003.pdf

Iowa Center on Health Disparities. (2003d). *Rural whites in Iowa: Fast facts on health disparity issues.* Retrieved from http://www.iowahealthdisparities.org/documents/ruralwhite.pdf

Iowa Department of Public Health. (2009a). *Center for Rural Health and Primary Care 2009 annual report: Iowa Chronic Disease Report.* Retrieved from http://www.idph.state.ia.us/apl/common/pdf/health_statistics/chronic_disease_report.pdf

Iowa Department of Public Health. (2009b). *Healthy Iowans: Iowa chronic disease report*. Retrieved from http://www.idph.state.ia.us/apl/common/pdf/health_statistics/chronic_disease_report.pdf

Iowa Newspaper Association. (2010). *You said it Iowa: Nothing works like newspaper advertising*. Retrieved from http://www.inanews.com/members/files/INAsurveybook.pdf

Iowa State University Extension. (2010). *Highlights from the 2010 farm poll*. Retrieved from http://www.soc.iastate.edu/extension/farmpoll/2010/population.html

Kaiser Family Foundation. (2010). *Iowa—Kaiser state health facts*. Retrieved from http://www.statehealthfacts.org/profileglance.jsp?rgn = 17

Linnan, L. A., Wildemuth, B. M., Gollop, C., Hull, P., Silbajoris, C., & Monnig, R. (2004). Public librarians as a resource for promoting health: Results from the Health for Everyone in Libraries Project (HELP) librarian survey. *Health Promotion Practice, 5*(2), 182–190.

McKay, D. L., Houser, R. F., Blumberg, J. B., & Goldberg, J. P. (2006). Nutrition information sources vary with education level in a population of older adults. *Journal of the American Dietetic Association, 106*(7), 1108–1111.

Minkler, M., Wallerstein, N., & Wilson, N. (2008). Improving health through community organization and community building. In K. Glanz, B. Rimer, & K. Viswanath (Eds.), *Health behavior and health education: Theory, research and practice* (4th ed.). San Francisco: Jossey-Bass.

Nothwehr, F., Snetselaar, L., Dawson, J. D., Hradek, C., & Sepulveda, M. (2010). Healthy option preferences of rural restaurant customers. *Health Promotion Practice, 11*(6), 828–836.

Nothwehr, F., Snetselaar, L., Dawson, J. D., & Schultz, U. (in press). Promoting healthy choices in non-chain restaurants: Effects of a simple cue to customers. *Health Promotion Practice*.

Pifalo, V., Hollander, S., Henderson, C. L., DeSalvo, P., & Gill, G. P. (1997). The impact of consumer health information provided by libraries: The Delaware experience. *Bulletin of the Medical Library Association, 85*(1), 16–22.

Rossman, M. (2003). *Agricultural behavioral health: In critical need. Partners in agricultural health, Module V*. Wisconsin Office of Rural Health. Retrieved from http://www.worh.org/files/AgHealth/ment.pdf

Schudson, M. (1989). The sociology of news production. *Media Culture Society, 11*, 263–282.

State of Iowa. (2010). *Final report. legislative commission on affordable health care plans for small businesses and families*. Retrieved from http://www.legis.state.ia.us/lsadocs/IntReport/2008/IPPAF001.PDF

United Health Foundation. (2010). *America's health rankings—Iowa*. Retrieved from http://www.americashealthrankings.org/SiteFiles/Statesummary/IA.pdf

University of Iowa and the Iowa Department of Public Health. (2011). *Iowa health fact book, 2011*. The University of Iowa College of Public Health, Iowa City, IA. Retrieved from http://www.public-health.uiowa.edu/factbook/

US National Institute of Health (NIH), National Cancer Institute. (2012). *Implementation science integrating science, practice, and policy. Reach effectiveness adoption implementation maintenance (Re-AIM)*. Retrieved from http://cancercontrol.cancer.gov/is/reaim/

Viswanath, K., Randolph Steele, W., & Finnegan Jr., J. R. (2006). Social capital and health: Civic engagement, community size, and recall of health messages. *American Journal of Public Health, 96*(8), 1456–1461.

Health Partnerships in Rural Communities

Part Three

Health Partnerships in
Rural Communities

Chapter 10

Health Assessment in Rural Communities

A Critical Organizing and Capacity-Building Tool

James N. Burdine   Bernard Appiah

Heather R. Clark   Chelsie N. Hollas

Lindsay J. Shea

Learning Objectives

- Describe the role of health assessment as a core function of public health.
- Identify the critical components of a health status assessment, particularly as they apply to a rural community.
- Explain the process of conducting a community health status assessment in a rural locale.

• • •

Assessing the health status of a population is one of the core functions of public health (Institute of Medicine, 1988). Done correctly, it can provide important insights into the factors influencing and producing health in a community. A **community health status assessment** is a powerful tool not only for identifying issues and circumstances that affect the health of a population, but also for community organizing and capacity building. In this chapter we present the basics of why and how to conduct a community health status assessment, particularly in the context of rural communities. We begin with definitions and a brief discussion of the theory underlying this process. Then we discuss specifics of an ideal community health status assessment and alternatives for when resources do not allow for the ideal.

Key Concepts

After reading this chapter, you should understand health status assessments from a theoretical perspective, the critical components of a health status assessment, and how to conduct an assessment. A few key points are critical to address up front. First, a health status assessment is not the same as a needs assessment. Perceived need is not a valid or useful measure if our goal is improving population health status or identifying factors influencing the health of a population (Burdine & Wendel, 2007). Finifter et al. (2005) concluded that using a single measure (i.e., need) as a proxy for the complex array of factors influencing health does not provide the information necessary for designing effective health interventions. Health status assessments also differs from health impact assessments (HIAs) in that HIAs focus on the health impact of particular policies, plans, or programs on various sectors of the community; both use a participatory, mixed-methods approach. By focusing on health status and examining the array of factors producing health or ill health in a specific community, we have evidence that can be used to draw conclusions that lead to actionable results.

Perhaps one of the easiest ways to grasp the community health status assessment concept is to reflect on your own experience with health status assessments—what happens when you visit your health care provider. Usually a provider will conduct an assessment of your health using a variety of methods such as taking a medical history, conducting a physical exam, and measuring your vital signs before making a diagnosis. The different methods used to gather health information from you are specifically designed to offer the provider the information needed not only to arrive at a diagnosis, but also to give you information and recommendations specific to your situation.

Although the general idea is the same, the doctor visit analogy falls short in that a community health status assessment does not focus on the individual nor does it emphasize a medical view. Rather it emphasizes the health of the broader community; public health looks beyond the individual patient and is broader than just medical or clinical factors. This population health status orientation requires thinking about community, health, and health status perhaps differently than your own experience as a health care consumer. Before we begin our exploration of assessment methods we will briefly discuss the basic concepts and definitions for *health* and *community*.

Definitions of Health

In 1946, the World Health Organization (WHO) reshaped thinking in health care by offering a new definition of *health* that addressed the whole person. That definition states, "Health is a state of complete physical, mental and social well-being and not merely the absence of disease or infirmity" (World Health Organization, 1946, p. 100). Since then, public health has recognized that other factors contribute to disease (e.g., risk factors such as smoking or obesity) and that there are underlying determinants of health such as education, income, housing, culture, and social systems that must be understood if we are to design effective interventions to maintain or improve health (Tarlov, 1996). Others have broadened the definition of health to include ideas such as functional capacity, quality of life, and population health (Felix & Burdine, 1995; Kindig & Stoddart, 2003), refocusing outcomes to groups of people and the broader population and environment rather than simply focusing on one individual's health or even the aggregate health of many individuals.

This perspective places an individual as an actor in a much larger system rather than existing in a vacuum on his or her own. Different system levels are considered to interact with one another affecting an individual's health in various ways with multiple and sometimes compounding outcomes. McLeroy and colleagues (1988) describe health behavior as being influenced by factors at the individual, interpersonal, institutional and organizational, community, and policy levels and emphasize the interaction of those levels in producing health behaviors and influencing those behaviors from a program planning perspective. This social ecological perspective provides a conceptual framework for thinking about the production of health behaviors. In thinking about broader determinants of health, we move beyond assessing individual characteristics and assess whole populations that have qualities that exist beyond the individual.

An appreciation of a population health focus and the broader determinants of health are fundamental to the rationale for and methods of community health status assessments as described in this chapter. This enlightened perspective on health status not only better informs assessment planning, but also dramatically increases the number of potential stakeholders in any community health improvement endeavor. This latter point is critical in rural communities where limited numbers of potential stakeholders make the participation of each more significant.

Definitions of Community

Communities have been defined in a variety of ways over time. Traditionally, *community* was defined on the basis of geography—those living within a geopolitical boundary. In the 1960s, Warren (1963), Sanders (1966), and others described communities on the basis of where goods and services are exchanged. Israel et al. (1998) describe community as a collective and characterized by "a sense of identification and emotional connection to other members, common symbols, shared values and norms, mutual influence, common interests, and commitment to meeting shared needs" (p. 178). This shared identity may be a family, cultural, or ethnic group. Yet, these may be spread out over many other types of communities or geographical areas. These perspectives encourage thinking in different ways about what it means to be part of a community and how membership in these communities might affect health (using our broader definition). Those of us living or working in rural communities, which can be structurally as complex as urban communities, need to pay particular attention to definitions of community.

Assessment Approaches

Similar to our example of a doctor visit, different approaches to community assessment can focus on specific problems or issues or take a broader perspective. Useful in many situations in which assessment is motivated by a response to some event that has brought public attention to or political pressure for solving a problem, a topic-oriented assessment takes advantage of that political and public interest to gather resources and enhance the likelihood of that action being taken.

The approach to a community health status assessment that is more broadly focused requires developing the kind of community interest that drives a specific problem-focused assessment but without that precipitating event's motivational influence. For example, a cluster of cancer in young children in a neighborhood or the diagnosis of an unusual disease in a prominent citizen can generate public interest in addressing that problem. Without that "event," organizing a community to conduct a community health status assessment requires identifying other motives and reasons for investing resources in this kind of activity. Although it is beyond the scope of this chapter, discussion of these community-organizing activities exists elsewhere (e.g., Wendel et al., 2009).

In addition, certain types of organizations within rural communities must conduct periodic health assessments. Federally qualified health centers, funded through the Health Resources and Services Administration, are required to demonstrate local need for services in order to obtain funding to operate in a particular community. State offices of rural health, which differ from state to state, also must document rural health needs and disparities to access federal funding. Nonprofit hospitals are required to conduct a community health status assessment every three years as part of health care reform.

Finally, the new move to accredit public health departments includes a require-ment to conduct a community health status assessment and community health improvement planning every five years. Although this is not specific to rural public health departments, the requirements may be disproportionately costly for them because of limited resources. The cost of conducting an assessment in rural communities actually promotes the collaborative model we will describe.

Regardless of the motivation for conducting a community health status assessment, one of the critical elements in the process is deciding to what extent developing community problem-solving capacity is tied to the purpose of the assessment. We argue that a tremendous opportunity is missed if a community health status assessment is conducted without recognizing and investing in capacity building as a part of that process. This approach to assess-ment does not just tackle the initial problems or only issues identified through the assessment but also addresses them in a longer term, more fundamental level. Here, results fuel the organizing process.

Theoretical Foundations

The type of community health status assessment we are describing in this chapter is built on the assumption that its goal is to improve, not just docu-ment, the overall health of the community. The approach we will discuss in the remainder of this chapter is built on two core elements: a community health development model and building community capacity for problem solving as an outcome of the process.

Community Health Development

Community health development can be defined as a process in which a com-munity identifies its needs and resources, develops goals and objectives, and builds capacity in order to develop a plan of action to address its needs with the goal of improving community well-being (Burdine, Felix, & Wendel, 2007; Steckler et al., 1993). Community health development is an approach that recognizes that social change occurs for a variety of reasons and can be influ-enced by different strategies that include facts and information, social forces, or being forced to change (Chin & Benne, 1976; Rothman, 1979).

When we bring together the concepts of population health, the social determinants of health, and community health development, we find that the community health status assessment is an incredibly powerful tool for generat-ing information and creating opportunities to address the health status of a population. These same concepts and tools force us to recognize that no single organization in a community can or should try to address major health

Therefore collaboration, community involvement, and community buy-in are critical to successful community health status assessments. This is particularly the case in rural communities where large institutions and human service organizations are less common.

problems without engaging the larger community. Therefore collaboration, community involvement, and community buy-in are critical to successful community health status assessments. This is particularly the case in rural communities where large institutions and human service organizations are less common.

Community Capacity Building

Building community capacity is also fundamental to our approach to sustaining the *process* and *products* of community health status assessments. Chavis, Florin, and Felix (1992) discuss the importance of building capacity through enabling mechanisms through actions such as (1) creating linkages between community members and organizations and externally to federal and state health-related agencies, (2) supplying and managing resources and removing barriers to success by (3) providing trainings to develop skills for planning, and (4) communication. The basic premise of community capacity building is helping communities to become more self-sufficient and more effective problem solvers at the end of the process (Goodman et al., 1998).

Partnerships and linkages are also critical to the assessment process. McKenzie, Neiger, and Thackeray (2009) state that the assessment advisory or planning committee must be composed of *doers* who are willing to roll up their sleeves to do the physical work and *influencers* who can mobilize others to take part, and new individuals need to be added periodically throughout the assessment process. Rural communities face the additional challenge of scarce human resources in terms of numbers as well as individuals with specific skills. This requires defining participants in the assessment process more broadly than those who are part of the formal health system and fostering collaboration and coordination among them.

An Ideal Community Health Status Assessment

So far this chapter has presented a background, theory, and general philosophy for conducting a community health status assessment. Now we present what we describe as the ideal or optimal community health assessment consisting of a *population-based survey, community discussion groups, key informant interviews,* and *secondary data analysis*. Although often beyond the scope of a small rural community, there are ways rural communities can adapt the assessment process or expand the pool of potential partners to support the effort to make an ideal assessment possible. The ideal community health status assessment is one that is comprehensive and optimally matches results with available resources.

Community Health Survey

The most costly element of a comprehensive assessment is a **community health survey** (a random-sample survey mailed to households in the community). A well-constructed survey implemented correctly yields useful information. This is also the one component that is also most likely to be implemented poorly. Although it is true that the subject matter of a community health status assessment seems straightforward, seemingly simple topics often require sophisticated methodology to gain a meaningful understanding. Take smoking behaviors as an example. The straightforward closed-ended question, "Do you smoke?" tells little about smoking in a population. How is smoking defined? Does it include cigarettes, pipes, cigars, or other things? What about nontobacco cigarettes (e.g., clove)? If I quit yesterday but I smoked for thirty years, does my answer of *no* correctly allow you to understand the potential impact of smoking on my health or in our community?

This example illustrates the importance of working with experienced survey researchers who are familiar with existing tools and resources in order to ensure that a household survey incorporates standardized, validated measures. The CDC, for example, conducts periodic household surveys, as does the National Cancer Institute and other state and federal agencies. All these surveys have question sets that are available to examine and adapt and adopt in part or in whole for use in your community.

In our ideal assessment, the major elements of the household survey include overall health status, medical history, health habits, physical activity, preventive screening, places where health care is obtained, perceptions around access to and quality of health care, transportation, food and nutrition, health insurance coverage, community perceptions of key local issues, social capital, human services needed and used, and demographic information. Community participation in development of the survey instrument may also suggest other factors to consider including which of the results is important to local ownership. Although there are many factors to consider, this list is suggested as most valuable based on the authors' collective experience of conducting community health status assessments in more than two hundred communities in forty states during the past twenty-five years.

Definition of Survey Boundaries

The scope of a community health survey generally is defined by the parameters of the community. Although we know there are multiple ways to define a community, fundamentally health surveys are conducted among people living within a designated area—most frequently a hospital's service area, a city, neighborhood, county, or cluster of any of these. Generally, the interaction of budget (limitations) and institutional politics determines the scope or area to be surveyed. For example, if an assessment is premised on building community capacity as a byproduct of the assessment, and little collaboration exists among local institutions (hospitals, clinics, health departments, United Way agencies, local churches, schools, etc.), engaging those institutions as cosponsors can begin to build some of the needed trust. The service areas of those institutions may serve as a possible scope or area for the assessment. Rural communities generally discover that working collaboratively at the county or regional level is the most cost-effective way to approach a household survey.

Survey Sample and Costs

Quality household surveys are expensive, so designing an assessment that requires the smallest number of respondents while still being able to generalize the findings to the entire community is beneficial. It is critical to have involvement from a survey expert in the survey development process to ensure that usable data are gathered. Often local colleges, universities, or state agencies will have personnel with this expertise. This is another reason to pursue broad participation in your assessment process (which will be discussed later in this chapter).

In our experience, between one thousand and two thousand surveys is the balance point of budget and methodology with which the average-sized community can live (aggregated population up to three hundred thousand). However, in smaller communities that cannot be aggregated into a region, this may not be realistic, and the target for number of surveys may be much smaller. For example, in a county of fifteen thousand, you may elect to survey 350, which will allow you to generalize to the population but limit your ability to break the results down into subpopulations by education, age, race and ethnicity, income, and so on. This is, again, why it is important to plan such a survey with an experienced researcher.

Although costs continue to increase, at the time of this writing it generally ends up costing about $50 per completed survey for good survey data. In this case, 1,500 surveys would cost us about $75,000 to collect. That doesn't include the analysis but it would include a basic summary report (item frequencies, response rates, etc.) from the vendor contracted to do the data collection. Split among a number of cosponsors, the cost becomes feasible for many organizations.

Survey Timeline

In planning a community health status assessment you should anticipate that the survey component will take at least six months from survey development through preliminary results, often longer. Processes that stretch out more than a year will likely lose community interest and require significant effort to regain momentum for doing anything with the assessment results, again based on our experience.

Survey Frequency

The question of how often to survey is a function of four factors:

- The type(s) of changes in health status you are looking for
- Resources available for assessment
- Success with efforts to affect community health status
- Regulatory or other policy requirements setting frequency parameters

On balance, three years is probably the minimum number of years between administrations that would effectively measure change.

An important but often overlooked component of a community survey is finding data for comparative purposes. Information such as the *Healthy People 2020* goals or previous assessments that provide baselines or external frames of reference allows the community to more easily interpret where it stands. Therefore *before* implementing a community survey, comparable data should be identified and acquired. Similarly, there are other important considerations to keep in mind when conducting a household survey as part of your community health status assessment, such as the following:

- If planning to compare characteristics such as race or age to national survey data, you should aim to collect local data from a similar proportion or percentage of that same characteristic.
- Avoid taking a convenience sample. Although it may be tempting to conduct surveys with people using a specific service or sitting in a waiting room, these results are not representative of the community at large and can only be discussed in terms of the population from which it was collected.
- Pilot test the survey instrument before administration begins with a variety of population groups in order to identify and eliminate inconsistencies, confusion, and colloquialisms within the survey.

- Include questions about the community itself to gather information beyond the individual. Questions may include gathering information on the physical environment, sense of belonging, feeling safe, and so on in order to understand a variety of resources, problems, social capital, or community capacity.

- You can increase your survey response rate by providing a personalized letter with recognizable local signatories, a postage paid return envelope, and a survey that is not overwhelming in terms of its length or content.

- Be sensitive to the culture of your population when determining your recruitment methodology. Knowledge of local culture and practices, even in places that seem very familiar, is a critical piece of your preassessment research and planning process.

Understanding your community's preferences (particularly subcultures within the larger community) can have a major impact on the success of your data-collection activities (surveys and qualitative methods).

Secondary Data

Secondary data are data that have been previously collected by other researchers for a different purpose and are often available in the public domain or for purchase. These data can be helpful as a supplement to primary data collection or can be the primary type of data used for assessments. They may be found in the form of interviews, questionnaires, and surveys that can come from sources such as a state health department, the CDC, the US Census Bureau, university consortia, and *Healthy People 2020* (Bickman & Rog, 2009; Boslaugh, 2007; Tashakkori & Teddlie, 2003). Although secondary data is readily available in most cases, it is important to remember that these data were gathered for a purpose other than your assessment. Therefore, careful attention must be paid to the how the data were collected, analyzed, and reported. Some reputable sources for secondary data can be found in Table 10.1.

Community Discussion Groups and Key Informant Interviews

Community discussion groups (CDGs) and key informant interviews (KIIs) are two effective methods for generating primary qualitative data. CDGs and KIIs are critical to our assessment process when using the guiding principles of community health development and community capacity building. Members of the community must be involved in the assessment process if they ultimately will be stakeholders who can improve their community's health status. For best effectiveness, community discussions should engage local intermediaries for organization, recruitment, and conducting of CDGs. Key

Table 10.1. Descriptions of Secondary Data Sources

Secondary Data Source	Description
Adolescent Health Survey	The National Longitudinal Study of Adolescent Health was mandated by Congress to collect data for the purpose of measuring the impact of social environment on adolescent health.
The Centers for Disease Control (CDC)	The CDC is recognized as the lead federal agency for providing credible information to enhance health decisions and promoting health through strong partnerships. CDC serves as the national focus for health promotion and education activities designed to improve the health of the people of the United States.
Behavioral Risk Factor Surveillance System (BRFSS)	The goals of the BRFSS are to gather scientific data from each state on adult behaviors that endanger health and to provide researchers with these data so that they can design programs that will encourage adults to stop these behaviors.
CDC WONDER	CDC Wide-ranging Online Data for Epidemiologic Research (WONDER) is an easy-to-use system that provides a single point of access to a wide variety of CDC reports, guidelines, and numeric public health data.
County Health Rankings	The County Health Rankings project (www.countyhealthrankings.org) provides data on a variety of measures and ranks state and individual counties by health outcomes and health factors.
HealthComm Key	HealthComm Key is a database that contains comprehensive summaries of more than two hundred articles about health communication research and practice. The database, developed by CDC's Office of Communication, is designed for researchers and program staff within CDC and also for professionals, students, and others outside of CDC who are interested in health communication.
National Center for Injury Prevention and Control	This website contains Injury Maps, CDC Injury Center's interactive mapping system that gives you access to the geographic distribution of injury-related mortality rates in the United States. Injury Maps allows you to create county-level and state-level maps of age-adjusted mortality rates.

(Continued)

Table 10.1. (*Continued*)

Secondary Data Source	Description
Youth Risk Behavior Surveillance System (YRBSS)	The goals of the YRBSS are to provide researchers and public health professionals with data about the health-risk behaviors of young people and to use the survey data as the basis for programs to help young people avoid or stop behavior that endangers their health now or when they are older.
Child Trends DataBank	The Child Trends DataBank is a one-stop-shop for the latest national trends and research on more than eighty key indicators of child and youth well-being, with new indicators added each month.
FedStats	This is a launchpad to get to databases and statistics from more than one hundred US federal agencies.
Joint Canada/United States Survey of Health (JCUSH)	Canada partnered with the US National Center Health Statistics (NCHS) for this one-time, random telephone survey performed in the United States and Canada that provides comparative data on the amount and distribution of illness, the effects of disability and chronic impairments, health-risk factors, and the kind of health services people receive.
National Center for Health Statistics (NCHS)	The National Center for Health Statistics is rich source of information about America's health. As the nation's principal health statistics agency, NCHS compiles statistical information to guide actions and policies to improve the health of our people.
Healthy People 2020	*Healthy People 2020* provides science-based, 10-year national objectives for improving the health of all Americans. For 3 decades, Healthy People has established benchmarks and monitored progress over time in order to: encourage collaborations across communities and sectors, empower individuals to make informed health decisions, and measure the impact of prevention activities.
US Census Bureau	The US Census Bureau provides an extensive selection of statistics for the United States, with selected data for regions, divisions, states, metropolitan areas, cities, and foreign countries from reports and records of government and private agencies.
World Health Organization (WHO)	The WHO Statistical Information System (WHOSIS) is the guide to health and health-related epidemiological and statistical information available from the World Health Organization.

Source: http://www.collegeboard.com/yes/ae/links.html

informant interviews should be conducted with a variety of people who may not participate in CDGs for various reasons, including lack of time and sensitivity to the topics being discussed.

the community must be involved in the assessment process if they ultimately will be stakeholders who can improve their community's health status.

Several factors must be considered when conducting community discussion groups. First, CDGs should target multiple segments of the population to engage a wide array of individuals who may not otherwise have opportunities to share their opinions of health in their community. In addition, community discussion groups should be held at appropriate times and venues for the targeted community segment. For instance, community leaders are generally available for lunch meetings compared to community residents who might be more able to attend an early evening discussion group after work.

The facilitator(s) of the discussion groups should also be experienced in conducting or leading meetings and groups, have background information on that specific community, and be trained in techniques that solicit input from a variety of participants. Open-ended questions are likely to generate rich information from participants. The question set we generally recommend solicits input from participants by asking them to do the following:

- Describe their community
- Identify resources available in their community
- Identify issues that are present in their community
- Describe the history of collaboration among organizations in their community
- Give their advice on how to most effectively work with their community if attempting to improve the community's health

Individuals selected for interviews are usually considered local champions or opinion leaders in their communities. Such individuals may include government officials, health and human service providers, and health care, education, and religious leaders.

Alternatives to the Ideal Assessment

One goal of this chapter is to provide an array of alternatives for conducting a community health status assessment in a manner that fits the financial, human, and political resources, expectations, and capacity to apply the resulting information. Depending on available resources, the ideal community health status assessment may not be feasible. That does not mean, however, that a high-quality assessment cannot be done. Secondary data and qualitative data from community discussion groups and key informant interviews can be the sources of information on your community population without conducting a costly population survey. Obviously this is a much less robust assessment, but performed thoughtfully, it can yield useful information and in a much shorter time frame (Bickman & Rog, 2009). Once secondary data sources have been identified, more detailed information specific to the community (primary data) can be gathered through community discussion groups and key informant interviews. Collecting qualitative data supplements the secondary data by providing context and insights into why the community's health status is as it is.

Using the Assessment Process as an Organizing and Capacity-Building Tool

There are a number of models for conducting a community health status assessment, including Mobilizing for Action Through Planning and Partnerships (MAPP), Assessment Protocol for Excellence in Public Health (APEXPH), and Planned Approach to Community Health (PATCH). Each of these models includes a significant community health status assessment component (Green, 1992; National Association of County and City Health Officials, n.d.) with underlying linkages to the community. These are not assessments *of* a community but *with* a community.

This "with the community" approach requires that you understand the characteristics and dynamics of the community you are assessing. These characteristics include the community's history and experience with collaboration, the economic environment, key organizations, and cultural elements, among many others. This information helps with decisions about with whom should you partner, how you define the boundary of your community and, very important, in what context organizationally you should do your assessment.

Because the nature of rural communities varies, it is not easy to briefly describe how to take into consideration all those factors. For example, residents of many rural communities obtain their medical care in a nearby city or regional hub, making access to health care organization partners in an assessment potentially more difficult to engage. Extremely rural or frontier areas may have such a low population density that traditional methods such as community discussion groups are difficult to organize. All this points to the importance of having a process within which to organize your community health status assessment.

The Partnership Approach

The **partnership approach** (Stunkard, Felix, & Cohen, 1985) is a model that focuses on community engagement and was developed as a community capacity-building approach. Briefly stated, the partnership approach frames a unique partnership strategy for each community used to engage and organize community stakeholders, partners, and sponsors of the assessment. The assessment is then conducted and interventions to address the assessment's findings are crafted based on the overall partnership strategy as well as findings from the assessment itself. The implementation of those interventions and their evaluation provide feedback to the partnership, guiding future activities (Wendel, Burdine, & McLeroy, 2007).

Partnership Participants

There are many stakeholders in the partnership approach and other models with a community health development emphasis. An essential tool in working with community stakeholders is called *enlightened self-interest* (de Tocqueville, 1997). Based on the assumption that people generally act in their own self-interest, this self-interest can be enlightened to build understanding of common interests. When this occurs, stakeholders can be encouraged to work together for the common good. By identifying the self-interests of key players in a particular community, a strategy can be developed that addresses multiple self-interests simultaneously. This increases the array of potential stakeholders or partners in the assessment and also the depth of their commitment to the process and outcome.

One of the challenges facing rural communities is that the key stakeholders and major institutions may be few in numbers and likely have limited resources. Often we find that a small group of people are on every board, chair every organization, and make most of the decisions. If that group is predisposed toward your assessment process, their support can be invaluable. If they are not, it may require a great deal of effort to persuade those leaders of the value of an assessment.

Presenting Data for Action

The groundwork already done throughout the assessment process (community and stakeholder engagement) dictates the format of how data are presented back to the assessment stakeholders and the community in general. Multiple venues are typically identified through the process to reach different subgroups of stakeholders with the findings. If community members and organizations have been involved in planning, conducting, and analyzing of data, their ownership of the results can be further enhanced by having them play a major role in presenting the results. In addition, as mentioned previously, sometimes what motivates a community health status assessment is some high-profile event; if this is the case, the presentation of the assessment findings should be organized around that galvanizing issue. What is important at this stage of the assessment is generating buy-in by stakeholders and the community of the assessment results.

Significant challenges exist when presenting assessment data. First, assessments conducted as we have presented in this chapter yield a significant volume of information to be analyzed and then to be presented. Second, any given community will have a wide variation of levels of understanding data presented. And, most important, you cannot present everything!

It may be useful to focus on information that is statistically different from an external reference point such as *Healthy People 2020* goals, some state or national rate, or information from the assessment that has the ability to be acted on locally. It is also important to consider what common denominators in the data are important to most people in the audience, for example, educational attainment or exposure to health statistics.

There are two goals for any assessment presentation: (1) reporting the data and (2) identifying next steps for improving health status. One effective approach to presenting data to a community is through a community health summit that occurs in two parts: (1) presentation of the data and (2) discussion around the major findings of the assessment with groups agreeing to work collaboratively toward solutions or priorities for affecting specific issues.

Conclusion

The ability to conduct a successful community health status assessment is a core function of public health and a key skill for health professionals—particularly those working with rural communities. Beyond the measures, techniques, and approaches to assessment, understanding how to balance the benefits with the costs and how to use local resources and develop local buy-in all contribute to a successful assessment. The goal of this chapter was to give the reader an overview of the theory and methods of an ideal community health status assessment with additional insights into how to adapt that ideal model to local community circumstances, particularly rural communities.

Summary

- Assessment is one of the three core functions of public health. The ability to plan and conduct an assessment, as well as use the findings to improve health status, is an essential skill.

- Community health status assessment is *not* a needs assessment. Needs assessment focuses on perceived need, and a community health status assessment identifies issues and resources and uses the process and the information to mobilize change and build capacity.

- Communities are unique. This demands that assessment strategies be tailored to the specific characteristics and dynamics of a community.
- Assessment in rural communities may be more difficult because of low population density, lack of resources, and health improvement not being valued as a high local priority.
- The three key components to an ideal community health status assessment are a household survey, community discussion groups and key informant interviews, and secondary data.
- Assessments should not be conducted if there is no plan to use the data for health improvement.
- The assessment process can be an effective tool in organizing and building capacity in communities.

For Practice and Discussion

1. With a colleague, identify how the key stakeholders for an assessment may differ between rural and urban communities.
2. With a colleague, discuss the strengths and weaknesses of each component of a community health status assessment (household survey, community discussion groups, key informant interviews, and secondary data).
3. In a small group, describe how community health status assessments fit with the other two core functions of public health. Why is an assessment a core function?

Key Terms

community discussion groups household survey
community health development partnership approach
community health status assessment secondary data

Acknowledgments

This chapter was supported in part by cooperative agreement number 5U48DP001924 from the Centers for Disease Control and Prevention. The findings and conclusions in this chapter are those of the authors and do not necessarily represent the official position of the Centers for Disease Control and Prevention.

References

Bickman, L., & Rog, D. (Eds.). (2009). *The Sage handbook of applied social research methods*. Newbury Park, CA: Sage.

Boslaugh, S. (2007). *Secondary data sources for public health: A practical guide*. New York: Cambridge University Press.

Burdine, J., Felix, M., & Wendel, M. (2007). The basics of community health development. *Texas Public Health Association Journal, 59*(1), 10–11.

Burdine, J., & Wendel, M. (2007). Framing the question: Needs assessment vs. health status assessment. *Texas Public Health Association Journal, 59*(1), 12–14.

Chavis, D. M., Florin, P., & Felix, M.R.J. (1992). Nurturing grassroots initiatives for community development: The role of enabling systems. In T. Mizrahi & J. Morrison (Eds.), *Community organization and social administration: Advances, trends and emerging principles*. Binghamton, NY: Haworth Press.

Chin, R., & Benne, W. (1976). Planned change in historical perspective. In W. G. Benne, K. D. Chin, & K. E. Corey (Eds.), *The planning of change*. New York: Holt, Rinehart, Winston.

Felix, M. R., & Burdine, J. N. (1995). Taking the pulse of the community. *Healthcare Executive, 10*(4), 8–11.

Finifter, D. H., Jensen, C. J., Wilson, C. E., & Koenig, B. L. (2005). A comprehensive, multitiered, targeted community needs assessment model: Methodology, dissemination, and implementation. *Family & Community Health, 28*(4), 293–306.

Goodman, R. M., Speers, M. A., McLeroy, K., Fawcett, S., Kegler, M., Parker, E., et al. (1998). Identifying and defining the dimensions of community capacity to provide a basis for measurement. *Health Education & Behavior: The Official Publication of the Society for Public Health Education, 25*(3), 258–278.

Green, L. W. (1992). PATCH: CDC's planned approach to community health, an application of PRECEED and an inspiration for PROCEED. *Journal of Health Education, 23*(3), 140–147.

Institute of Medicine. (1988). *The future of public health*. Washington, DC: National Academies Press.

Israel, B. A., Schulz, A. J., Parker, E. A., & Becker, A. B. (1998). Review of community-based research: Assessing partnership approaches to improve public health. *Annual Review of Public Health, 19*, 173–202. doi:10.1146/annurev. publhealth.19.1.173.

Kindig, D., & Stoddart, G. (2003). What is population health? *American Journal of Public Health, 93*(3), 380–383.

McKenzie, J. F., Neiger, B. L., & Thackeray, R. (2009). *Planning, implementing, and evaluating health programs: A primer* (5th ed.). San Francisco: Benjamin Cummings.

McLeroy, K. R., Bibeau, D., Steckler, A., & Glanz, K. (1988). An ecological perspective on health promotion programs. *Health Education Quarterly, 15*(4), 351–377.

National Association of County and City Health Officials. (n.d.). *Mobilizing for action through planning and partnerships (MAPP)*. Retrieved from www.naccho.org/topics/infrastructure/mapp/

Rothman, J. (1979). Three models of community organization practice, their mixing and phasing. In F. Cox, J. Ehrlich, J. Rothman, & J. Tropman (Eds.), *Strategies of community organization* (3rd ed.). Itasca, IL: F. E. Peacock.

Sanders, I. T. (1966). *The community: An introduction to a social system* (2nd ed.). New York: Ronald Press.

Steckler, A. B., Dawson, L., Israel, B. A., & Eng, E. (1993). Community health development: An overview of the works of Guy W. Steuart. *Health Education Quarterly, Suppl. 1*, S3–S20.

Stunkard, A. J., Felix, M.R.J., & Cohen, R. Y. (1985). Mobilizing a community to promote health: The Pennsylvania county health improvement project (CHIP). In J. Rosen & L. Solomon (Eds.), *Prevention in health psychology*. Hanover, NH: University of New England Press.

Tarlov, A. (1996). Health and social organization: Towards a health policy for the twenty-first century. In D. Blane, E. Brunner, & R. Wilkinson (Eds.), *Social determinants of health: The sociobiological translation*. New York: Routledge Press.

Tashakkori, A., & Teddlie, C. (2003). *Handbook of mixed methods in social & behavioral research*. Thousand Oaks, CA: Sage.

de Tocqueville, A. (1997). How the Americans combat individualism by the principle of self-interest rightly understood. *Democracy in America*. Charlottesville: University of Virginia. (Originally published in 1840.)

Warren, R. L. (1963). *The community in America*. Chicago: Rand McNally.

Wendel, M., Burdine, J., & McLeroy, K. (2007). The evolving role of partnerships in addressing community public health issues: Policy and ethical implications. *Organizational Ethics: Healthcare, Business, and Policy, 4*(1), 53–64.

Wendel, M., Burdine, J., McLeroy, K., Alaniz, A., Norton, B., & Felix, M. (2009). Community capacity: Theory and application. In R. DiClemente, R. Crosby, & M. Kegler (Eds.), *Emerging theories in health promotion practice and research* (2nd ed., pp. 277–302). San Francisco: Jossey-Bass.

World Health Organization. (1946, June 19–22). *Preamble to the Constitution of the World Health Organization*. New York: Author.

Chapter 11

Strategies for Building Coalitions in Rural Communities

Michelle C. Kegler
Frances D. Butterfoss

Learning Objectives

- Understand the rationale for collaboration and the reasons for building coalitions in rural public health practice.
- Be able to identify various types of coalitions.
- List and describe benefits of coalitions to rural public health.
- Understand the theoretical basis of using coalitions to improve rural public health and identify key elements of community coalition action theory.
- Describe the unique aspects and benefits of community coalition action theory when applied to rural communities.

•••

Rural populations are more likely to be uninsured, older, have lower income and educational achievement, higher rates of chronic illness and disability, and report poorer overall health status than urban communities (Behringer & Friedell, 2006; Harris et al., 2005). Geographical, personnel, infrastructure, and funding challenges contribute to these disparities (Pennel, Carpender, & Quiram, 2008). Furthermore, lack of public transportation, fewer health care providers, and lower levels of community services exacerbate the problem (Behringer & Friedell, 2006; Pennel et al., 2008). Numerous cultural issues in rural areas also influence the incidence of chronic disease, mortality rates, and care-seeking behavior. For example, in Appalachia, communication and use of screening and treatment for cancer is influenced by skepticism, a sense of fatalism toward health, distrust of health professionals, and fear of being taken advantage of by the health care system (Behringer & Friedell, 2006). In US-Mexico border areas, language issues lead to fewer visits with physicians, especially for preventive care (Ingram, Gallegos, & Elenes, 2005). For all of these reasons, **coalition building** (collaboration among diverse groups to reach a common goal) is essential, but often more difficult, in rural areas.

Fortunately, rural communities also have many characteristics that facilitate a collaborative approach to problem solving. These include an ability to reach a large proportion of residents with modest efforts; interconnected social networks; relatively accessible media, organizational leaders, and policy makers; a strong attachment to place; and a well-developed sense of community (Downey et al., Mahon & Taylor-Powell, 2007, 2010; Smith, Baugh Littlejohns, & Roy, 2003). In rural areas facing economic decline and **out-migration** (movement from rural to urban area) of young people, another factor motivating collaboration is a strong, shared commitment to invest in the future for the survival of the community.

Key Concepts

Collaboration begins when a perceived need exists and two or more organizations anticipate deriving a benefit that depends on mutual action (Gray & Wood, 1991). **Collaboration** is "a mutually beneficial and well defined relationship entered into by two or more organizations to achieve common goals" (Mattesich, Murray-Close, & Monsey, 2001, p. 7). These organizations often enter into a formal, sustained commitment to mutual relationships and goals, jointly developed structures, shared responsibility, mutual authority and accountability, and shared resources and rewards.

Collaboration represents the highest level of working relationships that organizations can experience. Collaboration changes the way organizations work together—it moves them from competing to building consensus; from working alone to including others from diverse cultures, fields, and settings; from thinking mostly about activities, services, and programs to looking for complex, integrated strategies; and from focusing on short-term accomplishments to broad, policy systems and environmental changes (Winer & Ray, 1994).

Despite its rewards, effective collaborations must acknowledge and respect each organization's self-interest (i.e., structure, agenda, values, and culture), relationships, linkages, and how power is shared and distributed (Gray, 1996). Three types of working relationships build on each other and may lead to collaboration: networking, cooperation, and coordination. These relationships exist across a continuum where (1) linkages become more intense and are influenced by common goals, tasks, rules, and resources; (2) purposes become more complex as information sharing gives way to joint problem solving; (3) agreements become more formal with operating procedures and policies; and (4) relationships take more time to develop and involve greater risks and rewards (Habana-Hefner et al., 1989; Himmelman, 2001; Kagan, 1991; National Network for Collaboration, 1996).

Coalitions: Effective Vehicles for Collaboration

Coalitions are collaborations that are formal, long-term, and composed of diverse organizations, factions, or constituencies who agree to work together to achieve a common goal (Butterfoss, Goodman, & Wandersman, 1993; Feighery & Rogers, 1990). A coalition is **action-oriented** (focused on outcomes) and focuses on reducing or preventing a community problem by analyzing the issue, identifying and implementing solutions, and creating social change. The best coalitions bring people together, expand resources, focus on issues of community concern, and achieve better results than any single group could achieve alone (Butterfoss & Kegler, 2002). Technically, partnerships assume a more businesslike arrangement and may involve as few as two partners, but the terms *coalitions* and *partnerships* are used interchangeably. Coalition members may be individuals, organizations, or groups. However, if a coalition is composed solely of individuals, then it should be classified as an organization or network. Membership size may vary but a coalition usually involves professional and grassroots organizations.

Coalitions are one of the most effective strategies for achieving community change. Through advocacy and education, coalitions are critical for mobilizing communities to develop and implement effective strategies and policies for the following reasons (CDC, 2008):

- Coalitions are versatile—they have been used effectively in all states; thousands of cities, towns, and counties; and many countries.

- Science supports coalitions as effective community interventions that change social norms and policies that lead to decreased morbidity and mortality (Crowley, Yu, & Kaftarian, 2000; National Cancer Institute, 2005; Roussos & Fawcett, 2000).

- Although the financial investment in coalitions is relatively low, they effectively leverage resources (e.g., members' services, time, and expertise) that enhance public health outcomes.

- Coalitions enhance the stability of public health programs by building political and public support, securing and maintaining funding, and advocating for policy change.

Types of Coalitions

Coalitions may be categorized by their patterns of formation, functions, or structures that accommodate these functions. However, most are typed according to membership or geographic focus. Three types of coalitions are based on membership (Feighery & Rogers, 1990):

- **Grassroots coalitions** are organized by advocates in times of crisis to pressure policy makers to act on an issue. They can be controversial but effective in reaching their goals and often disband when the crisis ends, such as when a group of residents pressures county officials to add shoulders and bike paths to rural roads to prevent injuries.

- **Professional coalitions** are formed by professional organizations or agencies to increase their power and influence, such as when health professionals pressure their state licensing board to establish more group homes for mental health patients. Although funding is provided to address community issues, the strategies usually come from professionals or institutions; local residents are secondary players (Wolff, 2001).

- **Community-based coalitions** of professional and grassroots members are formed to influence more long-term health and welfare practices for their community, such as obesity-prevention coalitions. Community ownership is higher in these groups but external funding is often required to provide needed resources.

Coalitions may also be classified by their geography—they may focus on community, regional, state, national, or international levels. Community coalitions operate in neighborhoods, towns, cities, or counties and usually serve a defined location that is recognized by local residents as representing and serving them (Clarke et al., 2006). Its members reflect the diversity and wisdom of that community at grassroots and "grasstops" (professional) levels (Butterfoss et al., 1993; Feighery & Rogers, 1990). These members have direct experience with the social or health problem of interest and are actively engaged in decision making and problem solving. In sparsely populated rural areas, community coalitions may coalesce at county or multicounty levels to maximize their reach and influence.

State coalitions develop to facilitate communication and develop strategies over larger geographic areas. Effective state coalitions immediately forge relationships with community coalitions or do so when they recognize the need to disseminate information and strategies widely. Likewise, community coalitions mobilize to form state coalitions when they realize the benefits of more widespread commitment and support for their issue. Both approaches work well—the key is to link local and state concerns and resources. Many community coalitions are funded through state-level public health initiatives that have statewide coalitions.

Benefits of Community Coalitions

Collaborative efforts in public health, such as coalitions, offer many direct and indirect benefits (Butterfoss, 2007):

- Serve as effective and efficient vehicles for exchanging knowledge and ideas
- Demonstrate and develop community buy-in or concern for issues
- Establish greater credibility, trust, and communication among community agencies and sectors
- Mobilize diverse populations, talents, resources, and strategies
- Share costs and associated risks
- Leverage resources to minimize duplication of efforts and services
- Negotiate potential conflict by sharing power
- Reduce the social acceptability of health-risk behaviors
- Advocate for policy change by enlisting political and constituent support
- Develop synergy that allows organizations to adopt new issues without having sole responsibility for them

When real community involvement exists, coalitions address community health concerns while empowering or developing capacity in those communities. Coalition membership may lead to increased community participation and leadership, skills, resources, social and interorganizational networks, sense of community, community power, and successful community problem solving (Goodman et al, 1998; Kegler et al., 1998).

The overarching benefits that coalitions provide are improved trust and communication among agencies and organizations, as evidenced by increased networking, information sharing, and access to ideas, materials, and resources. This may help coalitions deliver more consistent and reliable information to their priority populations. In turn, community members are more likely to support and use public programs and services when they have input into setting priorities and tailoring programs and services to local needs and services. Open and transparent communication that is facilitated through community coalitions may also increase public awareness of relevant policy and legislative issues and provide better evaluation of the impact of coalition strategies (Jackson & Maddy, 2001).

Although they usually arise from well-meaning motives to improve community conditions, coalitions may experience difficulties that are common to many types of organizations as well as some that are unique to collaborative efforts. Promised resources may not be made available, conflicting interests may prevent the coalition from having the desired community effect, and recognition for accomplishments may be slow in coming (Butterfoss, 2007). Because it involves an investment of time and resources, a coalition should not be built if a simpler entity will get the job done or if community support is lacking.

Coalitions are best suited to assessing community assets and needs, strategic and action planning, conducting social marketing campaigns, implementing policy and environmental change strategies, educating community members and policy makers, providing technical assistance or training, garnering financial and in-kind resources, and enhancing community buy-in and involvement. Coalitions should focus on promising or evidence-based strategies that are more likely to be effective and not as much one-on-one education and costly programs or services that compete with those offered by their members.

Although coalitions are used in health promotion and disease prevention efforts of every kind, the most effective coalition examples exist in tobacco control and prevention's nearly forty-year history of educating communities about the negative health effects of tobacco use and secondhand smoke exposure and advocating for evidence-based policy strategies. This has led to decreased tobacco consumption, prevention of tobacco use initiation, and decreased tobacco-related disease and mortality. Tobacco control coalitions have done the following (National Cancer Institute, 2005):

- Advocated for increased tobacco excise taxes at state and local levels
- Reduced and eliminated tobacco product advertising and promotion
- Established countermarketing campaigns to disseminate antitobacco media messages promoting the adoption of healthy behaviors and provide information on health risks
- Decreased the social acceptability of tobacco by educating diverse groups (e.g., faith-based, low-income, youth) to further relay messages and create social norm change

- Expanded smoke-free environments in work and public places
- Limited the availability of and access to tobacco products, particularly to persons under eighteen years

The most effective coalition examples exist in tobacco control and prevention's nearly forty-year history of educating communities about the negative health effects of tobacco use and secondhand smoke and advocating for evidence-based policy strategies.

Theoretical Basis for Community Coalitions

Coalitions are now a mainstay of community-based health promotion efforts. Although clear theoretical underpinnings have always existed for community coalitions, the practice of coalition building outpaced the development of coalition theory for many years. This has changed since the turn of the century. Once viewed as atheoretical with an insufficient conceptual and empirical base, the literature is now rich with case studies, evaluation and research findings, and conceptual frameworks to explain coalition functioning and how they are instrumental in creating community change. One theory in particular, the **community coalition action theory** (CCAT), attempts to synthesize and provide an overarching framework for what is known about coalitions empirically and from years of collective experiences. The theoretical underpinnings of CCAT, which is articulated in "practice-proven propositions," stem from prior work in community development, participation and **empowerment** (multidimensional social process that helps individuals and communities gain control over their lives), interorganizational relationships, and social capital (Butterfoss & Kegler, 2002).

The field of community development and related work in citizen participation articulate the underlying philosophy for community-driven approaches—that people deserve a voice in designing changes that affect and take place in their communities, that communities have the capacity to address their own problems, and that resident involvement and ownership in community change leads to greater sustainability (Brager, Sprecht, & Torczyner, 1987; Minkler, 2004). Theoretical advances in empowerment described the differences among individual, organizational, and community empowerment, each of which is relevant to coalition-based initiatives that build community capacity for change (Goodman et al., 1998; Israel et al., 1994).

Coalition theory also draws from work done in the fields of interorganizational relations and political science. The former helps explain why organizations enter collaborative relationships, such as the desire to acquire resources and reduce uncertainty. Interorganizational relations also contributed to the observation that collaboration occurs through stages and that benefits must outweigh costs to ensure continued participation (Alter & Hage, 1993; Gray, 1989; Gray & Wood, 1991; Provan & Milward, 1995). The notion that coalitions can be used to negotiate potential conflict and redistribute power to achieve a common goal is a key topic of interest in political science (Bazzoli et al., 1997). Social capital, described as the trust, networks, and norms of reciprocity that enable people to effectively work together, includes two operational levels (Kreuter & Lezin, 2002; Putnam, 2000). The CCAT recognizes both implicitly: **bonding social capital** creates group cohesion and a sense of belonging, which may result from a positive organizational climate within a coalition. **Bridging social capital** refers to factors that facilitate the linking of organizations within a community as well as connections to resources external to the community (Kreuter & Lezin, 2002).

CCAT has been described in detail elsewhere (Butterfoss & Kegler, 2002, 2009) and its propositions are listed in Table 11.1. Briefly, CCAT posits that coalitions advance through stages from formation to institutionalization, with regular loops back to earlier stages as new issues are tackled, new funding streams are added, and planning cycles are repeated. The theory acknowledges that contextual factors within the community such as geography, history, community values, and norms affect coalition success in each stage of development. Coalitions form when a **convener group** or lead agency brings together a core group to collaborate in addressing a health or social issue of mutual concern. The **lead agency** is the organization that has the vision or mandate to initially mobilize community members to form a coalition focused on a specific issue of concern. Effective coalitions expand to a broader group of individuals and organizations to marshal diverse resources, perspectives, and constituencies in assessing, planning, and implementing strategies to address priority issues.

Coalitions advance through stages from formation to institutionalization, with regular loops back to earlier stages.

In the formation stage, the coalition identifies key leaders and staff and creates structures such as work groups to accomplish specific tasks and operating procedures to promote coalition functioning. Well-designed structures and processes can help to create a positive organizational climate, an engaged and contributing membership, and the pooling of diverse member resources. The maintenance stage involves sustaining member engagement and creating collaborative synergy by mobilizing and pooling member and external resources. Collaborative synergy is what enables coalitions to achieve greater success than a single agency could accomplish on its own (Butterfoss & Kegler, 2009; Lasker, Weiss, & Miller, 2001). The pooling of diverse talents, perspectives, connections, skills, and concrete resources such as space and funding leads to creative, comprehensive strategies. These strategies build on the existing evidence base but are

Table 11.1. Constructs and Related Propositions, Community Coalition Action Theory

Constructs	Propositions
Stages of development	• Coalitions develop in specific stages and recycle through these stages as new members are recruited, plans are renewed, and new issues are added. • At each stage, specific factors enhance coalition function and progression to the next stage.
Community context	• Coalitions are heavily influenced by contextual factors in the community throughout all stages of development.
Lead agency, convener group	• Coalitions form when a lead agency or convener responds to an opportunity, threat, or mandate. • Coalition formation is more likely when the lead agency or convener provides technical assistance, financial or material support, credibility, and valuable networks and contacts. • Coalition formation is likely to be more successful when the lead agency or convener enlists community gatekeepers to help develop credibility and trust with others in the community.
Coalition membership	• Coalition formation usually begins by recruiting a core group of people who are committed to resolving the health or social issue. • More effective coalitions result when the core group expands to include a broad constituency of participants who represent diverse interest groups and organizations.
Processes	• Open and frequent communication among staff and members helps make collaborative synergy more likely through member engagement and pooling of resources. • Shared and formalized decision making helps make collaborative synergy more likely through member engagement and pooling of resources. • Conflict management helps make collaborative synergy more likely through member engagement and pooling of resources.
Leadership and staffing	• Strong leadership from a team of staff and members improves coalition functioning and makes collaborative synergy more likely through member engagement and pooling of resources. • Paid staff make collaborative synergy more likely through member engagement and pooling of resources.
Structures	• Formalized rules, roles, structures, and procedures improve collaborative functioning and make collaborative synergy more likely through member engagement and pooling of resources.
Member engagement	• Satisfied and committed members will participate more fully in the work of the coalition.

(Continued)

Table 11.1. (*Continued*)

Constructs	Propositions
Pooled member and external resources	• The synergistic pooling of member and external resources prompts comprehensive assessment, planning, and implementation of strategies.
Assessment and planning	• Successful implementation of effective strategies is more likely when comprehensive assessment and planning occur.
Implementation of strategies	• Coalitions are more likely to create change in community policies, practices, and environments when they direct interventions at multiple levels.
Community change outcomes	• Coalitions that are able to change community policies, practices, and environments are more likely to increase capacity and improve health and social outcomes.
Health and social outcomes	• The ultimate indicator of coalition effectiveness is the improvement in health and social outcomes.
Community capacity	• By participating in successful coalitions, community members and organizations develop capacity and build social capital that can be applied to other health and social issues.

Source: Butterfoss and Kegler (2009).

tailored to local contexts and thus have the greatest chance of leading to desired health or social outcomes. CCAT states that engaged coalition members and the acquisition of resources combined with comprehensive, multilevel planning and implementation lead to changes in community policies, practices, and environments that support health. These changes to organizational and community infrastructure, when implemented with sufficient reach, duration, and intensity, should lead to long-term outcomes, such as improved population health or substantive progress toward other social goals. Finally, CCAT predicts that a successful collaborative process has the potential to increase the capacity of local individuals and organizations to apply newly acquired or strengthened skills and resources to address additional issues of community concern.

Coalition Formation in a Rural Context

Although many aspects of coalition building are similar across various kinds of communities, rural settings present numerous unique challenges, such as fewer agencies; resource limitations that affect hiring of staff; limited office space, equipment, and space for coalition-sponsored activities; small population size that limits the pool of qualified staff and coalition leaders; isolation from others doing similar work; lack of diversity; and fewer well-established organizational networks (Downey et al., 2010; Kegler, Rigler, & Honeycutt, 2010; Mahon & Taylor-Powell, 2007). Coalitions typically form when a lead agency or convener group responds to an opportunity, such as new funding, a threat such as the closing of a rural hospital, or a mandate from higher levels of administration, such as state or federal government for local agencies or regional or national headquarters for other types of organizations. The lead agency initiates coalition formation by recruiting a core group of community leaders and providing initial support for the coalition. In rural communities, the pool of potential organizations to serve as a lead agency may be relatively small compared to urban areas. In county seats, a local government unit such as the county health department, county extension, a community-based organization, or a local hospital or clinic may be the obvious choice for a lead agency depending on the topic to be addressed. In outlying small towns or rural regions of a county, institutions may be especially limited in number. Elementary schools, small community-based organizations, or other community groups may serve as lead agencies, depending on the particular project and its required financial accountability systems. Some community groups may not have 501c(3) (nonprofit) status and therefore have difficulties accepting the grant funds that often support coalition formation. One model that has worked in some rural communities is for a larger agency from outside the immediate community to serve as the fiscal sponsor with the smaller, local organization taking responsibility for coalition building and programmatic aspects of an initiative.

Research on coalitions suggests that coalitions often evolve from other preexisting coalitions and networks (Butterfoss, LaChance, & Orians, 2006; Nezlek & Galano, 1993), which may accelerate their development. However, new initiatives can inherit past agendas, old ways of thinking, and grievances and conflicts that may limit coalition effectiveness (Kadushin et al., 2005). Rural coalitions may be especially vulnerable to this "organizational residue" because new partners are difficult to find and past collaborations may have long, complicated histories. On the positive side, small communities where everyone knows everyone can mobilize faster because trust is already established and agendas are well known.

Composition of the core group affects its ability to engage a broad spectrum of the community. Communities are often divided, sometimes by social class or race and ethnicity and sometimes by values and ideology. Rural communities also face divides because of distance between inhabited areas or features of the geography, such as mountains, rivers with few bridges, or dangerous roads. In rural communities, coalitions are often formed at the county level or even across multiple counties, even when little sense of community exists at this level. In many rural areas, sense of community, or bonding social capital, is strongest within the small towns scattered across a region. Wandersman and colleagues (1996) describe the struggles faced by an effort to form a regional coalition across geographically distant towns that considered themselves historical rivals.

According to CCAT, the core group must recruit those committed to the prioritized issue and a broad constituency of diverse groups and organizations, including community gatekeepers. This pooling of diverse views, perspectives, and resources is the hallmark of a coalition approach and enables them to address problems in ways that a single agency could not achieve on its own. Effective coalitions are deliberate in recruiting diverse members with specific expertise, constituencies, perspectives, backgrounds, and sectors. The latter can be especially challenging in rural areas where traditional community sectors may not exist (e.g., housing, local media) or only may have one or two viable representatives. For example, the recreation sector may be limited to the local Curves facility or the faith sector may be limited to a handful of churches with part-time pastors. Businesses may be limited to a gas station, convenience store, or chain restaurant out on the highway. Consequently, broad representation may need to be conceptualized differently, such as geographically or by types of livelihood (e.g., farmer, rancher, teacher).

Coalition leaders and staff organize the structures through which coalitions accomplish their work and are responsible for coalition processes, such as communication and decision making, which keep members satisfied and committed to coalition efforts. Practically speaking, coalitions accomplish much of their day-to-day work in small groups. Therefore, managing group processes such as decision making, communication, and conflict management is critical (Butterfoss et al., 2006; Florin et al., 2000; Kegler et al., 1998, 2005; Mayer et al., 1998; Rogers et al., 1993).

Another important task in the formation stage of coalition development is the selection of staff and leadership. Effective coalition leadership requires a collection of qualities and skills that are typically not found in one individual but rather in a team of committed leaders. A challenge often reported by practitioners in rural communities is that the pool of potential staff and leaders is small (Kegler, Rigler, & Honeycutt, 2010; Mahon & Taylor-Powell, 2007). As a result, staff of rural coalitions often wear multiple hats and are stretched very thin. Additionally, personal life events can have a significant impact when no one else is poised to transition into a leadership role, even temporarily. Coalitions are labor intensive in terms of cultivating and maintaining relationships and ensuring smooth and efficient group processes. Insufficient or poor leadership can easily lead to coalition failure through endless meetings with no real substance or infrequent meetings with no progress between meetings. Empirical research on coalitions shows a consistent relationship between leader competence and member satisfaction. Research also demonstrates relationships between staff competence and member satisfaction, member benefits, participation, action plan quality, resource mobilization, implementation of planned activities, and perceived accomplishments (Florin et al., 2000; Kegler et al., 1998, 2005; Rogers et al., 1993).

CCAT asserts that more formal coalitions are better able to engage members, pool resources, and assess and plan well. Research on the importance of formalization is mixed, however. One study documented that the existence of formal structures such as bylaws, agendas, and minutes was related to organizational commitment (Rogers et al., 1993) and another found no association between formalization and plan quality, scope of strategies, or perceived accomplishments (Florin et al., 2000). Rural coalitions, especially those with a high proportion of grassroots residents, may resist formalization, viewing it as inconsistent with local culture. The external trappings of formalization may not be essential (e.g., bylaws) but the underlying advantages of clarity of mission, continuity between meetings, and transparent processes usually are essential to success. Creating committees or task forces, which can be more challenging when numbers are small, is associated with increased resource mobilization, implementation of strategies, and progress in adopting evidence-based programs (Jasuja et al., 2005; Kegler et al., 1998).

Coalition Maintenance in Rural Communities

Following coalition formation, coalitions must plan, select, and implement actions to address their priority issues. At this point in a coalition's life cycle, members have been recruited, structures and processes are in place, and, ideally, members are enthused about their upcoming collaborative work. Members are the lifeblood of a coalition—they set its vision, course, and outcomes and represent the authentic voices of the community. Capable coalition members are sought after, recruited, trained, and valued. Member engagement is best defined as the process by which members are empowered and develop a sense of belonging to the coalition. Positive engagement is evidenced by commitment to the mission and goals of the coalition, high levels of participation in and outside of coalition meetings and activities, and satisfaction with the work of the coalition (Butterfoss & Kegler, 2009). Engaging members over time is more likely when the benefits of membership outweigh the costs and when members experience a positive coalition environment (Butterfoss, Goodman, & Wandersman, 1996).

To foster member engagement, coalitions should review their roster annually and ask for letters of commitment. However, members often participate in coalitions with varying levels of intensity—they can be core members who assume leadership roles or those who seek networking opportunities. Members rarely stay active throughout the coalition's life and may experience burnout if they do. Having different categories of membership provides flexibility that allows members to move into and out of activities depending on competing loyalties or demands from home or work. Categories of members for community coalitions include the following (Butterfoss, 2007):

- *Active members:* These people are involved in the work of the coalition, attend most meetings and events, serve on work groups, assume leadership roles, recruit members, and help fundraise.

- *Less active members:* These people lend their name and credibility to coalition efforts, publicly promote its work, and provide valuable connections to key organizations or populations, even if they only attend occasional coalition meetings or events. These members include community leaders, administrators, school officials, politicians, or religious leaders.

- *Inactive members:* These people are networkers or those who want to stay informed and receive mailings but rarely attend meetings. They may be asked to do specific tasks or become active later.

- *Shared members:* These people are appointed by lead organizations to alternately attend meetings and share responsibilities. The downside of this arrangement is that valuable time is spent in catching members up and they are often unprepared to make decisions.

Coalition maintenance also entails the ongoing pooling of resources and mobilization of talents and diverse approaches to problem solving. Given the relatively scarce human and material resources in rural communities, collaboration is a necessary and logical strategy for addressing health disparities. Disparities and inequities in health have multiple causes and consequences that require complex solutions from multiple disciplines and organizations. However, health and human service organizations in rural settings often are limited in addressing such issues due to fragmented services and unequal access to resources. By sharing their human and material resources, finances, and time, coalitions provide a multifaceted approach that can reverse the declining trend in civic engagement and reengage organizations to address local problems (Wolff, 2001).

Members are a coalition's greatest asset—they bring energy, knowledge, skills, expertise, perspectives, connections, and tangible resources to the table. As mentioned previously, the power to combine the perspectives, resources, and skills of a group of individuals and organizations has been termed *synergy* (Lasker, Weiss, & Miller, 2001). This pooling of resources ensures more effective assessment, planning, and implementation of comprehensive strategies that give coalitions unique advantages over less collaborative problem-solving approaches (Lasker et al., 2001; McLeroy et al., 1994). External resources may be raised to relieve some of the burden faced by rural communities and provide additional expertise and personnel. Internal and external partners can provide meeting facilities, mailing lists, referrals, loans or donations, equipment, supplies, and cosponsorship of events (Braithwaite, Taylor, & Austin, 2000).

Coalitions that possess high levels of synergy have leaders who promote productive interactions among diverse members and make good use of their participants' in-kind resources, financial resources, and time (Lasker et al., 2001). High levels of synergy also are related to more collaborative administration and management and the ability of coalitions to obtain sufficient nonfinancial resources from their participants (e.g., skills, information, connections, and endorsements). In short, the synergy that is created from collaborative work results in greater accomplishments than each group working on its own could ever achieve (Lasker et al., 2001).

Coalitions achieve their goals by pooling resources combined with assessing a situation and selecting actions that target the most critical determinants of a particular problem. Once a coalition is formed and has its structures and processes in place, one of its first priorities is often to conduct a community assessment. Community assessment is the process of understanding a community in terms of its strengths, needs, constituencies, history and politics, leadership structure, and related factors that affect community problem solving (Bartholomew et al., 2006). It also involves identifying a priority health issue or social issue, determining who it affects disproportionately, and assessing its behavioral and environmental determinants. According to CCAT, coalitions that conduct comprehensive community assessments are better positioned to select and implement strategies that will make a difference. As with other aspects of coalition performance, a rural environment has implications for the assessment, planning, and implementation processes that coalitions undertake. Kegler and colleagues (2010) noted that rural geography shaped assessment methods because reaching residents from varied locales within a region was difficult and often involved considerable distance. For example, one coalition used a map to identify each geographic pocket in its region where a cluster of people lived and personally invited one adult and youth from each of those areas to participate in the assessment and planning process.

Rural context also affects what is prioritized as a community concern. Isolation, lack of resources, and fragmentation due to geographic barriers were influential in selecting priorities for action by several rural sites in a coalition-based initiative that funded community-identified priorities (Kegler, Norton, & Aronson, 2008). Creation of community-gathering places, learning-enrichment opportunities for youth and adults, and economic development were prioritized by several coalitions, in large part because of the rural nature of these communities. Community norms and values also affect the planning process. Although present in metropolitan areas as well, the values of independence, privacy, and distrust of government are particularly strong in some rural areas. These values can limit engagement from some factions of the community. Negative views of government aid or social service provision can similarly limit participation in certain coalition activities (Kegler, Rigler, & Honeycutt, 2011).

Planning for Sustainability

All communities, especially rural ones, currently face a tough environment with limited and shorter funding cycles, increased competition for resources, and economic downturns. Sustainability often is misunderstood as involving only sustained funding because when the funding ends, so does the commitment. However, sustainability does not concern one strategy, policy, or approach but requires developing community understanding and leadership to embed new solutions in institutions, literally institutionalizing polices and organizational practices within community norms. With this understanding of sustainability, even if funding and efforts diminish, health priorities have been embedded and lasting change remains (Harris et al., 2010).

Despite their critical role in promoting health and preventing disease, many coalitions are unable to sustain their efforts long enough to change policies, systems, and environments. In order to create and build momentum to maintain communitywide change, coalitions must fulfill a continuing mission and be effectively managed and governed.

Sustainable coalitions accomplish the following:

- Develop strong, experienced leaders
- Have broad, deep organizational and community ties
- Coordinate efforts
- Implement evidence-based interventions
- Allow adequate time for sustainability planning (Feinberg, Bontempo, & Greenberg, 2008; Nelson et al., 2007)

Sustainability planning should begin early and continue throughout the life of the coalition. A sustained coalition will be more likely to attract varied funding sources and establish credibility among its constituency and policy makers (CDC, 2008).

Besides developing coalitions and partnerships, sustainability involves initiating a groundswell of community strategies that create change at the local level and assembling a wide range of disciplines to work with communities to improve their health. Sustainability can be considered from short- and long-term perspectives (Harris et al., 2010). Short-term sustainability deals with tasks that must be done to keep a strategy in place long enough to achieve its objectives. It means having buy-in and support from key decision makers and community volunteers, having sufficient leadership and funding and clear communications, and putting procedures in place to monitor results and modify strategies that are not working. Long-term sustainability is more proactive and future oriented. It involves the following:

- Having a long-term plan for ensuring the viability of an organization or a community-led initiative that manages several policy, systems, and environmental change strategies
- Developing a diverse funding portfolio, collaborative leaders, and marketing and branding strategies
- Ensuring that the community, its organizations, and strategies are ready to respond to changes in the environment

Future of Coalition Approaches in Rural Communities

Because of the limited organizational infrastructure and scarce resources in many rural communities, coalitions continue to be promising vehicles for creating community change. Rural coalitions face a number of unique challenges that affect their formation, maintenance, and sustainability. To deal with the geographic isolation and lack of transportation common in rural settings, coalitions must creatively build structures and procedures that make communication and networking easier, such as electronic communication and networking mechanisms (e-mail and social media) and meeting by conference call and webinar.

Another challenge is that volunteer burnout is more likely when fewer agencies are available for collaborative efforts. Rural coalitions might consider organizing coalitions at the county level with work groups that have a geographic focus on population clusters or towns within that county. Each work group could cover a broader set of issues identified by community assessments. For example, they might focus on populations (youth, older adults, or ethnic groups), diseases, or health issues (chronic diseases, substance abuse, preventive care, or oral health). In this way, less travel is required and work groups are more relevant for community partners.

Conservative attitudes and distrust of government may be more challenging to address head on. The best approach may be to collaborate with like-minded individuals or, if possible, to use personal connections to engage people around common goals that cross traditional lines, such as positive youth development or downtown restoration. To deal with possible distrust of outsiders and related communication issues, coalition staff and leaders must spend time getting to know and understand rural stakeholders and their issues. Before jumping into strategic initiatives, time must be spent cultivating relationships and meeting the needs of community-based organizations and agencies. Enlisting trusted professionals (e.g., faith leaders, agricultural extension agents, visiting nurses, and emergency medical personnel) in coalition work provides vital links to rural populations.

Additional recommendations from Mahon and Taylor-Powell's (2007) case studies of tobacco control coalitions in rural Wisconsin include training coalition leaders in rural areas to counter possible isolation and inadequate resources. They also suggest concerted efforts to create partnerships and communication linkages across rural coalitions to encourage sharing and dissemination of promising and evidence-based practices.

From a research perspective, additional case studies of rural coalitions would be useful. The accumulation of data on challenges faced by rural coalitions would help identify those that are common across a range of community types or are unique to certain types of rural communities (e.g., farm communities in decline versus rural areas with outdoor recreation destinations and vibrant tourist industries). Finally, evaluating various strategies to address rural barriers and documenting coalition success stories in rural settings and the factors that contributed to the success would add to the evidence base.

Conclusion

Rural communities face challenges to coalition building, such as smaller pools of qualified staff and coalition leaders and fewer agency and organizational partners. These challenges arise in part because of their lower population density. This same issue of reduced population, though, offers unique advantages that facilitate collaborative work, namely, interconnected social networks, fairly accessible media and policy makers, and a strong sense of community. Given the resource scarcity common in many rural communities, coalitions may be an especially effective strategy for addressing issues of community concern. For example, coalitions can minimize duplication of efforts by jointly coordinating the training of patient navigators to deliver services at a number of local clinics and hospitals. Coalitions also can share costs across member organizations, for example, by coordinating community assessments that provide useful information to a range of agencies and community groups. Moreover, coalitions allow organizations to adopt new or politically risky issues without having to take sole responsibility for them by jointly advocating for systems change. For example, a coalition might ask commissioners to routinely add bike lanes on county roads under construction to promote physical activity. Finally, coalitions can provide a voice to underrepresented segments of the community. For example, a coalition that represents several outlying small towns can increase the visibility and power of a particular region with county agencies in the county seat or with state government. Coalitions have been formed across the country and are quite common, even in rural areas.

CCAT provides practice-proven propositions that can guide rural practitioners as they develop and maintain coalitions. CCAT also may help researchers to identify research questions that contribute to our collective understanding of how to harness the strengths of rural communities to effectively address health disparities.

Summary

- Community collaboration provides a multitude of benefits such as consensus building, exchange of knowledge and ideas, establishing trust, and strategy, policy, and systems development; however, effective collaboration requires acknowledgment and respect of each organization's self-interest, relationships, and power distribution.

- Community collaboration in the form of coalitions provides an effective strategy for achieving community change and implementing policy through advocacy and education.

- The best coalitions bring people together, expand resources, focus on issues of community concern, and achieve better results than any single group could achieve alone.

- Tobacco control coalitions serve as the best examples of successful coalitions, having succeeded in decreasing tobacco consumption, preventing tobacco-use initiation, and decreasing tobacco-related disease and mortality.

- Maintenance and sustainability of coalitions are imperative and require member engagement, effective resource allocation, community assessment and strategy development, and early, thorough sustainability planning.

- Coalition approaches in rural communities face challenges in limited organizational infrastructure and scarce resources; however, through effective planning, communication, and collaboration, coalitions continue to be a promising vehicle for creating community change.

For Practice and Discussion

1. Working with one or two colleagues from class, identify and discuss strategies for engaging community members in rural health coalitions.

2. Identify some of the inherent problems when health coalitions consist of both rural and urban members? How might this prove a disadvantage for rural coalition members? How could you facilitate the coalition to encourage rural members to exercise their political voice?

Key Terms

action-oriented

bonding social capital

bridging social capital

coalition building

coalition maintenance

collaboration

community-based coalitions

community coalition action theory

convener group

empowerment

grassroots coalitions

lead agency

out-migration

professional coalitions

Acknowledgments

Funding for this project was made possible in part by cooperative agreement number U48 DP 000043 from the Centers for Disease Control and Prevention. We would also like to thank Amanda Wyatt for her work in obtaining background materials for this chapter.

References

Alter, C., & Hage, J. (1993). *Organizations working together: Coordination in interorganizational networks.* Newbury Park, CA: Sage.

Bartholomew, L., Parcel, G., Kok, G., & Gottlieb, N. (2006). *Planning health promotion programs: An intervention mapping approach* (2nd ed.). San Francisco: Jossey-Bass.

Bazzoli, G., Stein, R., Alexander, J., Conrad, D., Sofaer, S., & Shortell, S. (1997). Public-private collaboration in health and human service delivery: Evidence from community partnerships. *The Milbank Quarterly, 75*(4), 533–561.

Behringer, B., & Friedell, G. H. (2006). Appalachia: Where place matters in health. *Preventing Chronic Disease, 3*(4). Retrieved from http://www.cdc.gov/pcd/issues/2006/oct/06_0067.htm

Brager, G. A., Sprecht, H., & Torczyner, J. L. (1987). *Community organizing* (2nd ed.). New York: Columbia University Press.

Braithwaite, R., Taylor, S., & Austin, J. (2000). *Building health coalitions in the black community.* Thousand Oaks, CA: Sage.

Butterfoss, F. D. (2007). *Coalitions and partnerships for community health.* San Francisco: Jossey-Bass.

Butterfoss, F. D., Gilmore, L. A., Krieger, J. W., LaChance, L. L., Lara, M., Meurer, J. R., Nichols, E. A., Orians, C. E., Peterson, J. W., Rose, S. W., & Rosenthal, M. P. (2006). From formation to action: How Allies Against Asthma coalitions are getting the job done. *Health Promotion Practice, 7,* 34S–43S.

Butterfoss, F., Goodman, R., & Wandersman, A. (1993). Community coalitions for prevention and health promotion. *Health Education Research, 8*(3), 315–330.

Butterfoss, F., Goodman, R., & Wandersman, A. (1996). Community coalitions for prevention and health promotion: Factors predicting satisfaction, participation and planning. *Health Education Quarterly, 23*(1), 65–79.

Butterfoss, F. D., & Kegler, M. C. (2002). Toward a comprehensive understanding of community coalitions: Moving from practice to theory. In R. DiClemente, L. Crosby, & M. C. Kegler (Eds.), *Emerging theories in health promotion practice and research* (pp. 157–193). San Francisco: Jossey-Bass.

Butterfoss, F. D., & Kegler, M. C. (2009). Community coalition action theory. In R. DiClemente, L. Crosby, & M. C. Kegler (Eds.), *Emerging theories in health promotion practice and research* (2nd ed., pp. 236–276). San Francisco: Jossey-Bass.

Butterfoss, F. D, LaChance, L. L., & Orians, C. E. (2006). Building allies coalitions: Why formation matters. *Health Promotion Practice, 7,* 23S–33S.

CDC. (2008). *Best practices user guide—coalitions: State and community interventions.* St. Louis, MI: US Department of Health and Human Services, National Center for Chronic Disease Prevention and Health Promotion, Office on Smoking and Health. Retrieved from http://www.cdc.gov/tobacco/ stateandcommunity/bp_user_guide/pdfs/user_guide.pdf

Clarke, N. M., Doctor, L. J., Friedman, A. R., Lachance, L. L., Houle, C. R., Geng, X., & Grisso, J. A. (2006). Community coalitions to control chronic disease: Allies against asthma as a model and case study. *Health Promotion Practice, 7*(2 Suppl.), 14S–22S.

Crowley, K. M., Yu, P., & Kaftarian, S. J. (2000). Prevention actions and activities make a difference: A structural equation model of coalition building. *Evaluation and Program Planning, 23*(3), 381–388.

Downey, L. H., Castellanos, D. C., Yadrick, K., Threadgill, P., Kennedy, B., Strickland, E., et al. (2010). Capacity building for health through community-based participatory nutrition intervention research in rural communities. *Family and Community Health, 33*(3), 175–185.

Feighery, E., & Rogers, T. (1990). *Building and maintaining effective coalitions.* Palo Alto, CA: Health Promotion Resource Center, Stanford Center for Research in Disease Prevention.

Feinberg, M. E., Bontempo, D. E., & Greenberg, M. T. (2008). Predictors and level of sustainability of community prevention coalitions. *American Journal of Preventive Medicine, 34*(6), 495–501.

Florin, P., Mitchell, R., Stevenson, J., & Klein, I. (2000). Predicting intermediate outcomes for prevention coalitions: A developmental perspective. *Evaluation and Program Planning, 23*, 341–346.

Goodman, R. M., Speers, M., McLeroy, K., Fawcett, S., Kegler, M., Parker, E., Smith, S., Sterling, T., & Wallerstein, N. (1998). Identifying and defining the dimensions of community capacity to provide a basis for measurement. *Health Education and Behavior, 25*(3), 258–278.

Gray, B. (1989). *Collaboration: Finding common ground for multiparty problems.* San Francisco: Jossey-Bass.

Gray, B. (1996). Cross-sectoral partners: Collaborative alliances among business, government and communities In C. Huxham (Ed.), *Creating collaborative advantage.* London: Sage.

Gray, B., & Wood, D. (1991). Collaborative alliances: Moving from practice to theory. *Journal of Applied Behavioral Science, 27*(1), 3–22.

Habana-Hafner, S., & Reed & Associates. (1989). *Partnerships for community development: Resources for practitioners & trainers.* Amherst: University of Massachusetts Center for Organizational and Community Development.

Harris, J. R., Brown, P. K., Coughlin, S., Fernandez, M. E., Hebert, J. R., Kerner, J., et al. (2005). The Cancer Prevention and Control Network. *Preventing Chronic Disease, 2*(1). Retrieved from http://www.cdc.gov/pcd/issues/2005/jan/04_0059.htm

Harris, J. R., Brown, P. K., Coughlin, S., Fernandez, M. E., && Hebert, J. R. (2010). *A sustainability planning guide for healthy communities.* Atlanta: US Department of Health and Human Services, National Center for Chronic Disease Prevention and Health Promotion. Retrieved from http://www.cdc.gov/healthycommunitiesprogram/pdf/sustainability_guide.pdf

Himmelman, A. (2001). On coalitions and the transformation of power relations: Collaborative betterment and collaborative empowerment. *American Journal of Community Psychology, 29*(2), 277–284.

Ingram, M., Gallegos, G., & Elenes, J. (2005). Diabetes is a community issue: The critical elements of successful outreach and education model on the U.S.-Mexico border. *Preventing Chronic Disease, 2*(1). Retrieved from http://www.cdc.gov/pcd/issues/2005/jan/04_0078.htm/

Israel, B. A., Checkoway, B., Schultz, A., & Zimmerman, M. (1994). Health education and community empowerment: Conceptualizing and measuring perceptions of individual, organizational and community control. *Health Education Quarterly, 21*(2), 149–170.

Jackson, D., & Maddy, W. (2001). Introduction. *Ohio State University fact sheet CDFS-1.* Columbus: Ohio Center for Action on Coalitions. Retrieved from http://ohioline.osu.edu/bc-fact/0001.html

Jasuja, G., Chou, C., Bernstein, K., Wang, E., McClure, M., & Pentz, M. (2005). Using structural characteristics of community coalitions to predict progress in adopting evidence-based prevention programs. *Evaluation and Program Planning, 28*, 73–184.

Kadushin, C., Lindholm, M., Ryan, D., Brodsky, A., & Saxe, L. (2005). Why it is so difficult to form effective community coalitions. *City and Community, 4*(3), 255–275.

Kagan, S. L. (1991). *United we stand: Collaboration for child care and early education services* (pp. 1–3). New York: Columbia University Teachers College Press.

Kegler, M., Norton, B., & Aronson, R. (2008). Achieving organizational change: Findings from case studies of 20 California healthy cities and communities coalitions. *Health Promotion International, 23*(2), 109–118.

Kegler, M., Rigler, J., & Honeycutt, S. (2010). How does community context influence coalitions in the formation stage? A multiple case study based on the community coalition action theory. *BMC Public Health, 10*, 90.

Kegler, M., Rigler, J., & Honeycutt, S. (2011). The role of community context in planning and implementing community-based health promotion projects. *Evaluation and Program Planning, 34*(3), 246–253.

Kegler, M., Steckler, A., McLeroy, K., & Malek, S. (1998). Factors that contribute to effective community health promotion coalitions: A study of 10 Project ASSIST coalitions in North Carolina. *Health Education and Behavior, 25*(3), 338–353.

Kegler, M., Williams, C., Cassell, C., Santelli, J., Kegler, S., Montgomery, S., et al. (2005). Mobilizing communities for teen pregnancy prevention: Associations between coalition characteristics and perceived accomplishments. *Journal of Adolescent Health, 37*(3S), S31–S41.

Kreuter, M., & Lezin, N. (2002). Social capital theory: Implications for community-based health promotion. In R. DiClemente, L. Crosby, & M. C. Kegler (Eds.), *Emerging theories in health promotion practice and research* (pp. 228–254). San Francisco: Jossey-Bass.

Lasker, R., Weiss, E., & Miller, R. (2001). Partnership synergy: A practical framework for studying and strengthening the collaborative advantage. *Millbank Quarterly, 79*(2), 179–205.

Mahon, S., & Taylor-Powell, E. (2007). Case study of capacity building for smoke-free indoor air in two rural Wisconsin communities. *Preventing Chronic Disease, 4*(4), A104.

Mattesich, P., Murray-Close, M., & Monsey, B. (2001). *Collaboration: What makes it work—a review of the research literature on factors influencing successful collaboration* (2nd ed.). St. Paul, MN: Amherst H. Wilder Foundation.

Mayer, J., Soweid, R., Dabney, S., Brownson, C., Goodman, R., & Brownson, R. (1998). Practices of successful community coalitions: A multiple case study. *American Journal of Health Behavior, 22*(5), 368–377.

McLeroy, K., Kegler, M., Steckler, A., Burdine, J., & Wisotzky, M. (1994). Community coalitions for health promotion: Summary and further reflections. *Health Education Research, 9*(1), 1–11.

Minkler, M. (2004). *Community organizing and community building for health.* New Brunswick, NJ: Rutgers University Press.

National Cancer Institute. (2005). ASSIST: Shaping the future of tobacco prevention and control. *Tobacco Control Monograph no. 16.* Bethesda, MD: US Department of Health and Human Services, National Institutes of Health.

National Network for Collaboration. (1996). *Collaboration framework addressing community capacity.* Fargo, ND: Author.

Nelson, D. E., Reynolds, J. H., Luke, D. A., Mueller, N. B., Eischen, M. H., Jordan, J., Lancaster, R. B., Marcus, S. E., & Vallone, D. (2007). Successfully maintaining program funding during trying times: Lessons learned from tobacco control programs in five states. *Journal of Public Health Management and Practice, 13*(6), 612–620.

Nezlek, J., & Galano, J. (1993). Developing and maintaining state-wide adolescent pregnancy prevention coalitions: A preliminary investigation. *Health Education Research, 8*(3), 433–447.

Pennel, C. L., Carpender, S. L., & Quiram, B. J. (2008). Rural health roundtables: A strategy for collaborative engagement in and between rural communities. *Rural and Remote Health Research, Education, Practice and Policy, 8*, 1054. Retrieved from http://www.rrh.org.au/articles/subviewnew.asp?ArticleID = 1054

Provan, K., & Milward, H. (1995). A preliminary theory of interorganizational network effectiveness: A comparative study of four community mental health systems. *Administrative Science Quarterly, 40*, 1–33.

Putman, R. (2000). *Bowling alone: The collapse and revival of American community.* New York: Simon & Schuster.

Rogers, T., Howard-Pitney, B., Feighery, E., Altman, D., Endres, J., & Roeseler, A. (1993). Characteristics and participant perceptions of tobacco control coalitions in California. *Health Education Research, 8*(3), 345–357.

Roussos, S., & Fawcett, S. (2000). A review of collaborative partnerships as a strategy for improving community health. *Annual Review of Public Health, 21*, 369–402.

Smith, N., Baugh Littlejohns, L., & Roy, D. (2003). *Measuring community capacity: State of the field review and recommendations for future research.* Retrieved from http://www.ohcc-ccso.ca/en/webfm_send/218

Wandersman, A., Valois, R., Ochs, L., de la Cruz, D. S., Adkins, E., & Goodman, R. M. (1996). Toward a social ecology of community coalitions. *American Journal of Health Promotion, 10*(4), 299–307.

Winer, M., & Ray, K. (1994). *Collaboration handbook: Creating, sustaining, and enjoying the journey.* St. Paul, MN: Amherst H. Wilder Foundation.

Wolff, T. (2001). A practitioner's guide to successful coalitions. *American Journal of Community Psychology, 29*(2), 173–191.

Chapter 12

Capacity Building in Rural Communities

Monica L. Wendel

Angie Alaniz

Brandy N. Kelly

Heather R. Clark

Kelly N. Drake

Corliss W. Outley

Whitney Garney

Keli Dean

Lyndsey Simpson

Britt Allen

Hon. Pam Finke

Teresa Harris

Vicky Jackson

Hon. Dean Player

Albert Ramirez

Hon. Mike Sutherland

Camilla Viator

E. Lisako J. McKyer

Julie A. St. John

Kenneth R. McLeroy

James N. Burdine

Learning Objectives

- Define community capacity in relation to addressing rural health issues.
- Describe the dimensions of community capacity and how those dimensions may be manifested in rural communities.
- Explain strategies for building community capacity in rural communities.
- Articulate how capacity building in rural communities may differ from capacity building in urban communities.
- Specify advantages and disadvantages of using a partnership approach to building capacity in a rural community.

•••

In the past several decades, public health practitioners and researchers have demonstrated an increased focus on community-based approaches to health promotion and disease prevention. This shift can be attributed to several elements, including a growing understanding of the complex factors that produce health issues (Krieger, 2008), acknowledgment of the relationship between communities and their physical and social environments (DiClemente, Salazar, & Crosby, 2007), and recognition that health improvement strategies that focus solely on individuals have limited effectiveness (Udehn, 2002).

The attention to community in public health interventions seeks to address the problems within communities through input and action by the communities where the problem is situated. However, this input and action takes a variety of forms. Differing perspectives of community result in diverse methods for working with and intervening in communities to improve health. Broadly described, community-based public health research and practice seeks to encourage collaboration among sectors of society, thus enhancing the social responsibility and capabilities of all community members while incorporating knowledge by outside practitioners (McLeroy et al., 2003; Minkler & Wallerstein, 2003). In rural areas, the importance of organizing each segment of a community to improve, promote, protect, and restore the health of the population through collective action is increasingly important.

Community-based participatory research (CBPR, also known as participatory action research) has increased its importance in the public health field for nearly fifty years (Green & Mercer, 2001). As a collaborative approach to research, CBPR "combines methods of inquiry with community capacity-building strategies to bridge the gap between knowledge produced through research and what is practiced in communities to improve health" (Viswanathan et al., 2004, p. v). Researchers and practitioners have highlighted the importance of community members' perspectives on understanding problems and successfully implementing intervention strategies (Kreuter, Lezin, & Young, 2000; Schwab & Syme, 1997; Wendel et al., 2009). Furthermore, funding agencies have increased attention because they view capacity building as essential to sustaining programs and maintaining health improvements. Through capacity-building strategies, communities, institutions, families, and individuals are strengthened long after external funding ends (Wendel et al., 2009). Nevertheless, capacity building and collaboration requires a long-term commitment. Schwab and Syme (1997) noted this process requires collaboration from many different actors, practitioners, and community members. Although effective collaboration has its challenges, the outcome of increased community capacity may yield far-reaching effects that benefit residents for generations.

Community capacity, defined as the characteristics, resources, and patterns within a community that can be brought to bear to address local issues (Wendel et al., 2009), has been identified as a key component of greater health outcomes using a CBPR approach (Wallerstein & Duran, 2010). When communities evaluate their assets and issues, they are able to establish unique and dynamic relationships to solve systemic problems. Community capacity builds on the ecological framework that recognizes "health promotion interventions are based on our beliefs, understandings and theories of the determinants of behavior" (McLeroy et al., 1988, p. 355).

As the World Health Organization's definition of health suggests, health is not simply making sure communities are free from preventable disease and premature death, but that they are poised to solve problems that affect individuals' quality of life. This definition directs public health practitioners to community capacity building as a means of enhancing public health.

In this chapter, we will first define the dimensions of community capacity and then we provide a case study from a rural area in central Texas. In discussing community capacity, we draw on rural examples such as the shortage of health professionals, the influence of rural community values, and the participation of marginalized populations who traditionally have not had a political voice in their community.

Key Concepts

The idea of capacity building is not new. In fact, numerous programs seek to build individual capacity and organizational capacity to succeed in a variety of endeavors. The focus on community capacity hinges on understanding what characteristics of community are central to its ability to effectively address local priorities.

The Concept of Community

The concept of community capacity cannot fully be explained without first briefly discussing the notion of community. Geography is not as binding as it used to be; communities can now be defined largely in terms of what they have in common rather than just where they are located. Israel and colleagues (1998) describe **community** as a collective and characterized by "a sense of identification and emotional connection to other members, common symbols, shared values and norms, mutual influence, common interests, and commitment to meeting shared needs" (p. 178).

In examining different conceptualizations of community, one aspect that should always be considered is who is included and excluded from community membership. Also important is recognizing who has influence in the community and who has access to community networks and resources. Wendel and colleagues (2009) detailed these salient elements of community as the "social dynamics of membership" (p. 281).

Perspectives on Community Capacity

Community capacity is an integrative process that enables people to recognize and organize resources within their communities to create change. Given the complexity of communities and our ever-growing understanding of the dynamics at work, the theory driving community capacity building is always evolving.

Chaskin and colleagues (2001) proposed a definition of community capacity that also incorporates the influence of the different dimensions and understands the desired outcomes in context:

> Community capacity is the interaction of human capital, organizational resources, and social capital existing within a given community that can be leveraged to solve collective problems and improve or maintain the well-being of a given community. It may operate through informal social processes and/or organized efforts by individuals, organizations, and social networks that exist among them and between them and the larger systems of which the community is a part. (p. 295)

Goodman and colleagues (1998) cautioned that capacity is used interchangeably with other, similar concepts such as community empowerment, competence, and readiness. Whereas these terms have contributed to our current understanding of community capacity, the differences in what each of those constructs contributes individually to community capacity must not be diminished (Goodman et al., 1998). To that end, they defined the dual nature of community capacity as "the characteristics of communities that affect their ability to identify, mobilize, and address social and public health problems and the cultivation and use of transferable knowledge, skills, systems, and resources that affect community- and individual-level changes consistent with public-health related goals and objectives" (p. 259)

Because of different dimensions and definitions of community, approaches to solving problems, and the contexts in which problems are analyzed, building community capacity cannot follow a one-size-fits-all approach. Given the current understanding, Wendel and colleagues (2009) posed community capacity as a set of dynamic community traits, resources, and associated patterns that can be brought to bear for community building and community health improvement, making it clear that community capacity is a value-laden concept examined through individual and structural levels of analysis.

Dimensions of Community Capacity

Stemming from these definitions of community capacity, a great deal of research has sought to operationalize the concept. Synthesizing across a substantial body of literature exploring these ideas, Wendel and colleagues (2009) extracted a set of seven dimensions critical to building capacity. These seven dimensions include the following:

- Skills, knowledge, and resources
- Social relationships
- Structures, mechanisms, and spaces for community dialogue and collective action
- Quality of leadership and leadership development
- Civic participation
- Value system
- Learning culture

Level of Skills, Knowledge, and Resources

At the core of community capacity is the goal of improving a community's ability to address an identified problem. This complex approach requires skills, knowledge, and resources from individuals as well as organizations internal and external to the community. Important skills include leadership, organization, facilitation, and collaboration as well as basic skills in planning, resource development, and evaluation. These skills also require knowledge regarding the community as well as policies and protocols and how to access information and resources outside the community (e.g., evidence-based practices). Resources cover a large range of physical capital—items that form tools to facilitate production, such as machines, equipment, or other productive materials, social capital—the connectedness of community members to each other, and human capital, which is created by "changes in persons that bring about skills and capabilities that make them able to act in new ways" (Coleman, 1988, p. S100).

Nature of Social Relationships

The nature and extent of social relationships in a community are critical to its capacity for health improvement. These relationships form social networks through which a variety of resources flow, such as information, material support, social support, identity, and access to new contacts (Israel, 1985). In rural communities, many social relationship networks go back several generations and may be founded on familial ties. Often, these historical relationships form the basis of power structures in a community; alternately, they can also be the source of long-term dissention that hinders community cohesion and collaboration.

Social networks are also integral to social capital in a community, that is, the degree to which people experience social connectedness to their community, feeling that they are valued by the community. Social capital has been recognized as important to health in a community, particularly as shown in the strength of social relationships (Kilpatrick, 2009; Trickett, 2009). Grounded in the quality of these relationship ties, social capital includes norms of reciprocity, social trust, inter-network relationships, a sense of mutual commitment among its members, and a sense of community.

Structures, Mechanisms, and Spaces for Community Dialogue and Collective Action

Primarily highlighting the importance of relationships as a community asset, this dimension focuses on relationships and organizational networks and how they facilitate open, constructive community dialogue and action on community priorities. Networks are an important community resource because they are interwoven with other dimensions of capacity (Merzel et al., 2008). Formal and informal community structures may promote open dialogue and action, such as meetings of elected officials (commissioners' court, city council, or school board) or civic group activities, such as the Rotary or Lions clubs. Town hall meetings are sometimes held to obtain community input as well. Specific to rural communities, other social events may also provide a forum for collective conversation relative to a particular issue, for example, a Relay for Life event in a rural community may engage a diverse group of cancer survivors in dialogue about community resources needed for prevention and treatment.

The Prevention Research Center in Michigan focuses primarily on building community capacity to reduce health disparities in African American communities. Griffith and colleagues (2010) described their efforts as targeting intraorganizational, interorganizational, and extraorganizational capacity to engage and mobilize community members in systemic change. This construction of collaborative intra-, inter-, and extraorganizational structures provides a mechanism for community dialogue that can reduce the gap between those who have the greatest voice in community change as visible leaders and those who may be marginalized in their community.

Quality of Leadership and Leadership Development

Crossing multiple disciplines and held up as a cornerstone of human governance, **leadership** is a critical attribute of communities. Many dimensions of quality leadership have been identified: representation and communication, coordination and collaboration, structure and organization, accountability and feedback are all necessary for mobilizing communities for capacity building. Leadership is essential to not only mobilize and empower communities but also to promote positive relationships within and outside the community (El Ansari, Oskrochi, & Phillips, 2010).

Specific to health promotion, Goodman and colleagues have characterized quality leadership as inclusion of formal and informal leaders who provide direction and structure for diverse participants in the future. Participation from diverse networks in the community and implementing procedures for ensuring that there are multiple voices represented is imperative for enhancing community capacity. Quality leadership also facilitates sharing of information and resources by participants and organizations shaping and cultivating the development of new leaders.

In addition to developing leadership skills in a community, another significant aspect of capacity building is the creation of new leadership opportunities. Particularly in rural communities, positions of leadership may be limited and those who fill those positions may be incumbent for extended periods. This phenomenon actually inhibits leadership development in communities; thus, the creation of new opportunities is especially important for rural communities.

Recent work focuses on youth leadership development (Sullivan & Larson, 2010). In a community youth development framework, young people are involved in engaging and challenging activities that enhance youth voice and participation that fosters community involvement and cohesion (Perkins et al., 2010). Community youth development relies on a strengths-based model in which the assets and resources of young people are acknowledged to promote positive relationships.

According to Wendel and colleagues (2009), communities with greater capacity not only draw on the quality leadership of those who are in positions of leadership but also are critically aware of the changing demographic of communities and the need to develop new leaders. As communities grow and change, leadership in communities should reflect the increasing diversity.

Extent of Civic Participation

As Robert Putnam (2000) stated, the national myth of an individualistic American society "often exaggerates the role of individual heroes and understates the importance of the collective effort" (p. 24). The importance of the collective effort or civic participation is an essential dimension in community capacity and a cornerstone of social policy change. **Civic participation** encompasses participation in voluntary associations that are community based to national organizations or institutions that extend beyond the community level. It includes voting behavior in local and national elections as well as the involvement of youth voice in policy and social change. Described by Norris and colleagues (2008) as "citizen participation," civic engagement affects community bonds, roots, and commitments that will influence the engagement and opportunities for individuals as well as the structure and relationship of their roles that contribute to community resilience.

Recognizing the variety of ways residents participate and the diversity among social networks and organizations, community leaders must establish and cultivate a mutual trust and collaboration that highlights each member's role.

Intensity of Value System

Community capacity is not a value-free construct. Understanding the complexity and the interconnected value system within communities is central to the effectiveness of capacity-building efforts. Individuals, families, organizations, and institutions that comprise communities each come with their standards, norms, values, and belief systems, which may highlight commonalities or may lead to conflict and tension. Particularly in rural settings, communities are more likely to publicly uphold more homogenous values and to engage in a system that matches their needs and reinforces their values (Kilpatrick, 2009). A community's ability to articulate a clear set of values that the community as a whole can agree on is an important goal but Goodman and colleagues (1998) cautioned that these recognized values within communities should not contradict the value of social justice. In some situations, conflict in communities may be an important part of building capacity. For example, in a rural southern community, a predominant value may be framed as solidarity but rooted in racism. To build community capacity, bringing that value to public light and engaging in dialogue around it may result in conflict but may also yield positive community change.

Learning Culture

This dimension can be explained in terms of three dynamic phases that are constantly feeding back into one another in a cyclical process. This process entails a community's ability to do the following:

- Think critically about complex problems and situations and reflect on ideas and actions
- Consider alternate ways of thinking and doing
- Determine key lessons from one's actions

Similarly, Norris and colleagues (2008) discussed community resilience as an important aspect of the reflection and learning culture of a community. In rural communities, history and tradition sometimes overrule change that could benefit local residents. A community's willingness to evaluate the impact of its efforts and incorporate that information into future planning, potentially altering its course, is a central component to improving capacity for ongoing and sustainable improvement.

By being conscious of a community's history, values, and interest, where failures and successes are used as resources for learning, communities have a greater ability to reflect on their future outcomes. Having confidence to draw on past situations in a community and identifying local and individual strengths for potential change in the future improves a community's ability to sustain and improve its health.

Capacity Building

Capacity building, particularly in terms of health improvement, is primarily done through training, technical assistance, and facilitated experience. Technical assistance has become "a popular vehicle in the prevention field to improve community program capacity and enhance outcomes" (Hunter et al., 2009, p. 810). The capacity-building process begins with the identification of specific needs and resources that can meet those needs. Those engaging in community capacity building must make a long-term commitment. Their efforts initially are focused on demonstrating and modeling for communities and then progress to facilitating experiences that provide hands-on skill building, which also improves community members' confidence in their ability to perform those actions again. The importance of having a skilled facilitator in this role cannot be overemphasized; this role requires someone who can rapidly identify learning opportunities (teachable moments) and understand social dynamics that may be capitalized on to more effectively transfer skills to the community in a relevant and appropriate way. These activities gradually shift to teaching, assisting, and advising. Capacity-building efforts can tie back to any and all of the dimensions of capacity, understanding that they are interrelated and that changes in one area inherently affects the others. By working with communities to identify areas of needed assistance and then enabling them to do for themselves, changes in community capacity have greater potential to extend beyond the original effort.

Case Study: The Brazos Valley, Texas

The Center for Community Health Development at the Texas A&M School of Rural Public Health has worked with many communities in an effort to develop community capacity. Funded by the Prevention Research Centers Program at the Centers for Disease Control and Prevention, capacity building is the center's main focus. Since its inception in 2001, one of the center's partner communities has been the Brazos Valley, a seven-county region in central Texas consisting primarily of rural communities. The region is home to Texas A&M University, with the twin cities of Bryan-College Station located approximately ninety miles northwest of Houston and a population of just over 180,000 residents (including nearly 50,000 students). Six rural counties ranging in population from thirteen thousand to thirty thousand surround Brazos County, which encompasses Bryan-College Station.

The partnership between the Center for Community Health Development and the Brazos Valley community began with the joint endeavor to plan and conduct a regional health assessment in 2001. Community response to the assessment findings resulted in the creation of the Brazos Valley Health Partnership (BVHP), composed of health and social services providers, key community leaders, academicians, elected officials, and area nonprofit organizations. The center served as the facilitator of this partnership whose mission was to increase access to care and improve health status throughout the region.

Through the collaboration between the BVHP and the center, and the center's technical assistance, four of the rural counties in the region expanded their local capacity to address their health care priorities through the development of health resource centers and county-appointed health resource commissions. Key leaders in Madison, Burleson, Leon, and Grimes Counties committed local funds, facilities, and in-kind resources to open health resource centers where providers could co-locate, share overhead costs, and simultaneously offer a wide variety of health and ancillary care to local residents. In an effort to ensure ongoing community involvement, the county commissioners' courts (the chief governing body of a county) appointed residents to serve on county health resource commissions.

As the center worked with these four rural communities to build their capacity to deal with local issues, the communities emerged as the new leaders of the Brazos Valley Health Partnership. In 2009, the health partnership reorganized as a small community-based nonprofit organization whose mission was "to support the health resource commissions and their communities in improving health and well-being. Through centralized representation, the Brazos Valley Health Partnership will develop collective strategies that, implemented locally, will leverage and cultivate resources to improve access to services in the Brazos Valley" (http://www.bvhp.org/#!about-us).

Since 2000, the center has provided the necessary training, facilitation, and technical assistance to support these local efforts. On behalf of the health partnership, the center secured the funding in 2003 to initiate the development of the resource centers and the volunteer-based transportation program. Once funding was obtained, the center worked as a facilitator in each community as health resource commissions were appointed. Working with the local commissions and other key leaders, the center provided technical assistance in the documentation of a health resource center development process, crafting bylaws, policies, and procedures for county-appointed health resource commissions, authoring health resource center operation protocols, creating resources for data collection, and creating facility-use agreements between service providers working in the health resource centers and the county health resource commissions. As each county health resource commission increased its capacity, it has been able to hire executive directors or other staff. Over time, the center's support became focused on resource development, evaluation of activities, and developing the Brazos Valley Health Partnership.

Most of the literature on community capacity has been written from an academic perspective by those who seek to assist communities to improve their ability to address local needs. To provide deeper insight and an alternative perspective, this case study is written by the Brazos Valley Health Partnership board members who are leaders in their respective communities. Members include one county judge, two county commissioners, three health resource center executive directors, and two county health resource commission members.

Skills, Knowledge, and Resources

Through the regional health assessments conducted with the center, Burleson County was able to prioritize health-related needs and identify barriers inhibiting service accessibility. Prior to the first assessment in 2002, there was no convenient central location for residents to seek out available services. Instead, community members likely had to travel into the Bryan-College Station area, oftentimes hindered by a lack of transportation.

Although many groups had various pieces of information, the 2002 assessment consolidated the health status and condition of Burleson County residents into one report. The Burleson Health Resource Center (BHRC) was then opened as a single place where linkages to health and human services could be provided in an easily accessible location. The BHRC became a network of providers, through which resources were pulled together and duplicative efforts eliminated.

Numerous services and activities offered through the BHRC are available for the Burleson County community to take advantage of—services that were previously inaccessible. For example, the BHRC's transportation program offers free rides to medical services. Parent education and anger management classes are now offered at the BHRC to area residents and counselors are now providing affordable services to the population segment falling outside of the state-supported mental health and mental retardation's area of responsibility.

In Burleson County, a person with good communication skills was hired to act as an advocate and ultimately to offer a positive image of the BHRC to the community. His primary role was providing service coordination, a comprehensive case management approach that addresses each individual's multiple needs. The nature of case management requires that the service coordinator work simultaneously with multiple health and social services organizations. Eventually, he was named the executive director of the Burleson County Health Resource Commission and manages the commission and the daily operations of the BHRC.

Leon County learned how to bring together available services and people in need because they were fragmented across its perimeters. The Leon County Health Resource Commission is now able to better identify countywide current issues because its members represent all Leon County communities. The commission meetings have become a valuable forum for communication and partnering. As a result, coordination efforts have transpired that otherwise might not have happened.

The center brought many ideas from other rural communities in hopes of transferring the success to the community. Most important, through the assessment they brought focus out of an array of fragmented data for the commission to use as justification for service needs and the pursuit of funding to develop local programs.

Madison County now has access to resources from regional organizations and providers. One example is that the Brazos Valley Council of Governments Area Agency on Aging (AAA) provides funding to support a transportation program so that older adults are provided with rides to health-related appointments. AAA also contracts with the county to operate a senior congregate meal and home-delivered meal program.

Burleson County embraced the theme of **community health development** as can be seen by the center's leading many public discussions on the issues at hand. Once a focus was developed among community leaders, the commission was then able to create awareness among the community with the actual resources. This work created buy-in from the local government (county, city, and school districts), whose involvement was extremely crucial to its success.

The BHRC has been able to pull in even more services to the community and an increasingly steady amount of people have been able to access services as a result. Furthermore, resources that previously existed were given the opportunity to have a larger presence in the county through the BHRC as well as providers who were offering additional services for the first time. These were services that have been receiving funding to serve rural areas but were being conducted at a regional hub with the expectation that people needing the services would travel to the hub. Of course, transportation was often a barrier. Advocacy from local leaders and the health resource commission is what ultimately brought providers to the table to begin serving clients in Burleson County.

Quality Leadership and Leadership Development

Through the health resource commission and the executive director, Madison County now has another forum for developing leadership. There are people in the community who have stepped up and realized that community engagement is vital in addressing health care needs. These people have become leaders and are always taking care of something, often before even being asked.

Leaders like this are hard to come by but a concerted effort was made to develop these leaders through education and training. The degree to which the leaders are committed has paid off for the community substantially. As the larger community continues to witness the progress being made, there has been a stronger desire for others to participate. This led to recruiting new folks who are willing to be trained as leaders.

Civic Participation

County participation is essential in establishing and maintaining a health resource center. As evident in local communities, citizens of small rural areas throughout Texas often engage through volunteering, sharing knowledge, and advocating for interests. One example is the transportation programs operated through all five health resource centers. Volunteer drivers' donation of time makes this vital resource possible.

Another example of civic involvement is the county health resource commissions, which are the groups that set the priorities of the health resource centers. These commissions are made up solely of citizen volunteers who represent different interests within the county, and who not only attended scheduled meetings, but also promote services and advocate for the well-being of the health resource center in their free time. In Madison County, the executive director periodically has to present progress reports to the county commissioners' court as a key step in annually securing local funds to support the center.

The Burleson County Health Resource Commission members do a very good job of distributing knowledge of activities and services within the community, which has led to increased civic participation. The local government took the lead in the implementation of the health resource centers and the community followed its lead. The office managers of two BHRC locations have gone above and beyond their job responsibilities and have contributed many extra hours of volunteer time to lead local health fair efforts, organize outings for seniors, and promote the resource center.

The Leon Health Resource Center has the largest health resource commission of the four counties. The twenty-three-member commission strategically represents each pocket of Leon County, and there is a quorum at every meeting. These members have recruited volunteer drivers for the transportation program and for local health fairs. They have donated their time and their money in promoting the health resource center.

Community Values

Each community has core values that influence how a community collectively responds to opportunities and adversity. The values of a community are

The values of a community are often evident in the activities citizens engage in and the initiatives they support.

often evident in the activities citizens engage in and the initiatives they support. Values common among all of our communities include personal responsibility and self-reliance.

One value exemplified by Burleson County citizens is charity. Community members donate their money and time to reach out to the less fortunate through the health resource center as well as through local faith-based and social service initiatives. This value is balanced, though, with the value of self-reliance and personal commitment. As citizens donate money and time toward the cause of the center, they expect that their contributions be used in a way that furnishes people with skills and resources that will expedite their path to self-sufficiency. These donors trust in the mission of the health resource center and never question if their donations are being misused in a way that promotes dependence.

Madison County values education as a tool for encouraging personal responsibility among all residents regardless of age, race, or socioeconomic status. They embrace access for all and promote the resource center as benefit not only for the disadvantaged residents but rather the entire community. This had led to the Madison Health Resource Center's educational seminars being standing-room-only events at times.

Social Relationships

A great example is found in Leon County. Once they had the resource center and commissioners on board, the center took on the role of being a coach and providing support. The center helped find resources. A $540,000 federal grant was received as a direct result of this support. The county has a large commission that brings people together to discuss priorities. These meetings have resulted in strong relationships. Leon County is divided by I-45 and by design it is a challenge for one area to share the needs of another point in the county. Health professionals have to work through the churches if they want to get information out but that strategy still does not reach everyone.

Structures and Mechanisms for Community Dialogue

In Burleson County, the establishment of the health resource centers and the health resource commission has shifted community perceptions. For example, individuals with mental health issues are increasingly more aware of the purpose of the BHRC and are beginning to view the health resource center as a place where they can be ensured of advocacy and assistance. There is also more openness in the community in dealing with people experiencing mental health issues.

The health resource centers and commission have also provided a common thread among the cities, the hospital district, and the school districts. There is a communitywide recognition across sectors that the BHRC functions to integrate a multidisciplinary response to the health-related needs of county residents. Once the awareness was there, there was a good deal of cooperation among the city, the county, and others. The county and the hospital district collaborated to purchase the building that would become the resource center's new home and worked together to promote the new location and services available. Purchased the building that would become the resource center and the city and county worked together to get the road to the center and the parking lot paved.

The county and the hospital district collaborated to purchase the building that would become the resource center's new home and worked together to promote the new location and services available.

Learning Culture

In Madison County, there has been a big change in how the county commissioners' court views the county health resource commission. The health resource commission's main purpose is to oversee the operations of the health resource center but the county commissioners did not realize the full value of the health resource commission beyond their primary responsibility. Eventually, however, the commissioners' court recognized that the commission and the executive director can advise on how to maximize opportunities to the benefit of Madison County. For example, when the county had the opportunity to subsidize the health resource center transportation program, the county judge sought advice from the commission's executive director prior to signing an agreement that stipulated the number of rides that must be given in order to receive the funding.

Lessons and Challenges

Despite the many stops and starts throughout the process and challenges in gaining and sustaining momentum at times, the communities are experiencing real change. The relationships in these counties have been strengthened through the health assessment process—particularly community discussion groups that brought schools, county and city officials, and others into a room together. It helped to acknowledge the fragmentation within the community and helped the community conclude that they must unite in their efforts to improve the well-being of its residents. They realize that they must seek assistance from the whole community because no one group can take care of this on its own. That is a huge step forward. Now new networks of folks are addressing problems in their communities. There is also increased awareness that there are problems and that the health resource centers can help.

Members of the BVHP have been able to learn about best practices and see what has worked or has not worked elsewhere. Fellow board members provide each other with great support and advocacy. Board members know that they can go to the other members for support and advice.

Board members also have designed services so they can measure effectiveness to justify continued support. The implementation of the health resource centers, service coordination, and the volunteer-based transportation system in the communities are tangible services that are improving access for its citizens. This also means the commission has to continue to build and use advocacy skills and keep the resource centers and their impact at the forefront; the partnership with CCHD is so critical in this aspect. Without them the commission would not have been able to build a case for developing health resources the way it has. Leaders have become more willing to consider investing now in order to achieve a more long-term payoff. The commitment of these leaders has been tremendous to the network. The counties are light years away from where they were in 2004 and 2005. There is much left to be done, but they have laid a good foundation to continue the work.

Conclusion

Communities are increasingly recognized as appropriate places and partners for health improvement strategies. Through community-based participatory research and practice, advances are being made in prevention and health promotion. Because communities are complex, their activities must take into account their unique characteristics, history, structures, assets, and challenges. One aspect of communities that can enhance effectiveness of health-promotion activities is local community capacity. Building capacity should be a goal of any community-based work, leaving the community better off than it was before and better able to address its own needs. This provides the best chance for lasting improvements in a community.

Summary

- Communities are complex systems with unique characteristics that must be considered when attempting to implement health interventions and programs.

- Community capacity refers to a community's collective ability to address its own issues.

- Elements of community capacity include knowledge, skills and resources, leadership, structures for community dialogue, social relationships, civic participation, community values, and a learning culture.

- Capacity building in communities is largely accomplished through training and technical assistance.
- Community capacity is an input and an outcome of community-based efforts for health improvement.
- Building local capacity offers considerable promise for sustainable change in communities.

For Practice and Discussion

1. With a colleague, discuss the nature of community in the place where you live. What characteristics stand out to you as being important in relation to efforts for health improvement?
2. With a small group, discuss how a rural community may differ in dimensions of community capacity compared to an urban community. How would those differences affect implementation of a health program or intervention?

Key Terms

civic participation

community

community capacity

community health development

leadership

social networks

Acknowledgments

Support for this publication was made possible in part through the Prevention Research Centers Program, Centers for Disease Control and Prevention, cooperative agreement number 5U48DP001924.

References

Chaskin, R. J., Brown, P., Venkatesh, S., & Vidal, A. (2001). *Building community capacity*. New York: Aldine de Gruyter.

Coleman, J. S. (1988). Social capital in the creation of human capital. *American Journal of Sociology, 94 Supplement*, S95–S120.

DiClemente, R. J., Salazar, L. F., & Crosby, R. A. (2007). A review of STD/HIV preventive interventions for adolescents: Sustaining effects using an ecological approach. *Journal of Pediatric Psychology, 32*(8), 888–906.

El Ansari, W., Oskrochi, R., & Phillips, C. J. (2010). One size fits all partnerships? What explains community partnership leadership skills? *Health Promotion Practice*, *11*(4), 501–514.

Goodman, R. M., Speers, M. A., McLeroy, K. L., Fawcett, S., Kegler, M., Parker, E., Smith, S., Sterling, I. T., & Wallerstein, N. (1998). Identifying and defining the dimensions of community capacity to provide a basis for measurement. *Health Education and Behavior*, *25*(3), 258–278.

Green, L. W., & Mercer, S. L. (2001). Community-based participatory research: Can public health researchers and agencies reconcile the push from funding bodies and the pull from communities? *American Journal of Public Health*, *91*(12), 1926–1929.

Griffith, D. M., Allen, J. O., DeLoney, E. H., Robinson, K., Lewis, E. Y., Campbell, B., Morrel-Samuels, S., Sparks, A., Zimmerman, M. A., & Reischl, T. (2010). Community-based organizational capacity building as a strategy to reduce racial health disparities. *Journal of Primary Prevention*, *31*, 31–39.

Hunter, S. B., Chinman, M., Ebener, P., Imm, P., Wandersman, A., & Ryan, G. W. (2009). Technical assistance as a prevention capacity-building tool: A demonstration using the Getting to Outcomes® framework. *Health Education and Behavior*, *36*(5), 810–828.

Israel, B. A. (1985). Social networks and social support: Implications for natural helper and community-level interventions. *Health Education Quarterly*, *12*(1), 65–80.

Israel, B. A., Schulz, A. J., Parker, E. A., & Becker, A. B. (1998). Review of community-based research: Assessing partnership approaches to improve public health. *Annual Review of Public Health*, *19*, 173–202.

Kilpatrick, S. (2009). Multi-level rural community engagement in health. *The Australian Journal of Rural Health*, *17*(1), 39–44.

Kreuter, M. W., Lezin, N. A., & Young, L. A. (2000). Evaluating community-based collaborative mechanisms: Implications for practitioners. *Health Promotion Practice*, *1*(1), 49–63.

Krieger, N. (2008). Proximal, distal, and the politics of causation: What's level got to do with it? *American Journal of Public Health*, *98*, 221–230.

McLeroy, K. L., Bibeau, D., Steckler, A., & Glanz, K. (1988). An ecological perspective on health promotion programs. *Health Education Quarterly*, *15*(4), 351–377.

McLeroy, K. R., Norton, B. L., Kegler, M. C., Burdine, J. N., & Sumaya, C. V. (2003). Community-based interventions. *American Journal of Public Health*, *93*(4), 529–533.

Merzel, C., Moon-Howard, J., Dickerson, D., Ramjohmn, D., & VanDevanter, N. (2008). Making the connections: Community capacity for tobacco control in an urban African American community. *American Journal of Community Psychology*, *41*(1–2), 74–88.

Minkler, M., & Wallerstein, N. (2003). *Community-based participatory research for health*. San Francisco: Jossey-Bass.

Norris, F. H., Stevens, S. P., Pfefferbaum, B., Wyche, K. F., & Pfefferbaum, R. L. (2008). Community resilience as a metaphor, theory, set of capacities, and strategy for disaster readiness. *American Journal of Community Psychology*, *41*, 127–150.

Perkins, D. F., Feinberg, M. E., Greenberg, M. T., Johnson, L. E., Chilenski, S. M., Mincemoyer, C. C., & Spoth, R. L. (2010). Team factors that predict to sustainability indicators for community-based prevention teams. *Evaluation and Program Planning, 34*(3), 283–291. doi:10.1016/j.evalprogplan.2010.10.003:1–10.

Putnam, R. D. (2000). *Bowling alone: The collapse and revival of American community*. New York: Simon & Schuster.

Schwab, M., & Syme, S. L. (1997). On paradigms, community participation, and the future of public health. *American Journal of Public Health, 87*(12), 2049–2051.

Sullivan, R., & Larson, R. (2010). Connecting youth to high-resource adults: Lessons from effective youth programs. *Journal of Adolescent Research, 25*, 99–123.

Trickett, E. J. (2009). Multilevel community-based culturally situated interventions and community impact: An ecological perspective. *American Journal of Community Psychology, 43*, 257–266.

Udehn, L. (2002). The changing face of methodological individualism. *Annual Review of Sociology, 28*, 479–507.

Viswanathan, M., Ammerman, A., Eng, E., Gartlehner, G., Lohr, K. N., Griffith, D., Rhodes, S., Samuel-Hodge, C., Maty, S., Lux, L., Webb, L., Sutton, S. F., Swinson, T., Jackman, A., Whitener, L. (2004, July). Community-based participatory research: Assessing the evidence. *Evidence Report/Technology Assessment No. 99* (Prepared by RTI—University of North Carolina Evidence-based Practice Center under Contract No. 290-02-0016). AHRQ Publication 04-E022-2. Rockville, MD: Agency for Healthcare Research and Quality.

Wallerstein, N., & Duran, B. (2010). Community-based participatory research contributions to intervention research: The intersection of science and practice to improve health equity. *American Journal of Public Health, 100*(Supp. 1), S40–S46.

Wendel, M. L., Burdine, J. N., McLeroy, K. R., Alaniz, A., Norton, B., & Felix, M.R.J. (2009). Community capacity: Theory and application. In R. DiClemente, R. Crosby, & M. Kegler (Eds.), *Emerging theories in health promotion practice and research: Strategies for improving public health* (2nd ed.). San Francisco: Jossey-Bass.

Part Four

Evidence-Based Practice in Rural Communities

Chapter 13

Promoting Adolescent Health in Rural Communities

E. Lisako J. McKyer   Jamilia J. Blake
Corliss W. Outley   Brandy N. Kelly

Learning Objectives

- Describe contextual factors that contribute to adolescent health behavior in rural communities.
- Identify disparities among rural adolescents regarding substance use.
- Explain how a strengths-based model of community youth development can be used to prevent substance use in rural communities.
- Describe 4-H program strategies to engage youth in civic activities to prevent substance use and promote healthy choices.

●●●

Adolescents. Teenagers. Teens. Youth. Each term is used to describe humans undergoing the transitional phase between puberty and adulthood (Medline-Plus, 2011). In the United States, dating, driving, and other privileges are important milestones usually reached during this developmental stage. Ask adolescents what it means to be a "teen" and they will respond by discussing the importance of decreased adult supervision, increased independence, and being given additional responsibilities (although not all new responsibilities may be welcome). In short, adolescence is about increasingly feeling like and being perceived as an adult.

Adolescence is the window of opportunity that sets the health trajectory for the next generation of adults.

Adolescence is critical because it is during this stage that health behaviors and practices typically become lifelong habits. Hence, adolescence is the window of opportunity that sets the health trajectory for the next generation of adults.

Health issues of concern among rural adolescents include **alcohol, tobacco, and other drugs** (ATOD) use, mental health, sexual health, and increased risk of obesity (Curtis, Waters, & Brindis, 2010). Smoking tobacco and drinking alcohol, in particular, are of concern for several reasons: (1) onset of use usually occurs during adolescence (MedlinePlus, 2011) and (2) both are gateway drugs (Torabi et al., 2010). In other words, adolescents who use tobacco or drink alcohol greatly increase their risk for a life complicated with disease, addictions, or even early death.

Adolescence

Adolescence is a human physical, psychological, and social developmental period marked by the onset of puberty and ending at early adulthood (MedlinePlus, 2011). The concept of adolescence and its duration varies around the world (Brown, Larson, & Saraswathi, 2002). Some cultures (e.g., Maasai) have a very brief period when children are prepared for adult roles, and in other areas of the world (e.g., Europe) the period is extended until around twenty-five years of age. In the United States, adolescence is a protracted period of time lasting at least a decade; the transition to adulthood can continue through twenty to twenty-four years old (MacKay & Duran, 2007). Therefore rural adolescent issues covered in this chapter may be unique to the context of rural United States.

Social changes for adolescents include increased independence and autonomy (Brown et al., 2002) because parents and guardians allow more freedom to adolescents. As this stage progresses, adults allow teens to travel further from home for longer periods of time with less adult supervision. This period is also marked by increased reliance on friends and peers for social support. Indeed, approval and acceptance from their friends become increasingly important to adolescents. Friend and peer groups, therefore, wield tremendous influence on adolescents' health behaviors.

Issues Unique to Adolescents in Rural Settings

As made evident from previous chapters in this text, rural settings are not just less dense versions of cities and suburbs. For adolescents growing up in rural areas, the setting provides a unique context and set of challenges deserving of special attention. Yet, there is very limited research about rural adolescent health. We need to study and understand adolescent health in the proper context—in this case, rurality—in order to have effective positive effects on rural adolescents' health.

The chapter on capacity building in rural communities highlights some challenges for adolescents from rural communities. For example, travel distance to access resources (e.g., shopping, health care) is a barrier, particularly in areas with little or no public transportation. Although lack of transit is a communitywide issue, adolescents may suffer the burden disproportionately by feeling more isolated than adults and having limited power to constructively address transportation barriers (e.g., lack of a driver's license or not owning a car).

For example, one study used a qualitative approach (interviews) to assess rural adolescents' perception of rural communities. The term *isolation* emerged and was conceptualized in three dimensions: (1) difficulty with accessing transportation, (2) dearth of social and cultural events, and (3) limited exposure to cultural and ethnic diversity (Hedlund, 1993). Even if the last two issues were addressed, rural youth still were left to cope with the first issue— lack of transportation. Rural youth are highly dependent on parents and other trusted adults to be available, financially able, and cooperative toward their need for travel assistance. In order to have even a minimal social life outside of the school setting, rural youth are at the mercy of others, more so than urban and suburban youth who are more likely to be within safe walking or biking distance of places to socialize.

This example highlights the issue that although adolescents are part of the rural community, they may not be actively engaged in capacity-building efforts. They may not have a voice and therefore their concerns might not be heard. For rural youth, it may further compound a sense of isolation, which may contribute to other problems (e.g., smoking, drinking, mental health issues).

Critical Adolescent Health Issues

Many believe that health issues related to adolescent sexual activity are most critical. Teen sex, after all, is linked to the spread of sexually transmitted infections (both curable and noncurable), pregnancy, and all the commensurate consequences. Yet, if we take a broader perspective and consider long-term and wide-scale impact on our health, using tobacco would rank higher in importance. Among the leading causes of death and chronic diseases (e.g., diabetes, hypertension), the associations among diabetes, hypertension, and heart attack and tobacco use and alcohol misuse are striking (see Table 13.1).

Table 13.1. Morbidity and Mortality Linked to Tobacco Use and Alcohol Misuse

	Morbidity				Mortality		
	Heart disease	Emphysema	Hypertension	Diabetes	Heart attack	Stroke	Lung cancer
Tobacco use	X	X	X		X	X	X
Alcohol misuse			X	X			

For example, smoking tobacco is linked to increased risk for heart and lung diseases. As a result, smokers are more likely to die from heart attacks, strokes, emphysema, and lung cancer than nonsmokers (CDC, 2010). A study published in the *Journal of the American Medical Association* noted that tobacco ranks highest as the actual cause of death in the United States because of its contribution to various medical conditions that lead to death (McGinnis & Foege, 1993). Although not specific to adolescents, Chapter Twenty in this book is detailed and informative on tobacco prevention and control.

Adolescents in general face a variety of issues related to their growing need for and experience of independence. Rural adolescents specifically face different or heightened challenges from accessing jobs or recreational activities to obtaining services for mental health, learning disabilities, or domestic violence because community resources are scarce. These challenges perpetuate some behaviors into adulthood that greatly affect health. Rural adolescent tobacco and alcohol use has been linked to lack of recreation opportunities, poor employment prospects, mental health issues, and as a strategy to cope with stress, among other influences.

In this chapter, we explore aspects of tobacco smoking specific to rural adolescents as well as examine factors of successful programs designed to prevent rural adolescent ATOD use. It is important to note, however, that tobacco and alcohol use are merely one of many health issues faced by adolescents in rural communities. Furthermore, the strategies we present to enhance adolescent rural health provide a comprehensive approach to improving adolescent health and will yield gains across multiple developmental domains (e.g., physical, psychological, academic, and social).

Key Concepts

There are illicit substances more easily accessible by adolescents than tobacco and alcohol because these substances have proof-of-age requirements to purchase. So why is tobacco of particular concern when it comes to rural adolescent health? There are two main reasons. First, it is considered a gateway drug (Torabi et al., 2010). **Gateway drugs** (e.g., tobacco, alcohol, and marijuana) increase an adolescents' risk for using more illicit drugs such as cocaine or heroin. Second, research shows that adolescents living in rural areas are at increased risk for tobacco use than nonrural youth (Lutfiyya et al., 2008). When considered together, it is clear that preventing tobacco use, in particular, will go a long way toward preventing a host of health issues over the lifespan.

Gateway Drugs and Rural Adolescents

It is not likely that a teen who never engaged in any illicit behaviors would wake up one day and decide to try an extremely high risk and serious substance like heroin. Smoking tobacco, a gateway drug, is usually the first step of a progression toward other riskier behaviors. That is, adolescents who smoke are significantly more likely to have problems with hard drugs and multiple drugs as young adults (Lewinsohn, Rohde, & Brown, 1999).

Disparities in Rural Adolescents' Substance Use

There has been a decline nationally in ATOD use since 2000. Nevertheless, adolescent tobacco use and alcohol misuse are still considered major public health concerns (Torabi et al., 2010). Additionally, there are disparities in prevalence rates of smoking and other substances between rural and other (urban and suburban) adolescents (Gfoerer, Larson, & Colliver, 2007; see Table 13.2). More rural adolescents as compared to urban and suburban adolescents smoke, drink, and use other illicit drugs regularly. Higher use rates of these substances by rural youth suggest that these health-risk behaviors, particularly smoking, are a public health issue warranting attention.

Case Study: 4-H Programs and Rural Adolescent Smoking Prevention

There is a plethora of programs touting their effectiveness in preventing problems among youth. Most programs, however, have been developed and tested on urban or suburban youth, simply due to pragmatics. It is costly to develop and test programs. Therefore, it makes sense to do so in highly dense settings with access to large numbers of adolescents. Rural settings usually do not fit the criteria.

An exception to this approach is the establishment of 4-H programs in rural settings. The 4-H mission is to "empower youth to reach their full potential, working and learning in partnership with caring adults" (4-H, 2011). The 4-H program began as clubs for young girls and boys interested in farming and agricultural techniques. The primary premise of the 4-H program was to teach youth research-based agricultural information to pass on to their parents and

Table 13.2. Significant Disparities in Substance Use Among Youth Ages Twelve to Seventeen

	Percent of Users	
Substance	Rural	Urban
Tobacco		
Monthly use (any type)	20.5	13.7
Cigarettes	16.4	11.6
Smokeless tobacco	5.7	1.6
Cigars	5.5	5
Alcohol		
Monthly use	20.4	17.2
Binge	13.8	10.3
Other substances		
Stimulants	3.0	2.2
Methamphetamine	1.1	0.7

Note: Table modified from Gfroerer et al. (2007).

Table 13.3. Sample 4-H Programs

Science	Citizenship	Healthy Living
4-H National Youth Science Day	4-H Youth in Governance	Fantastic Foods
Environmental Science and Alternative Energy Programs	Financial Champions	Keeping Fit and Healthy
Filmmaking Studio and Workshop	Citizenship Washington Focus	Youth Voice: Youth Choice
Robotics	Rural Youth Development	Health Rocks
Winning Investigative Network for Great Science	Service Learning	Building Partnerships for Youth

members of the local community. As a publicly funded program, 4-H reaches youth in community settings in order to address pressing issues that affect their development.

4-H has more than one type of program divided into three categories: science, citizenship, and healthy living. Table 13.3 shows some examples of the various 4-H programs under each category.

All 4-H programs are designed to facilitate optimal youth development by reducing risk and by promoting factors leading to positive youth development

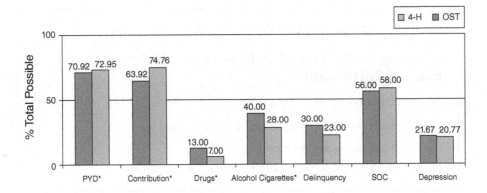

Figure 13.1. Longitudinal Group Analyses: Developmental Outcomes in Grade 10
Source: Reprinted from Lerner et al. (2009).
Note: PYD refers to positive youth development; SOC refers to a measurement model of selection, optimization, and compensation. Statistically significant differences: *$p < .05$.

(Lerner et al., 2009). For example 4-H's Health Rocks program is designed specifically to reduce smoking using a curriculum that addresses intrapersonal factors (e.g., knowledge, attitudes, self-efficacy) as well as interpersonal factors (e.g., relationships with friends, peers). It targets pre- and early adolescents (ages eight to fourteen years). Health Rocks is just one of several programs designed to modify factors at varying socioecological levels (i.e., individual, interpersonal, organizational, community, policy, environment, and culture) respective to adolescent development.

Evidence from evaluations of 4-H programs show that participants of 4-H are less likely to use tobacco, alcohol, or drugs than nonparticipants (Lerner et al., 2009). Additionally, youth who participated in the 4-H program were less likely to exhibit depressive symptoms than nonparticipants, which is an important predictor of alcohol and drug use (see Figure 13.1).

Specific to smoking, participating in 4-H is linked to lower odds of smoking and to other smoking-related risks (see Box 13.1).

The 4-H program teaches children to make healthy lifestyle choices and provides information about the consequences of tobacco and other substances. Outside of providing youth with information about healthy living, the program also encourages youth to develop partnerships with adults and participate in community-enhancing activities, all aimed toward fostering healthy lifestyles.

What may contribute to the success of this particular program is that it is nested within a set of activities designed to deal with problems at multiple ecological levels. For example, the programs under Healthy Living provide

---

Box 13.1. 4-H Program Participants Smoking Outcomes

Smoking Attitudes and Behaviors of 4-H Versus non-4-H Participants

Nonparticipants are

- 0.6 times as likely to have smokers in the home
- 0.3 times as likely to smoke
- 0.5 times as likely to expect to smoke in the future

---

participants with the opportunity to recognize that there are multiple contexts in which to promote health and well-being by examining the relationships that exist between themselves and their families, friends, schools, neighborhoods, and communities.

What Works for Smoking Prevention with Rural Adolescents?

Younger adolescents engage in fewer and less serious health-risk behaviors than do older adolescents. Most early adolescents (ages twelve to fourteen years) do not engage in multiple risk behaviors at one time, due in part to limited opportunities but often also due to developmental status. In other words, most adolescents are not ready to handle multiple risk behaviors. Instead, they replace one behavior with another and often of a more serious nature (Brener & Collins, 1998). Therefore, efforts to delay initiation of smoking results in a domino effect; that is, delay of youth being exposed to and engaging in other risk behaviors. The further smoking initiation is delayed, the less likely an adolescent will engage in smoking and the health-risk behaviors that tend to follow. This strategy is relevant to adolescents irrespective of setting. However, given the lifelong health consequences for rural adolescents, the impact of successfully delaying smoking initiation is much more profound for rural populations.

Get Youth Actively Involved in Capacity Building

Children and adolescents in a community are often considered as consumers of community resources and as recipients of the benefits of capacity-building efforts rather than contributors toward solutions. Few communities think to include their youth in the formation of ideas for community capacity building. Yet, we can argue that adolescents (and younger youth) might have more at stake than adults in any community-changing effort. After all, adolescents will likely live with the outcomes of such efforts longer than their parents and grandparents.

Sullivan et al. (2010) highlight the growing scholarship that looks at increasing community capacity by enhancing the capacity of youth in rural areas to become active contributors to the social capital of their communities. In the growing field of community-based participatory research, organizations, funders, and communities are starting to realize that youth must be involved in the leadership and decision-making process—not simply as an outcome of positive community change but also as an input. Research has shown that the more adolescents are engaged in civic activities, the less likely they are to engage in problem behaviors such as smoking (Brennan, Barnett, & Lesmeister, 2008; Shears, Edwards, & Stanley, 2006). Even for those youth who are not actively involved, simply being aware that they have a voice and that their concerns are being represented by one of their peers may serve to strengthen to social bonds between adolescents and adult community members. Stronger bonds between adolescents and adults result in a lower likelihood of youth smoking and other problem behaviors (Shears et al., 2006).

The more adolescents are engaged in civic activities, the less likely they are to engage in problem behaviors.

In addition to promoting community change among adults, capacity building also has dimensions of positive youth development in the area of quality leadership, involving youth as agents as well as recipients of change. This dimension represents a collection of strategies that are critical for the community as a whole. In a **community youth development** framework, young people are involved in engaging and challenging activities that enhance youth voice and participation fostering community involvement and cohesion (Wong, Zimmerman, & Parker, 2010).

Community youth development relies on a **strengths-based model** in which the assets and resources of young people are acknowledged to create environments that promote positive relationships. Sullivan and colleagues' (2010) research addresses issues of loss of industry, high unemployment, eroding infrastructure, and high levels of out-migration in an already geographically spread-out environment, akin to many rural areas, and has identified that the most vulnerable populations are youth who are left behind. Focusing on building the capacity of the youth in these areas by shaping their understanding and role in social policy, their research finds this participation and involvement "maximizes the sustainability of such communities in the future" (Sullivan et al., 2010, p. 2).

Following the definition of community capacity as emphasizing strengths and abilities within the community (rather than being overcome by powerlessness), a youth development approach focuses on the strengths and abilities of the often untapped and underused leadership skills of youth within a community. This involvement enhances community capacity and promotes a sense of place and belonging (Sullivan et al., 2010). It is important to make the distinction between engaging adolescents in coalitions that target them and their issues from including youth in coalitions serving a broader segment of the community. Adolescents should be included in all aspects of capacity building, not just those with direct relevance to youth.

The Roles of Rural Schools

Due to the remoteness of some rural communities, schools provide a social context where youth can interact with their same-age peers and also engage in civic and community activities. Research indicates that adolescents who feel bonded or connected to their schools have better academic performance, fewer problem behaviors, and are less likely to engage in substance use such as smoking (Simons-Morton et al., 1999). Specific to rural adolescents, evidence suggests that the importance of adolescents feeling bonded to their schools becomes more important as a protective factor for more remote (i.e., more rural) communities (Shears et al., 2006). Therefore, efforts to enhance adolescents' positive bonds to their schools are an important strategy for preventing health-risk behaviors such as smoking and for overall positive adolescent development.

In rural communities, schools can be the nexus of community, providing key avenues for entertainment (e.g., athletic events) and other activities key to the stability of the community. A study comparing rural towns with schools to those without schools showed that those with schools fared better across several socioeconomic indicators (Lyson, 2002). Rural towns with schools have higher housing values than those without, which translates to tax revenue available to the communities. Although there were no differences in household and per capita income, there was a greater disparity in income in rural towns without schools as compared to those with schools (Lyson, 2002). In other words, the difference between the richest and poorest in rural towns with schools was smaller than for rural communities without schools.

The way public schools are funded is an important dimension to note when discussing the role of rural schools in adolescent health. Funding for public schools derives primarily from state funds and from property taxes within the school district. Because property values in rural communities are lower, the smaller revenue for schools generated through property tax perpetuates the educational disparities facing these communities. Several court cases have attempted to have school funding redesigned in the United States—even stemming back to the four cases consolidated into *Brown* v. *Board of Education* (1954), which focused on desegregation, but have been unsuccessful (see also *Abbeville County School District* v. *State of South Carolina*, 1999).

Despite funding disparities, rural schools are still critical to the social and economic health of rural communities because they serve multiple purposes. They serve as symbols of the communities' current capacity to be autonomous, as symbols of tradition and history, as well as a sign of hope for the future. Rural schools that provide health services have an additional resource in their arsenal against adolescent substance use. Studies show that rural adolescents are willing to use school-based health care services (Rickert et al., 2009), and schools may include prevention counseling in their services to augment other existing prevention programs.

Conclusion

Adolescents in rural communities live in a context that is not merely a less-dense version of suburban and urban youth. Rural settings present a unique set of challenges. As a result, rural adolescents require prevention and intervention programs specific to their situation.

Although adolescent tobacco use was featured in this chapter, it is merely one of several health issues faced by rural adolescents. However, what can be learned through the experience of tobacco prevention programs in rural communities is that programs and efforts designed to enhance adolescents' involvement in community and civic activities appear to yield strong and positive results. Programs such as 4-H, designed to help build and strengthen community bonds, appear to create positive results across several dimensions: better physical and psychological health, higher academic achievement, lower engagement in risk behaviors, and so on. In other words, adolescents who feel needed are treated like important contributors to their communities and in turn are academically and socially successful.

Summary

- Adolescents in rural settings have higher prevalence rates for smoking tobacco and drinking alcohol compared to their urban and suburban counterparts.
- Smoking tobacco, in particular, functions as a gateway drug, and increases risk of engaging in a variety of other health-risk behaviors, which may have major and adverse consequences to adolescent health and beyond.

- Rural adolescents' dependence on their parents and their positive perception of their communities are critical factors that can serve as resources to be used in programs.

- Principles learned from community capacity-building efforts should be leveraged to actively include youth and their perspectives. Adolescents have a lot at stake in the successful development and improvement of their communities. They should have their voices heard on issues affecting them.

- Programs (such as 4-H) that use strategies to intervene in multiple ecological levels are likely to be most effective and have an impact beyond preventing tobacco smoking.

- Schools serve a special role in rural communities. In addition to addressing the needs of youth, schools also function as a nexus to all community residents at some point during their lifetime. For adults, schools are institutions entrusted with the most valuable community resource: children.

For Practice and Discussion

1. With a group, discuss the potential benefit of preventive programs focusing on the adolescent stage of development (rather than other stages) as a way to alter future health risk.

2. With a small group of classmates, develop a health prevention program focusing on tobacco use among adolescents. What age would you target? What intervention components would you include? How would you intervene?

3. With a colleague, describe reasons why it is important for adolescents to contribute toward and participate in rural community capacity-building efforts.

Key Terms

adolescence

alcohol

community youth development

gateway drugs

strengths-based model

tobacco and other drugs

References

4-H. (2011). *About 4-H: 4-H mission.* Retrieved from http://www.4-h.org/about

Brener, N. D., & Collins, J. L. (1998). Co-occurrence of health risk behaviors among adolescents in the United States. *Journal of Adolescent Health, 22,* 209–213.

Brennan, M. A., Barnett, R. V., & Lesmeister, M. K. (2008). Enhancing local capacity and youth involvement in the community development process. *Community Development: Journal of the Community Development Society, 38*(4), 13–27.

Brown, B., Larson, R., & Saraswathi, T. S. (Eds.). (2002). *The world's youth: Adolescence in eight regions of the globe.* New York: Cambridge University Press.

CDC. (2010, September 15). *Smoking and tobacco use: Health effects of cigarette smoking.* Retrieved from http://www.cdc.gov/tobacco/data_statistics/fact_sheets/health_effects/effects_cig_smoking/

Curtis, A.C., Waters, C. M., & Brindis, C. (2010). Rural adolescent health: The importance of prevention services in rural communities. *The Journal of Rural Health, 27*(1), 60–71.

Gfroerer, J. C., Larson, S. L., & Colliver, J. D. (2007). Drug use patterns and trends in rural communities. *Journal of Rural Health, 23*(s1), 10–15.

Hedlund, D. (1993). Listening to rural adolescents: Views on the rural community and the importance of adult interactions. *Journal of Research in Rural Education, 9*(3), 150–159.

Lerner, R. M., Lerner, J. V., Phelps, E. & colleagues. (2009). *Waves of the future 2009: Report of the findings from the first six years of the 4-H study of positive youth development.* Institute for Applied Research in Youth Development, Tufts University. Retrieved from http://www.4-h.org/uploadedFiles/About_Folder/Research/Tufts_Data/4-H-Positive-Youth-Development-Study-Wave-6.pdf

Lewinsohn, P. M., Rohde, P., Brown, R. A. (1999). Level of current and past adolescent cigarette smoking as predictors of future substance use disorders in young adulthood. *Addiction, 94*(6), 913–921.

Lutfiyya, M., Shah, K. K., Johnson, M., Bales, R. W., Cha, I., McGrath, C., Serpa, L., & Lipsky, M. S. (2008). Adolescent daily cigarette smoking: Is rural residency a risk factor? *Rural and Remote Health, 8,* 875. Retrieved from http://www.rrh.org.au/articles/subviewnew.asp?ArticleID = 875

Lyson, T. A. (2002). What does a school meant to a community? Assessing the social and economic benefits of schools to rural villages in New York. *Journal of Research in Rural Education, 17*(3), 131–137.

MacKay, A. P., & Duran, C. (2007). *Adolescent health in the United States.* Hyattsville, MD: National Center for Health Statistics.

McGinnis, J. M., & Foege, W. H. (1993). Actual causes of death in the United States. *Journal of the American Medical Association, 270,* 2207–2212.

MedlinePlus. (2011, January 25). *Puberty and adolescence.* Retrieved from http://www.nlm.nih.gov/medlineplus/ency/article/001950.htm

Rickert, V. I., Davis, S. O., Riley, W., & Ryan, S. (2009). Rural school-based clinics: Are adolescents willing to use them and what services do they want? *Journal of School Health, 67*(4), 144–148.

Shears, J., Edwards, R. W., & Stanely, L. R. (2006). School bonding and substance use in rural communities. *Social Work Research, 30*(1), 6–18.

Simons-Morton, B. G., Crump, A. D., Haynie, D.L.K., & Saylor, K. E. (1999). Student-school bonding and adolescent problem behavior. *Health Education Research, 14*(1), 99–107.

Sullivan, E. M., Sullivan, N. E., Cox, D. H., Butt, D., Dollemont, C., & Shallow, M. (2010). "You are taking who?! to a national conference on social policy?": A place for youth in the social policy life of their communities. *Community Development Journal*, pp. 1–15.

Torabi, M. R., Jun, M. K., Nowicke, C., de Martinez, B. S., & Gassman, R. (2010). Tobacco, the common enemy and a gateway drug: Policy implications. *American Journal of Health Education*, *41*(1), 4–13.

Wong, N. T., Zimmerman, M. A., & Parker, E. A. (2010). A typology of youth participation and empowerment for child and adolescent health promotion. *American Journal Community Psychology*, *46*, 100–114.

Chapter 14

Rural Food Disparities

Availability and Accessibility of Healthy Foods

Wesley R. Dean
Cassandra M. Johnson
Joseph R. Sharkey

Learning Objectives

- Understand the nature of rural food environments and how these environments lead to rural food disparities.
- Articulate the importance of rural food insecurity and its association to negative nutrition and health outcomes.
- Describe the three As related to community and household food environments as well as consumer characteristics: accessibility, availability, and affordability.
- Recognize why rural communities are characterized by the term *food deserts.*

• • •

Food access is largely dependent on the food environment or the food resources potentially accessible by an individual. Understanding the sources of food potentially available to rural residents, here referred to as **rural food environments,** is critical to addressing **rural food disparities,** which are the differences in food access between rural and nonrural households. Rural food disparities parallel place-based health disparities such as access to health care, chronic-disease prevalence, and mortality risk (Ricketts, 1999). Rural residents often drive greater distances to food stores and have higher food acquisition

Rural residents often drive greater distances to food stores and have higher food acquisition costs, including food price, transportation, and time, and have less selection in terms of variety and quality.

costs, including food price, transportation, and time, and have less selection in terms of variety and quality (Smith & Wright Morton, 2009).

The rural food environment is changing because of the loss of smaller, locally owned stores and the consolidation of larger chain food stores (Sharkey, 2009; Smith & Wright Morton, 2009). Rural areas have a wider range in the variety of types of food stores and service places than urban areas, although these food stores are more sparsely distributed, especially in areas with low population densities (Sharkey, 2009; Sharkey & Horel, 2008; Smith & Wright Morton, 2009). Rural households face unique challenges in accessing sufficient quantities of the healthy and affordable foods needed to promote good nutrition and health. One challenge is smaller store size. This results in an environment with less variety of available foods, poorer food quality, and more expensive foods than those available to urban households (Dean & Sharkey, 2011; Dunn et al., 2011; Kaufman, 1998; Morris, Neuhauser, & Campbell, 1992; Smith & Wright Morton, 2009). Greater variety, higher quality, and lower cost of fruit and vegetables are associated with their increased consumption, an important correlate of positive health outcomes including reductions in cancer and cardiovascular diseases (Bazzano et al., 2002; Dean & Sharkey, 2011; Eikenberry & Smith, 2004; Mushi-Brunt, Haire-Joshu, & Elliott, 2007; Sharkey, Johnson, & Dean, 2010; Smith & Wright Morton, 2009; World Health Organization, 1990; Zenk et al., 2005).

Inadequate access to enough food to maintain a healthy and active lifestyle among all members of a household has been defined as **food insecurity** (Nord et al., 2010). Food insecurity has been associated with a host of negative outcomes including diminished consumption of fruit, vegetables, fiber, and potassium, and obesity (Adams, Grummer-Strawn, & Chavez, 2003; Kendall, Olson, & Frongillo, 1996). Food insecurity has been slightly more prevalent in urban settings than nonmetropolitan areas (Nord et al., 2010). However, the factors that contribute to rural food insecurity are distinct. They include isolation, which is a disparity that takes the form of greater travel distances to food stores and other sources of food, and limited or no access to a personal vehicle or public transportation (De Marco, Thorburn, & Kue, 2009; Gross & Rosenberger, 2010; Smith & Wright Morton, 2009).

Key Concepts

Establishing Context

The ability to access food is shaped by an individual's location within his or her food environment, a nested set of environmental contexts that operate at the household and community levels (Dean & Sharkey, 2011; Glanz, 2009; Liese, Weis, & Pluto, 2007; McKinnon et al., 2009; Powell et al., 2007; Sharkey, 2009). The relationship shown in Figure 14.1 between consumers' realized food access and their potential access to food within the household and community food environments is a useful model for discussing rural food disparities (Sharkey, Horel, & Dean, 2010).

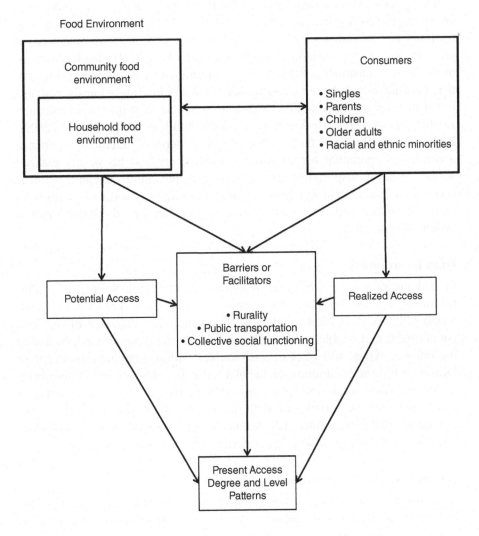

Figure 14.1. Conceptual Model for Rural Food Disparities
Source: Sharkey, Horel, and Dean (2010).

Conceptual Model Overview

Individuals and households are located within the community food environment, which links individual food choice through the household to the larger food environment (French et al., 2008; Sharkey, Horel, & Dean, 2010). The community food environment provides the universe of potential access for individuals and families within that community. Figure 14.1 shows the household food environment nested within the larger community food environment. This reflects a hierarchy with households located within communities. The community and household food environments provide potential access to a variety of food stores, eating places, and other sources of food. However, food access depends on potential access (availability) and realized access (actual use) and the consumer's ability to interact with the food environment based on individual and household characteristics (Sharkey, 2009). Realized access, or the food a consumer actually uses, is determined by consumer characteristics. Consumers may have a supermarket or smaller food store locally available but if they do not have regular access to a vehicle they may have difficulty reaching these stores (De Marco et al., 2009; Smith & Wright Morton, 2009). Barriers and facilitators refer to community characteristics that mediate between a consumer's potential access within a community and his or her realized access. Public transportation provides an example. Rural residents without access to a private vehicle report the lack of public transportation diminishes their access to community food resources (De Marco et al., 2009; Smith & Wright Morton, 2009).

Food Environment

Individuals must have accessible, available, and affordable sources of healthful, nutrient-dense foods to achieve and maintain health (Laraia et al., 2004; Sharkey, 2009). Accessibility refers to the spatial characteristics of the food environment that enable or hinder households from obtaining food, including the number, types, and sizes of food sources within a community and their location within a community or in relation to individual households. Availability describes food store offerings, such as the presence (or absence of certain items), their variety, and their quality. Affordability is the relative cost of food at retail food outlets. Affordability is dependent on other costs including child care, transportation, convenience, and time spent shopping.

Community Food Environment

In addition to retail food venues, potentially accessible food sources also include redistributive food resources and reciprocal food economies. Retail food environments include food stores and food service places. Many types of food stores exist in rural areas. These include traditional food stores such as supercenters, supermarkets, and small grocery stores; convenience stores; and nontraditional food stores including dollar stores, mass merchandisers or discounters, pharmacies, mobile food vendors, flea markets or *pulgas*, farmers' markets, fruit and vegetable stands, bakeries and bread shops or *panaderias*, *tortillerias*, butcher shops or *carnicerias*, and household food stands or *puestecitos en casa* (Dean, Sharkey, & Johnson, 2011; Dean, Sharkey, & St. John, 2011; Sharkey et al., 2009; Sharkey & Horel, 2008). The term *food service place* refers to venues that sell prepared foods, snacks, and beverages for onsite consumption and to go; these places may be full service or limited service, such as fast food restaurants, and be fixed (stationary location) or mobile (traveling food truck or stand) (Bustillos et al., 2009). Redistributive food resources are institutionalized food and nutrition assistance programs (Wright Morton et al., 2008), including federal and state-run food assistance programs such as the Supplemental Nutrition Assistance Program (SNAP), the Special Supplemental Nutrition Program for Women, Infants, and Children (WIC), the school breakfast program, the free or reduced-cost school lunch program, the summer food program for children, senior nutrition programs, food banks and food pantries, and community gardens. Reciprocal food economies are informal or noninstitutionalized food sources including neighbors, friends, or relatives; food from gardening, hunting, and fishing; and churches, although church-run food distribution can be highly institutionalized (Wright Morton et al., 2008).

Household Food Environment

Individual households are located at varying points within a community food environment and their distance to particular food sources shapes their disparate access to healthy foods (Dean & Sharkey, 2011; De Marco et al., 2009; Smith & Wright Morton, 2009; Wright Morton et al., 2008). The material status of the household is of primary importance. A key concept here is material hardship, a conception of poverty that incorporates income yet also accounts for household access to essential housing, food, clothing, transportation, and medical care (Beverly, 2001). Material hardship accounts for the condition of home infrastructure. For example, if a household does not have safe and secure storage that is resistant to vermin or sufficient refrigeration to keep perishable items such as fruits and vegetables or meats and dairy then household members may have difficulty keeping sufficient staples and fruits and vegetables on hand (Beverly, 2001; Campbell, 1991).

Consumer Characteristics

Many characteristics of individual consumers may explain their food use within the household and their access to food within the community. For example, limited personal vehicular access is one obstacle to obtaining food and other domestic items (De Marco et al., 2009; Smith & Wright Morton, 2009; Wright Morton et al., 2008). Characteristics that account for material hardship and the overall availability of resources to spend on food acquisition such as home ownership, employment, and income also contribute to household food insecurity (Kaiser et al., 2003; Kendall et al., 1996; Nord et al., 2010). Health also affects the ability to adequately acquire, prepare, and feed oneself and other family members (Lee & Frongillo, 2001; Sharkey, 2002; Sharkey, 2003). Poverty and poor health limit all individuals in their ability to access food but these factors are disproportionately distributed among rural residents, especially the rural poor (Kusmin, 2008; Ricketts, 1999). Meal-preparation skills and individual and cultural food preferences affect the behaviors within a home in regards to food choice (Abarca, 2006; Charles & Kerr, 1988; Dean et al., 2010; DeVault, 1994; Johnson, Sharkey, et al., 2010; Murcott, 1983). Travel and activity patterns including work, recreation, school location, and food acquisition may also be determinants of access (Kestens et al., 2010).

Barriers and Facilitators

Characteristics of the built and social environment function as barriers or facilitators between the individual household and the community food environment in rural settings. Isolated communities will have difficulty accessing a range of services including food stores (Pearce et al., 2008). Also, the distance between many rural households and larger retail food outlets limits the consumption of healthy foods (Dean & Sharkey, 2011). The limited access of rural residents to public transportation also contributes to disparities in the accessibility of healthy foods (De Marco et al., 2009; Smith & Wright Morton, 2009; Wright Morton et al., 2008). Other problematic aspects of rural settings are limitations in collective cultural, social, and historical characteristics that may constrain or enable access to food resources. Common community characteristics such as neighborhood safety and the social ties through which individuals exchange food, transportation assistance, and information about food resources may increase access (Wright Morton et al., 2008). The perception that these communal characteristics are not present may also be a barrier to food access (Dean, Sharkey & Johnson, 2011).

The Food Environment in Rural Areas

Rural environments have unique features that make evaluating and addressing rural food disparities challenging. Many rural communities have lost locally owned food stores (Bailey, 2010; Bitto et al., 2003; Gross & Rosenberger, 2010; Sharkey, 2009; Smith & Wright Morton, 2009; Walker, Keane, & Burke, 2010). Rural areas have more varied food sources including traditional and nontraditional food venues and natural resources than urban areas (Bustillos et al.,

---

Box 14.1. Economic Research Service Food Desert Locator Description

---

To learn more about food deserts in the United States, we encourage you to visit the US Department of Agriculture's Economic Research Service Food Desert Locator website at http://www.ers.usda.gov/data/fooddesert/index.htm.

The three primary objectives of the food desert locator are as follows:

- To present a spatial overview of where food desert census tracts are located

- To provide selected population characteristics of food desert census tracts

- To offer data on food desert census tracts that can be downloaded for community planning or research purposes

The website allows users to create maps illustrating food deserts at the census tract level, view statistics on select population characteristics in food deserts, and download data from food desert census tracts.

2009; De Marco et al., 2009; Hoisington, Shultz, & Butkus, 2002; Larson, Story, & Nelson, 2009; Liese et al., 2007; Sharkey, 2009; Sharkey et al., 2009; Sharkey & Horel, 2008; Smith & Wright Morton, 2009). Food stores are also unevenly distributed (Sharkey & Horel, 2008; Smith & Wright Morton, 2009) and frequently not identified in available lists (see Box 14.1) (Liese et al., 2007, 2010; Sharkey, 2009). Scholars have described many rural neighborhoods with poor food access as *food deserts* (Bitto et al., 2003; Blanchard & Lyson, 2006; Furey, Strugnell, & McIlveen, 2001; Gross & Rosenberger, 2010; Walker et al., 2010; Wright Morton & Blanchard, 2007; Wright Morton & Smith, 2008; Wrigley, Warm, & Margetts, 2003).

Rural areas also have few food stores with limited healthful options, more small stores, and higher prices (Kaufman, 1998; Larson et al., 2009). Direct methods for measuring food environments use existing lists of food venues and in-person audits or ground-truthing, identifying destinations by systematically driving all major roads (Sharkey, 2009). Intermediate methods use existing lists of food venues.

Very few lists provide an accurate census of rural food stores and eating places. A handful of studies have compared the validity of using intermediate methods with existing public and commercial lists to direct measurements. Results indicated available lists included places that were no longer present and omitted other locations, which misrepresented residents' food access

(Liese et al., 2010; Sharkey & Horel, 2008). Results from large mostly rural areas in South Carolina and Texas reported that 11 to 35 percent of food stores and food service places were missing from available lists (Creel et al., 2008; Liese et al., 2010; Sharkey & Horel, 2008).

Types of Food Outlets

There is a significant association between the rural food environment and adverse health outcomes (Boehmer et al., 2006; Casey et al., 2008) and an association between increased distance to the nearest supermarket or supercenter and decreased fruit and vegetable intake among rural residents (Dean & Sharkey, 2011; Sharkey, Johnson, & Dean, 2010). Unfortunately, there are few descriptive studies of rural food environments in the United States. Much of the published research on rural food disparities including food environment and rural food access is attributed to Sharkey and colleagues in Texas (Bustillos et al., 2009; Creel et al., 2008; Dean & Sharkey, 2011; Dean, Sharkey, & St. John, 2011B; Dunn et al., 2011; Johnson, Sharkey, & Dean, 2010; Sharkey, 2009; Sharkey et al., 2009, 2010 2011; Sharkey, Horel, & Dean, 2010), with other work in Oregon (De Marco, Thorburn, & Kue, 2009; Gross & Rosenberger, 2010), North Carolina (Jilcott et al., 2009), South Carolina (Liese et al., 2010; Liese, Weis, & Pluto 2007), and national studies (Kaufman, 1998).

There is a significant association between the rural food environment and adverse health outcomes.

The paucity of research is attributable to the intensive time, travel, and labor costs associated with identifying and geospatially locating all food venues and inventorying available foods (Sharkey, 2009). Descriptive research of the food environment typically reports the type, number, and distribution of food stores and service places based on geographic location. The type of food destination is an important consideration especially when evaluating rural food access. Similar to urban findings, rural supermarkets also offer a better variety of quality, healthful foods than smaller food stores (Bustillos et al., 2009; Morland et al., 2002). Rural areas usually have fewer food outlets (Powell et al., 2007), very few chain supermarkets, and a greater number of smaller and nontraditional foods stores, including dollar stores, than urban areas (Liese et al., 2007). With a dearth of supermarkets and grocery stores, rural residents depend on smaller food stores with less selection and higher food prices (Kaufman, 1998).

Rural residents perceive they have few food venues including supermarkets and fast food restaurants, lower quality of food, and higher food prices especially for healthy food (Dean & Sharkey, 2011; Garasky, Morton, & Greder, 2004; Jilcott et al., 2009; Morris et al., 1992; Peterson et al., 2010; Smith & Wright Morton, 2009). Although few studies include dollar stores, they offer rural residents an opportunity to purchase a variety of healthful foods (Bustillos et al., 2009; Sharkey, Horel, & Dean, 2010). Qualitative research reveals rural residents are relying more on dollar stores for routine food purchases (Webber, Sobal, & Dollahite, 2010). This may be related to food affordability, although there is little research documenting the affordability of foods at traditional and nontraditional food outlets in rural areas (Dunn et al., 2011).

Proximity and Coverage

Geocoding food outlets or identifying the geographic location of food outlets can be used to objectively measure rural residents' food access (Sharkey, 2009). Rural neighborhoods are often located much farther from the nearest super-market or grocery store than the nearest convenience stores, and relatively closer to the nearest fast food opportunity (Sharkey & Horel, 2008; Sharkey et al., 2011). Rural food stores and service places are typically located near major roads and communities with higher population densities, which further constrains residents who either cannot or do not live in more populated areas with better coverage (Sharkey & Horel, 2008; Sharkey et al., 2009).

Multidimensional Accessibility

Rural residents have adapted to economic, environmental, and social changes affecting their surroundings and created strategies to maintain food security (De Marco et al., 2009; Gross & Rosenberger, 2010; Olson et al., 2004; Peterson et al., 2010; Sano et al., 2011; Smith & Wright Morton, 2009; Swanson et al., 2008; Webber et al., 2010). In addition, rural residents may travel longer distances, plan trips based on the geospatial distribution of destinations, or decide to frequent more convenient "one-stop" outlets such as a supercenter. These activity travel patterns are influenced by community and household environments, household characteristics, and by family, employment, and social responsibilities (Bitto et al., 2003; Jilcott et al., 2009). Accessibility is multidimensional and includes factors related to the individuals, the environment, and their interactions. Traditional approaches that discount individual behavior and values or rely on limited definitions of food venues or accessibility provide inadequate explanations for rural food disparities (Salze et al., 2011; Sharkey, 2009; Webber et al., 2010). Future work will benefit from incorporating existing knowledge and methodologies and looking for innovative ways to understand how rural residents interact with and experience local food environments (Salze et al., 2011; Sharkey, 2009).

Conclusion

Economic, environmental, and social changes have resulted in a loss of local food venues in rural areas. These same changes have also led to disparities between rural and urban residents and their ability to access local sources of healthful food. These disparities place rural residents at risk of food insecurity. Thus an important principle in rural public health is that an individual's ability to access food is dependent on the food environment and larger social structures. The rural food environment has more sources and an uneven distribution of food venues. Compared to urban areas, rural areas have fewer food stores and food service places, very few supermarkets, and higher food prices. Consequently, understanding and addressing rural food disparities requires a multidimensional approach that considers unique features of rural environments, rural residents, and individual environmental interactions.

Summary

- Rural communities are faced with challenges in accessing sufficient quantities of the healthy and affordable foods needed to promote good nutrition and health, such as having poor food quality, selection, accessibility, and higher food acquisition costs.

- Food insecurity in rural areas is distinct from urban areas in that isolation plays a major role because of greater travel distances to food sources and limited access to transportation.

- The community food environment provides the basis for food accessibility for individuals and families; however, food access depends further on the characteristics of the individuals and households as to whether or not there is a means of transportation or sufficient monetary resources.

- There is a significant association between the rural food environment and adverse health outcomes.

- Because of the intensive time, travel, and labor costs associated with the rural food environment and access, research and descriptive studies are scarce; however, future work will benefit from integrating existing methodologies and knowledge to innovating ways to understand how rural residents interact with local food environments.

Key Terms

food deserts

food insecurity

rural food disparities

rural food environment

For Practice and Discussion

1. Describe three features of rural environments that exacerbate differences in food disparities between urban and rural residents.

2. Using no more than two pages, explain the concepts of food access and food availability and how these concepts might be included in strategies to alleviate rural health disparities.

3. Find someone with training in public health who is willing to listen to you talk about rural health. Explain to this person the distinct components of the rural food disparities conceptual model, paying special attention to the dynamic between potential and realized access. Use an example to describe the interaction between these distinct components with rural food acquisition as an outcome of the process.

Acknowledgments

This research was supported in part with funding from the National Institutes of Health (NIH) and National Center on Minority Health and Health Disparities (number 5P20MD002295) and by cooperative agreement number 1U48DP001924 from the Centers for Disease Control and Prevention (CDC), Prevention Research Centers Program through Core Research Project and Special Interest Project Nutrition and Obesity Policy Research and Evaluation Network. The content is solely the responsibility of the authors and does not necessarily represent the official views of the NIH and CDC.

References

Abarca, M. (2006). *Voices in the kitchen: Views of food and the world from working-class Mexican and Mexican American women*. College Station: Texas A&M University Press.

Adams, E., Grummer-Strawn, L., & Chavez, G. (2003). Food insecurity is associated with increased risk of obesity in California women. *Journal of Nutrition, 133*(4), 1070.

Bailey, J. M. (2010). *Rural grocery stores: Importance and challenges*. Lyons, NE: Center for Rural Affairs, Rural Research and Analysis Program.

Bazzano, L., He, J., Ogden, L., Loria, C., Vupputuri, S., Myers, L., et al. (2002). Fruit and vegetable intake and risk of cardiovascular disease in US adults: The first national health and nutrition examination survey epidemiologic follow-up study. *American Journal of Clinical Nutrition, 76*(1), 93–99.

Beverly, S. (2001). Measures of material hardship. *Journal of Poverty, 5*(1), 23–41.

Bitto, E., Wright-Morton, L., Oakland, M., & Sand, M. (2003). Grocery store access patterns in rural food deserts. *The Journal for the Study of Food and Society, 6*(2), 35–48.

Blanchard, T., & Lyson, T. (2006). *Food availability and food deserts in the nonmetropolitan South.* Mississippi State, MS: Southern Rural Development Center.

Boehmer, T. K., Lovegreen, S. L., Haire-Joshu, D., & Brownson, R. C. (2006). What constitutes an obesogenic environment in rural communities? *American Journal of Health Promotion, 20*(6), 411–421.

Bustillos, B., Sharkey, J., Anding, J., & McIntosh, A. (2009). Availability of healthier food alternatives in traditional, convenience, and nontraditional types of food stores in two rural Texas counties. *Journal of the American Dietetic Association, 109*(5), 883–889.

Campbell, C. C. (1991). Food insecurity: A nutritional outcome or a predictor variable? *Journal of Nutrition, 121*(3), 408.

Casey, A. A., Elliott, M., Glanz, K., Haire-Joshu, D., Lovegreen, S. L., Saelens, B. E., et al. (2008). Impact of the food environment and physical activity environment on behaviors and weight status in rural U.S. communities. *Preventive Medicine, 47*(6), 600–604.

Charles, N., & Kerr, M. (1988). *Women, food and families.* Manchester, UK: Manchester University Press.

Creel, J. S., Sharkey, J. R., McIntosh, A., Anding, J., & Huber Jr., J. C. (2008). Availability of healthier options in traditional and nontraditional rural fast-food outlets. *BMC Public Health, 8*(395), 9.

Dean, W., & Sharkey, J. (2011). Rural and urban differences in the associations between characteristics of the community food environment and fruit and vegetable intake. *Journal of Nutrition Education and Behavior, 43*(6), 426–433.

Dean, W., Sharkey, J., Cosgriff-Hernández, K., Martinez, A., Ribardo, J., & Diaz-Puentes, C. (2010). "I can say that we were healthy and unhealthy": Food choice and the reinvention of tradition. *Food, Culture and Society, 13*(4), 573–594.

Dean, W., Sharkey, J., & Johnson, C. (2011). Food insecurity is associated with community and familial social capital and perceived personal disparity among older and senior adults in a largely rural area of Central Texas. *Journal of Nutrition in Gerontology and Geriatrics, 30*(2), 169–186.

Dean, W. R., Sharkey, J. R., & St. John, J. A. (2011). Pulga (flea market) contributions to the retail food environment of colonias in the South Texas border region. *Journal of the American Dietetic Association, 111*(5), 705–710.

De Marco, M., Thorburn, S., & Kue, J. (2009). "In a country as affluent as America, people should be eating": Experiences with and perceptions of food insecurity among rural and urban Oregonians. *Qualitative Health Research, 19*(7), 1010.

DeVault, M. (1994). *Feeding the family: The social organization of caring as gendered work.* Chicago: University of Chicago Press.

Dunn, R., Sharkey, J., Lotade-Manje, J., Bouhlal, Y., & Nayga, R. (2011). Socio-economic status, racial composition and the affordability of fresh fruits and vegetables in neighborhoods of a large rural region in Texas. *Nutrition Journal, 10*(1), 6.

Eikenberry, N., & Smith, C. (2004). Healthful eating: Perceptions, motivations, barriers, and promoters in low-income Minnesota communities. *Journal of the American Dietetic Association, 104*(7), 1158–1161.

French, S., Shimotsu, S., Wall, M., & Gerlach, A. (2008). Capturing the spectrum of household food and beverage purchasing behavior: A review. *Journal of the American Dietetic Association, 108*(12), 2051–2058.

Furey, S., Strugnell, C., & McIlveen, M. (2001). An investigation of the potential existence of `food deserts" in rural and urban areas of Northern Ireland. *Agriculture and Human Values, 18*(4), 447–457.

Garasky, S., Morton, L. W., & Greder, K. (2004). The food environment and food insecurity: Perceptions of rural, suburban, and urban food pantry clients in Iowa. *Family Economics & Nutrition Review, 16*(2), 41–48.

Glanz, K. (2009). Measuring food environments: A historical perspective. *American Journal of Preventive Medicine, 36*(4, S1), S93–S98.

Gross, J., & Rosenberger, N. (2010). The double binds of getting food among the poor in rural Oregon. *Food, Culture and Society, 13*(1), 47–70.

Hoisington, A., Shultz, J. A., & Butkus, S. (2002). Coping strategies and nutrition education needs among food pantry users. *Journal of Nutrition Education and Behavior, 34*(6), 326–333.

Jilcott, S. B., Laraia, B. A., Evenson, K. R., & Ammerman, A. S. (2009). Perceptions of the community food environment and related influences on food choice among midlife women residing in rural and urban areas: A qualitative analysis. *Women & Health, 49*(2), 164–180.

Johnson, C., Sharkey, J., & Dean, W. (2010). Eating behaviors and social capital are associated with fruit and vegetable intake among rural adults. *Journal of Hunger and Environmental Nutrition, 5*(3), 302–315.

Johnson, C., Sharkey, J., McIntosh, A., & Dean, W. (2010). "I'm the momma": Using photo-elicitation to understand matrilineal influence on family food choice. *BMC Women's Health, 10.*

Kaiser, L., Melgar-Quiñonez, H., Townsend, M., Nicholson, Y., Fujii, M., Martin, A., et al. (2003). Food insecurity and food supplies in Latino households with young children. *Journal of Nutrition Education and Behavior, 35*(3), 148–153.

Kaufman, P. (1998). Rural poor have less access to supermarkets, large grocery stores. *Rural Development Perspectives, 13*(3), 19–26.

Kendall, A., Olson, C., & Frongillo, E. (1996). Relationship of hunger and food insecurity to food availability and consumption. *Journal of the American Dietetic Association, 96*(10), 1019–1024.

Kestens, Y., Lebel, A., Daniel, M., Thériault, M., & Pampalon, R. (2010). Using experienced activity spaces to measure foodscape exposure. *Health & Place, 16*(6), 1094–1103.

Kusmin, L. (2008). *Rural America at a glance 2008.* Economic Information Bulletin no. EIB-40. Washington, DC: US Department of Agriculture, Economic Research Service.

Laraia, B. A., Siega-Riz, A. M., Kaufman, J. S., & Jones, S. J. (2004). Proximity of supermarkets is positively associated with diet quality index for pregnancy. *Preventive Medicine, 39*(5), 869–875.

Larson, N. I., Story, M. T., & Nelson, M. C. (2009). Neighborhood environments: Disparities in access to healthy foods in the U.S. *American Journal of Preventive Medicine, 36*(1), 74–81.

Lee, J., & Frongillo Jr., E. (2001). Nutritional and health consequences are associated with food insecurity among U.S. elderly persons. *Journal of Nutrition, 131*(5), 1503–1509.

Liese, A., Weis, K., & Pluto, D. (2007). Food store types, availability and cost of foods in a rural environment. *Journal of the American Dietetic Association, 107,* 1916–1923.

Liese, A. D., Colabianchi, N., Lamichhane, A. P., Barnes, T. L., Hibbert, J. D., Porter, D. E., et al. (2010). Validation of 3 food outlet databases: Completeness and geospatial accuracy in rural and urban food environments. *American Journal of Epidemiology, 172*(11), 1324–1333.

Liese, A. D., Weis, K. E., Pluto, D., Smith, E., & Lawson, A. (2007). Food store types, availability, and cost of foods in a rural environment. *Journal of the American Dietetic Association, 107*(11), 1916–1923.

McKinnon, R., Reedy, J., Morrissette, M., Lytle, L., & Yaroch, A. (2009). Measures of the food environment: A compilation of the literature, 1990–2007. *American Journal of Preventive Medicine, 36*(4S), 124–133.

Morland, K., Wing, S., Roux, A. D., & Poole, C. (2002). Neighborhood characteristics associated with the location of food stores and food service places. *American Journal of Preventive Medicine, 22*(1), 23–29.

Morris, P. M., Neuhauser, L., & Campbell, C. (1992). Food security in rural America: A study of the availability and costs of food. *Journal of Nutrition Education & Behavior, 24*(S1), 52S–58S.

Murcott, A. (1983). Women's place: Cookbooks' images of technique and technology in the British kitchen. *Women's Studies International Forum, 6*(1), 33–39.

Mushi-Brunt, C., Haire-Joshu, D., & Elliott, M. (2007). Food spending behaviors and perceptions are associated with fruit and vegetable intake among parents and their preadolescent children. *Journal of Nutrition Education and Behavior, 39*(1), 26–30.

Nord, M., Coleman-Jensen, A., Andrews, M., & Carlson, S. (2010). *Household food security in the United States, 2009.* Washington, DC: US Department of Agriculture, Economic Research Service.

Olson, C. M., Anderson, K., Kiss, E., Lawrence, F. C., & Seiling, S. B. (2004). Factors protecting against and contributing to food insecurity among rural families. *Family Economics & Nutrition Review, 16*(1), 12–20.

Pearce, J., Witten, K., Hiscock, R., & Blakely, T. (2008). Regional and urban-rural variations in the association of neighbourhood deprivation with community resource access: A national study. *Environment and Planning A, 40*(10), 2469–2489.

Peterson, S. L., Dodd, K. M., Kim, K., & Roth, S. L. (2010). Food cost perceptions and food purchasing practices of uninsured, low-income, rural adults. *Journal of Hunger & Environmental Nutrition, 5*(1), 41–55.

Powell, L., Slater, S., Mirtcheva, D., Bao, Y., & Chaloupka, F. (2007). Food store availability and neighborhood characteristics in the United States. *Preventive Medicine, 44*, 189–195.

Ricketts, T. (1999). *Rural health in the United States.* New York: Oxford University Press.

Salze, P., Banos, A., Oppert, J.-M., Charreire, H., Casey, R., Simon, C., et al. (2011). Estimating spatial accessibility to facilities on the regional scale: An extended commuting-based interaction potential model. *International Journal of Health Geographics*, p. 16.

Sano, Y., Garasky, S., Greder, K., Cook, C., & Browder, D. (2011). Understanding food insecurity among Latino immigrant families in rural America. *Journal of Family and Economic Issues, 32*(1), 111–123.

Sharkey, J. (2003). Risk and presence of food insufficiency are associated with low nutrient intakes and multimorbidity among homebound older women who receive home-delivered meals. *Journal of Nutrition, 133*(11), 3485.

Sharkey, J. (2009). Measuring potential access to food stores and food service places in rural areas in the United States. *American Journal of Preventive Medicine, 36*(4S), S151–S155.

Sharkey, J., Dean, W., St. John, J., & Huber, J. (2010). Using direct observations on multiple occasions to measure household food availability among low-income Mexicano residents in Texas colonias. *BMC Public Health, 10*(445), 44.

Sharkey, J., & Horel, S. (2008). Neighborhood socioeconomic deprivation and minority composition are associated with better potential spatial access to the food environment in a large rural area. *Journal of Nutrition, 138*, 620–627.

Sharkey, J., Horel, S., & Dean, W. (2010). Neighborhood deprivation, vehicle ownership, and potential spatial access to a variety of fruits and vegetables in a large rural area in Texas. *International Journal of Health Geographics, 9*(1), 26.

Sharkey, J., Johnson, C., & Dean, W. (2010). Food access and perceptions of the community and household food environment as correlates of fruit and vegetable intake among rural seniors. *BMC Geriatrics, 10*, 32.

Sharkey, J. R. (2002). The interrelationship of nutritional risk factors, indicators of nutritional risk, and severity of disability among home-delivered meal participants. *The Gerontologist, 42*(3), 373.

Sharkey, J. R. (2009). Measuring potential access to food stores and food-service places in rural areas in the U.S. *American Journal of Preventive Medicine, 36*(4, S1), S151–S155.

Sharkey, J. R., & Horel, S. (2008). Neighborhood socioeconomic deprivation and minority composition are associated with better potential spatial access to the ground-truthed food environment in a large rural area. *Journal of Nutrition, 138*(3), 620–627.

Sharkey, J. R., Horel, S., Han, D., & Huber, J. (2009). Association between neighborhood need and spatial access to food stores and fast food restaurants in neighborhoods of colonias. *International Journal of Health Geographics, 8*(1), 9.

Sharkey, J. R., Johnson, C., & Dean, W. R. (2010). Food access and perceptions of the community and household food environment as correlates of fruit and vegetable intake among rural seniors. *BMC Geriatrics, 10*(32), 12.

Sharkey, J. R., Johnson, C. M., Dean, W. R., & Horel, S. A. (2011). Focusing on fast food restaurants alone underestimates exposure to fast food in a large rural area. *Nutrition Journal, 10*(10), 14.

Smith, C., & Wright Morton, L. (2009). Rural food deserts: Low-income perspectives on food access in Minnesota and Iowa. *Journal of Nutrition Education and Behavior, 41*(3), 176–187.

Swanson, J., Olson, C., Miller, E., & Lawrence, F. (2008). Rural mothers' use of formal programs and informal social supports to meet family food needs: A mixed methods study. *Journal of Family and Economic Issues, 29*(4), 674–690.

Walker, R., Keane, C., & Burke, J. (2010). Disparities and access to healthy food in the United States: A review of food deserts literature. *Health & Place, 16*(5), 876–884.

Webber, C. B., Sobal, J., & Dollahite, J. S. (2010). Shopping for fruits and vegetables. Food and retail qualities of importance to low-income households at the grocery store. *Appetite, 54*(2), 297–303.

World Health Organization. (1990). *Diet, nutrition and the prevention of chronic diseases.* Geneva: Author.

Wright Morton, L., Bitto, E., Oakland, M., & Sand, M. (2008). Accessing food resources: Rural and urban patterns of giving and getting food. *Agriculture and Human Values, 25*(1), 107–119.

Wright Morton, L., & Blanchard, T. (2007). Starved for access: Life in rural America's food deserts. *Rural Realities, 1*(4), 1–10.

Wright Morton, L., & Smith, C. (2008). Accessing food in rural food deserts in Iowa and Minnesota. *The Great Plains Sociologist, 19*, 57–82.

Wrigley, N., Warm, D., & Margetts, B. (2003). Deprivation, diet and food retail access: Findings from the Leeds "food deserts" study. *Environmental Planning A, 35*, 151–188.

Zenk, S., Schulz, A., Hollis-Neely, T., Campbell, R., Holmes, N., Watkins, G., et al. (2005). Fruit and vegetable intake in African Americans: Income and store characteristics. *American Journal of Preventive Medicine, 29*(1), 1–9.

Chapter 15

Promoting Oral Health in Rural Communities

Nikki Stone
Baretta R. Casey

Learning Objectives

- Understand that rural underserved populations with low socioeconomic status and low health literacy are less likely to receive oral health.
- Understand the importance of preventive dental services for rural populations.
- See the benefits of public health efforts to educate and raise awareness of oral health within communities.
- Understand the benefits of a multidisciplinary team approach to oral health.
- Gain knowledge of model programs in preventive oral health, such as school-based programs.

•••

Oral health and general health are inseparable. The term *oral health* refers to the teeth and gums but it extends further to include the entire craniofacial complex, which is inextricably linked to the entire body in myriad ways that have yet to be fully explained. The World Health Organization has made it clear to the world that being healthy is not just the absence of disease but a state of wellness biologically, socially, and mentally (WHO, 2012). Oral health has often been overlooked as a significant health issue. Since the 2000 surgeon general's report entitled *Oral Health in America: A Report of the Surgeon General* was published, a landslide of oral health surveys and publications have swept the nation (US Department of Health and Human Services, 2000). In 2003, the surgeon general followed up with another publication, *A National Call to Action to Promote Oral Health* (US Department of Health and Human Services, 2003). Oral health was featured prominently in *Healthy People 2010* including seventeen objectives to be met by 2010 (US Department of Health and Human Services, 2000). In 2007, the nation's community health centers benefited from the *Health Centers' Role in Addressing the Oral Health Needs of the Medically Underserved,* providing guidance to community health centers seeking to improve the oral health of their communities (Ruddy, 2007).

Key Concepts

Oral health is linked with and integral to overall health and well-being and, as stated by the surgeon general, "You can't be healthy without oral health" (US Department of Health and Human Services, 2000). There are two main oral **diseases**: caries (tooth decay) and periodontal (gum) disease. There are also oral and pharyngeal cancers and other less common diseases of the oral cavity and supporting tissues. Proper oral hygiene and access to oral health care can prevent the majority of these diseases (US Department of Health and Human Services, 2000).

Oral health can affect overall health in many ways. Much has been done since 2000 to try to describe the oral-systemic links between periodontal (gum) disease and cardiovascular disease, diabetes, stroke, preterm and low-birth-weight babies, and possibly even Alzheimer's disease. Most researchers explain these linkages as being related to the inflammatory mediator cascade that circulates through the blood system as well as whole bacteria that can also travel through the blood and settle in vulnerable areas of the body (Barnett, 2006; US Department of Health and Human Services, 2000).

Tooth decay is the single most-common chronic childhood disease in the United States, more common than hay fever or asthma (US Department of Health and Human Services, 2000). The bacteria causing tooth decay actually colonizes the oral cavity before the first tooth even erupts (Berkowitz, 2006). It is a bio-psychosocial disease, with physical and emotional affects ranging from pain and infection to impaired nutrition, impaired speech, impaired growth and development, poor self-image and confidence, and inability to learn in school.

Tooth decay and gum disease can be painful and may lead to very serious infections in children and adults. In 2007, a young Maryland boy named Deamonte Driver died from an abscessed tooth. The infection spread through his sinus cavities into his brain (Casamassimo et al., 2009). Poor oral health in the elderly, especially those in nursing home care, has been linked with pneumonia, a leading cause of death in the elderly (Barnett, 2006).

Untreated tooth decay or gum disease may lead to the loss of teeth, which can have multiple poor health outcomes including difficulty chewing and digesting food properly and therefore poor nutrition and overall poor health. Loss of teeth may also affect a person's ability to talk and communicate properly. Furthermore, tooth loss and visible cavities may have psychological effects such as poor self-esteem for children and result in difficulty obtaining and maintaining employment in adults (ASTDD, 2010).

Children with poor oral health have trouble learning and concentrating in school and may miss many hours of school from pain or dental appointments. A child with a toothache is unlikely to perform well on school work and examinations (Casamassimo et al., 2009). According to the National Maternal & Child Oral Health Resource Center, an estimated fifty-one million school hours per year are lost because of dental-related illnesses. Furthermore, poor children had almost twelve times as many days missed because of dental issues than their more affluent peers (NMCOHRC, 2003).

A dental outreach program in rural eastern Kentucky (described later in this chapter) found that, out of ten elementary schools, the two with the lowest untreated tooth decay rates were the same two schools with the highest standardized test scores (see Figure 15.1).

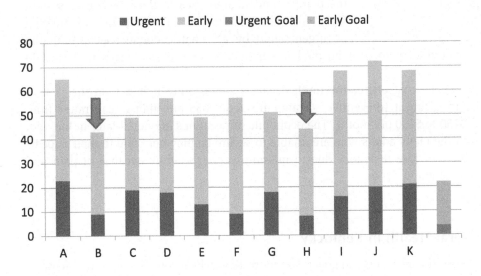

Figure 15.1. Untreated Tooth Decay, Perry County Elementary Schools, 2006–2007
Note: The two schools with the lowest decay rates are the two schools with the highest standardized test scores.

Children are often unable to verbalize their dental pain and may express their discomfort in other ways such as anxiety, fatigue, irritability, depression, or being withdrawn from their normal activities. Poor oral health can cause impairments to children's general health such as lowered height and weight gains and even failure to thrive (ASTDD, 2010).

Poor oral health during pregnancy may be a contributing factor to preterm and low-birth-weight babies, preeclampsia, gestational diabetes, and fetal loss. Poor maternal oral health is linked with childhood caries because the bacteria that causes tooth decay, streptococcus mutans, is transferred from mother to child within the first few months of life (Buerlein, Peabody, & Santoro, 2010).

Profound **disparities** (differences) still exist in America with regards to oral health. Low socioeconomic status and certain racial and ethnic minorities suffer a heavier burden of disease and are less likely to receive care. Early childhood caries disproportionately affect those who are **underserved,** who for a variety of reasons receive insufficient and inadequate health services. This is especially prevalent in populations who are poor, rural, and who have low health literacy. More than twice as many Americans lack dental insurance as lack medical insurance (US Department of Health and Human Services, 2003, 2000).

Early childhood caries disproportionately affects those underserved populations that are poor, rural, and with low health literacy.

The final economic consequences of poor oral health begin early with children missing school for pain and dental visits, parents missing work to take the child to the dentist, and higher costs to the health care system from emergency room use. The expense of treating an urgent child by a pediatric dental specialist in the operating room of a hospital under general anesthesia ranges from $4,000 to $8,000.

The cost of treating tooth decay is significantly higher than the cost of preventing it (preventive sealants are about $35 and fillings can range from $150 to $200 per tooth). The economic implications are noted later in life, too, in the many adults who are unable to secure employment due to their appearance or lose their jobs due to missing work frequently because of pain and infection.

Oral Health in Kentucky

After the 2000 surgeon general's report, Kentucky's dental community likewise responded with its own efforts toward improving oral health beginning with a dental access summit in 2001, statewide data collection profile in 2001, strategic planning meetings in 2004, and dissemination of documents such as the

2006 *Healthy Kentucky Smiles: A Lifetime of Oral Health* published by the state dental director (Cecil, 2006).

Kentucky has consistently ranked number one or number two in edentulism among older adults over sixty-five years old (42.3 percent of Kentuckians were toothless in 2003 according to the *Mortality and Morbidity Weekly Report* (Centers for Disease Control, 2003) compared to the state rate of 37 percent and the national rate of 33 percent (Kentucky Institute of Medicine, 2007). Furthermore, oral cancer, periodontal disease, and early childhood caries are well above *Healthy People 2010* goals (Wrightson & Stone, 2009).

The causes are many and include lack of access to dental care for poor, rural, elderly, and otherwise vulnerable populations in this state. Lifestyle choices such as smoking and poor dietary choices, a cultural acceptance of poor oral health, poor oral health literacy, as well as having a family history of poor oral health are other potential causes. Finally, a lack of dental **preventive** services (aimed at preventing disease before it begins such as fluoride treatments and sealants) early in life, including prenatally, leads to poor oral health outcomes throughout the life span (Wrightson & Stone, 2009).

One factor influencing low access to dental services in Kentucky is the fact that only 35 percent of Kentucky dentists participate in Medicaid, one of the lowest rates in the country. The effect of this low rate is compounded by a regional shortage of dentists and dental professionals. The state of Kentucky ranks twenty-ninth with 54.5 dentists per one hundred thousand population; however, this ratio is lower in the Appalachian counties of southeastern Kentucky where there are approximately 27.6 dentists per one hundred thousand residents.

There are only 0.29 dentists per one thousand serving the Appalachian residents of southeastern Kentucky (Saman, Arevalo, & Johnson, 2010). The report notes that one of the biggest challenges for Kentucky is dental and oral health care. Beyond basic dental services, specialty dental providers are sparse. Of greatest consequence, Kentucky has very few pediatric dental specialists and most are located in more urban areas of the state, virtually inaccessible to rural poor.

A 2007 article in the *New York Times* concluded that these dismaying statistics are likely due to a shortage of dentists in rural areas, limited access to free or subsidized dental clinics, historically low rates of Medicaid payment for dental care, and poor oral hygiene compounded by high rates of tobacco use (Urbina, 2007) (Herbert, 2007). Until August 2006, when Medicaid rates were raised, the reimbursement rate in Kentucky was one of the lowest in the country. Even with this increase, which was funded by cutting orthodontic benefits, reimbursement fees remain about 50 percent below market rate, and for adults, they are 65 percent below market.

Tooth decay, like other poverty-related health disparities, is rampant among Kentucky's poor children. In fact, 80 percent of the decay is found in 20 percent of the population (US Department of Health and Human Services, 2000). It is a disease of poverty and begins early in life with the transmission of the infective bacteria streptococcus mutans from mother to child. A parent with multiple large cavities has a much higher level of aggressive bacteria, and the bacteria is transferred through kissing and sharing food.

The 2001 *Kentucky Children's Oral Health Survey* revealed that Kentucky's children had higher rates of untreated tooth decay than national reports, 28.7 percent versus 21 percent nationally according to the 1999–2002 National Health and Nutrition Examination Survey (Hardison, 2003).

Oral Health in Rural Eastern Kentucky

The 2001 *Kentucky Children's Oral Health Profiles* ranked the eastern region of Kentucky worst on all of the following measures: percent of children with caries experience (60.5), percent of children with untreated tooth decay (32.6), and percent of children with need for urgent dental care within twenty-four hours (7.7). Third- and sixth-graders in eastern Kentucky experienced more toothaches than those in metropolitan areas (Hardison, 2003).

In some isolated pockets of rural Appalachian counties, over 70 percent of students suffer from untreated tooth decay (Stone et al., 2007). Furthermore, urgent dental needs in eastern Kentucky were nearly 20 percent for preschool and elementary children, significantly higher than the state average of around 4 percent (Stone et al., 2010).

Despite their poor oral health status, residents of eastern Kentucky counties are less likely than other Kentuckians to have visited a dentist recently. According to the 2002 Kentucky Adult Oral Health Survey, 16.7 percent of adults in the Appalachian counties of eastern Kentucky reported that it had been greater than five years since their last dental visit, the highest rate reported in the state (KCHFS, 2003).

Inextricably linked to eastern Kentuckian's failure to seek dental care is a lack of health care coverage. According to the 2000 surgeon general's report, medical insurance is a strong predictor of access to dental care. Uninsured children are two and one-half times less likely than insured children to receive dental care. Children from families without dental insurance are three times more likely to have dental needs than children with either public or private insurance (US Department of Health and Human Services, 2000).

In eastern Kentucky, even the availability of dental insurance does not necessarily translate into accessed care. Although the majority of children are eligible for dental benefits through Medicaid or the Kentucky Children's Health

Insurance Program (KCHIP). Only 58 percent of children ages zero to seventeen received even a single dental visit in 2002 in Perry County (KKCCDB, 2007).

There are a variety of other reasons for eastern Kentucky's oral health disparities. A leading contributor is limited access to the public water supply and, consequently, community water fluoridation. Studies have found that this water treatment technique can reduce tooth decay by up to 40 percent among children and by more than 30 percent among adults. According to the surgeon general's 2000 report, optimally fluoridated water was unavailable to approximately one-third of the US population (US Department of Health and Human Services, 2000). Despite several waterline extension projects in recent years, much of rural eastern Kentucky still does not receive this public service, leaving hundreds of households to rely on private wells void of fluoridation.

Although the University of Kentucky's dental outreach programs reach many children statewide, the burden of oral disease is undeniably focused in the poor counties of rural eastern Kentucky.

A Promising Program in Rural Eastern Kentucky

The data and messages in all of these publications are consistent:

- Access to oral health care is a critical issue in the United States, particularly for poor children, the elderly, and other vulnerable populations such as minority groups.
- Kentucky may well be the worst state in the nation for oral health.
- The rural eastern region of Kentucky fares the worst in nearly every measure evaluated, putting rural Appalachian southeastern Kentucky counties at the epicenter of the poorest oral health in America.

Fortunately, several factors came together to make it possible to implement a dental outreach program in four of these rural counties, targeting preschool and early elementary school children. The program has worked so well that it has been listed as one of five model dental programs by the Kentucky Institute of Medicine and data from the program have been presented locally, regionally, nationally, and internationally at a variety of venues.

Description of the Organization

One promising children's oral health outreach program in rural eastern Kentucky was initiated by the University of Kentucky at the Center for Excellence in Rural Health—Hazard (UK CERH-H). This center was established in 1990 by legislative mandate and serves the unique role of acting as a conduit between rural needs and university resources. The UK CERH-H is a fifty-seven-thousand-square-foot modern facility physically located two hours away from the Lexington campus in rural eastern Kentucky. It houses the University of Kentucky North Fork Valley Community Health Center (UK NFVCHC), a federally qualified community health center that serves as the clinical component of the UK CERH-H and helps fulfill all facets of the UKCERH-H's fourfold mission of education, service, research, and community engagement. The UK NFVCHC provides health care for the whole family (medical, dental, mental, pharmacy) and hosts family medicine and dental residency programs that provide a training ground for medical and dental school graduates seeking to serve in rural areas.

Description of the Dental Program

The medical program has been a part of the center since its inception in 1990 but the dental program was added in summer 2004 when the University of Kentucky Colleges of Medicine and Dentistry collaborated to open UK's first regional dental program in Hazard in the form of a five-chair dental clinic suite on the first floor of the new building. In May 2005, Ronald McDonald House Charities Global donated a Ronald McDonald Care Mobile to the program, a two-chair dental office on wheels.

The school-based preventive dental outreach program began in area schools and Head Start centers. Nearly every recommendation nationally had suggested that one of the only oral health interventions that works is school-based sealant programs or population-based fluoride programs (ASTDD, 2010). The dental outreach program operates by committing full efforts to providing only evidence-based preventive clinical care to underserved low-income children, focusing on reaching children at the youngest possible age in Head Start and WIC programs, daycare centers, and preschool classrooms and providing the most aggressive clinical protocols described in the available literature. Implementing these preventive services at the earliest ages possible allow for maximum long-term impact.

Even more unusual than the mobile unit is the innovative Head Start program which serves Letcher, Knott, Leslie, and Perry counties (LKLP). It is unusual because the dental care is provided without a mobile unit or portable dental equipment of any kind. Because many of the rural Head Start classrooms are located in areas away from school yards with parking for buses and mobile units, a more practical approach was needed. Children in the eighteen separate Head Start centers receive their care in a lap-to-lap position in which the dentist and dental assistant sit facing each other and the child literally uses their combined laps as the dental chair on which to lay down and be treated.

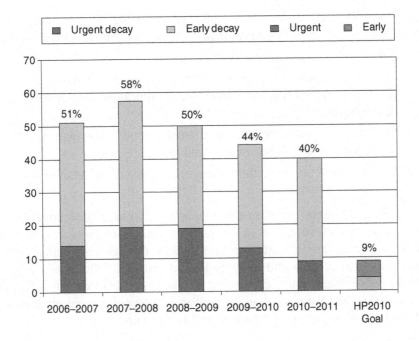

Figure 15.2. LKLP Head Start Centers

Supplies are prepackaged in bags that are transported and then sent home with the child holding a new toothbrush and toothpaste.

A front-page article in the *Lexington Herald* newspaper on November 9, 2008, entitled "State's Dental Disaster Begins at an Early Age" described the treatment position as follows: "Dr. Stone's lap formed half the dental chair and her assistant's made the other half" (Vos, 2008).

Children are very comfortable receiving care in this model and often gather around to watch each other. They are rarely if ever fearful because the treatment is enjoyable and provided in the child's environment with supportive peers and familiar teachers close by. Infants and babies are often held and if one or two teeth are erupted, fluoride varnish is applied.

The first year of baseline data was discouraging but (as shown in Figure 15.2) the subsequent five years have shown a steady improvement in untreated tooth decay rates, progressively dropping year by year from a high of 58 percent untreated decay in preschool children down to 40 percent. A drop of 18 percentage points is promising but there is still more to be done to reach the *Healthy People 2010* goal of 9 percent in this young age group.

The dental outreach program piloted in the Hazard area was presented at a series of statewide trainings during the development of the Kentucky Oral

Health Network and is now being replicated statewide. The mission of the eastern Kentucky dental outreach program is to serve the underserved through the following efforts:

- Provide prevention in an evidence-based preventive dental care program to reverse the trend in eastern Kentucky toward poor dental health

- Provide education to children and families about the importance of dental care in overall health and well-being

- Increase awareness in communities about this critical health issue for eastern Kentucky

This mobile dental program provides evidence-based preventive dental care to infants, preschool, and elementary low-income children in four rural Appalachian counties in southeastern Kentucky through contractual agreements with area schools and early childhood programs. The coverage area includes twenty elementary schools and eighteen Head Start centers in Leslie, Knott, Letcher, and Perry counties, as well as a variety of community festivals and events, daycare centers, churches, and health fairs.

Description of Services Provided

Provided services include comprehensive oral exams, child prophylaxis (cleanings), topical fluoride varnish, and sealants (on permanent molars). The program also provides science-based classroom education at each elementary school visited. Efforts are focused not only on population-based prevention of oral disease but also great emphasis is placed on the coordination of individual-based follow-up emergency and comprehensive care.

Potential solutions and recommendations for improving oral health are also consistent throughout the published literature, recommending school-based oral health programs as one of the most effective actions a community can take. The American Dental Association has two published evidence-based clinical recommendations: topical fluoride application and preventive dental sealants. Both of these clinical procedures can best be delivered to a population through a school-based dental program.

Fluoride Varnish

Fluoride has been recognized as a necessary component for good oral health for years. Fluoride supplementation of community water supplies has been heralded as one of the greatest public health achievements of the twentieth century (US Department of Health and Human Services, 2000). Those who provide care to newborns and young children are familiar with prescribing fluoride supplements to families without community water or whose water source is deficient in fluoride. Dentists have long recognized the benefits of topical fluoride applications in the health management of their children and adult patients.

The application of fluoride varnish is a relatively new form of topical fluoride aimed at reducing the incidence of childhood caries. This chronic disease is a process ranging from early enamel demineralization (white spots) to frank cavitations (holes in teeth). The disease occurs within the interplay of several potential coexisting negative forces: streptococcus mutans bacteria infection, sugar substrate causing acid formation, and teeth at risk due to poor oral hygiene or other factors such as tooth morphology or defects (Featherstone, 2008).

Fluoride helps maintain and improve tooth health. It alters bacterial metabolism to prevent acid formation, it prevents demineralization of the enamel and promotes remineralization, particularly in areas already damaged. These effects are mostly topical and are also seen with the use of fluorinated water, toothpastes, and fluoride varnish (Featherstone, 2008).

Children at moderate to high risk for early childhood caries should receive fluoride varnish applications twice a year from the eruption of their first tooth, starting somewhere between six and twelve months of age. At-risk children include those at lower socioeconomic status (including all children with state Medicaid insurance or no insurance), those with already demonstrated early childhood caries, children with poor dietary habits (bottle at bed time, bottle propping, drinks other than milk or water in the bottle, excessive use of sippy cups or sugary, sticky snacks), or family history of multiple caries or lost teeth from caries or periodontal disease. These applications should continue in the medical office until the establishment of a dental home (Wrightson & Stone, 2009).

The application of fluoride varnish is simple and relatively quick. It can be applied by physicians, other clinicians, nurses, or medical assistants. The materials required are gauze, a toothbrush, and the fluoride varnish. With the child lying on the exam table or with his or her head in the lap of the health care provider, the teeth are first cleaned of debris with the toothbrush. The teeth are then dried with the gauze and the fluoride is painted on the teeth, usually to one quadrant at a time (Wrightson & Stone, 2009).

Multiple European and Canadian studies have demonstrated the benefit of fluoride varnish application on children. In a study performed in San Francisco on low-income Chinese and Hispanic children, Weintraub and colleagues demonstrated that even a single fluoride varnish application reduced the incidence of early childhood caries. Weintraub found the incidence of caries significantly decreased over a two-year period from 12 percent to 6 percent with the application of fluoride varnish (Weintraub et al., 2006).

Sealants

Sealants are thin plastic coatings that can be applied with little effort to the chewing surfaces of back teeth (molars) to protect them from decay. Back teeth have grooves and pits where food and germs often get caught. The sealant covers those areas leaving a smooth surface that is easy to clean.

Applying sealants is easy and painless and is a short procedure that can be performed in a dental office or with portable dental equipment that can be moved from school to school. Ideally, a mobile dental unit is the easiest way to provide sealants at schools because it is easier to move and set up than portable equipment.

The scientific evidence shows that school-based sealant programs work. In fact, the Task Force on Community Preventive Services recommends school sealant programs and issued a strong endorsement in 2001. Then in 2003, the Association of State and Territorial Dental Directors published a best practice approach report presenting examples and providing the scientific evidence that school sealant programs work to stop tooth decay.

The Data

Data collected as part of outreach efforts have revealed that the untreated dental decay rates of elementary school children in these rural eastern Kentucky counties were 59 percent, significantly above those of white (26 percent), black (36 percent), and Hispanic (43 percent) populations and second only to the Native American and Alaskan Native populations (69 percent) (Beltran-Aguilar et al., 2005; Stone et al., 2007) (see Figure 15.3).

During the 2007–2008 school year, nearly six hundred Head Start children were examined and treated in the fall and again in the spring. Each child was assessed and categorized as low, moderate, or high risk of caries (tooth decay) and a letter was sent home to parents describing their child's oral status as urgent, early, or no obvious dental needs. Nearly 20 percent of children two to five years old were described as having urgent dental needs (compared to a 4 percent state rate), defined as having seven or more cavities, pain, and visible infection (abscessed teeth, swelling, etc.). All parents were encouraged by the dental staff and Head Start staff to seek follow-up care (Stone et al., 2010).

Six months later, at the spring visit, only six out of seventy-eight children (a mere 8 percent) had received complete follow-up care, another 14 percent had received some follow-up care (typically only one or maybe two of the multiple cavities had been filled), and the remaining 80 percent had not received any follow-up care at all or were not available to reexamine. Most disturbing of all, of those who did not receive any follow-up care, 40 percent

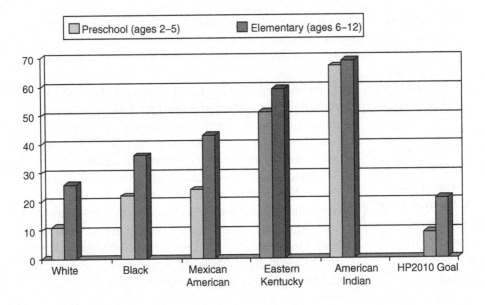

Figure 15.3. Percentage of Untreated Tooth Decay, Eastern Kentucky Versus National Ethnic Data

had progressively worse conditions with multiple new cavities, at an average of four new cavities per child, with one child having fourteen new cavities that had developed within that six-month period (Stone et al., 2010).

Multiple children were found to have all twenty decayed teeth (children have only twenty deciduous [baby] teeth until age six). When compared with national norms, these low-income, high-risk children have untreated decay rates second only to the Native American and Alaskan Native populations. Because eastern Kentucky's population is predominantly Caucasian, to compare these children to national norms reveals a difference of 48 percent (National Health and Nutrition Examination Survey [NHANES] reported 10 percent untreated decay for white children ages two to four, and eastern Kentucky children have 58 percent) (Stone et al., 2010).

The potential cost of treating all seventy-eight of the urgent Head Start children discovered during the 2007–2008 school year would be $546,000. Although the majority (66 percent) of these children qualify for free dental care through Kentucky Children's Health Insurance Program (KCHIP) and Medicaid (Stone et al., 2010), most parents do not access dental care for their children until there is an emergency situation. Without a mobile dental service provided for the children at their daycare or school site, most of these children will not have any dental care until about age five when they are brought in most often for a painful emergency visit. By contrast, the American Academy of Pediatric Dentistry now recommends that the first dental visit occurs by the first birthday.

Furthermore, many parents reported poor oral health for themselves, and because Kentucky ranks number one nationally in edentulism (adults with no remaining natural teeth), it is obvious that this is a critical health issue for eastern Kentucky, one for which limited resources are available for low-income adults.

Low-income adults in this area frequently report dental fear and anxiety, inability to afford dental care, and behavior patterns of seeking emergency care only, sometimes with multiple year spans between visits.

Anecdotally, low-income adults in this area frequently report dental fear and anxiety, inability to afford dental care, and behavior patterns of seeking emergency care only, sometimes with multiple year spans between visits. Until families in poverty become more comfortable with and place higher priority on dental care, this cycle will continue with the same devastating results.

Program Successes and Accomplishments

The University of Kentucky's dental outreach programs have grown to four mobile dental units operating all around the state, providing over six thousand dental visits each year, now linked through the Kentucky Oral Health Network. This groundwork provides an exceptional foundation to quickly develop and implement new projects by building on the successes of our existing programs and affords the assurance of sustainable long-term programs that will benefit the children of Kentucky for many years to come. Part of the infrastructure development by the University of Kentucky for the Kentucky Oral Health Network includes the development of an electronic dental information system to support dental outreach programs (Kentucky Children's Oral Health Information System). This has provided opportunities for collecting and sharing data with key research, education, and policy groups to improve the oral health of children across Kentucky and the nation.

The oral health service and research team at the UK Center for Oral Health Research has been available to provide oral health and training expertise and grant opportunities as may be appropriate. Additionally, the existing mobile dental program located at the UKCERH-H as part of the UKNFVCHC has proven to be financially sustainable due in large part to the health center's status as a federally qualified health center, receiving a higher reimbursement rate for Medicaid services and some federal funds to offset the sliding-fee services.

The Mobile Dental Program at UK North Fork Valley Community Health Center has been in successful operation since 2005, and has partnered with a variety of community members; those partnerships have been essential to the success of the program. To date, the mobile dental program has served over eight thousand children and provided over thirteen thousand preventive dental care visits. The program has also provided science-based classroom education at elementary schools and has sent home educational material to all parents and families.

The mobile dental program has consistently visited the same schools and Head Start centers on an annual basis and is therefore able to provide consistent care to a large population of children from infancy in the early Head Start program through their third grade of elementary school when the six year molars have erupted and are sealed.

The program's accomplishments so far include exceeding the *Healthy People 2010* goal for dental sealants every year and decreasing the untreated and urgent dental needs of these rural children by 18 percent and 11 percent respectively (Stone et al., 2010).

These efforts have been successful in increasing Medicaid use rates in these counties. The mobile dental program serves only underserved children, those who are uninsured or who qualify for Medicaid or KCHIP dental benefits. Participation rates at individual schools range from 40 to 78 percent (58 percent of Perry County children qualified for Medicaid or KCHIP in 2006). Further emphasis and collaboration with a local pediatric dentist have led to one of the greatest successes of the program: increasing access to comprehensive treatment for urgent Head Start children from 8 to 33 percent via a partnership with a local pediatric dentist providing care in the local hospital emergency room.

Clearly, there is an extremely heavy burden of dental decay in this population group, from early childhood through old age, and the only way to reverse the trend is to provide primary preventive services as early as possible to as many children as possible and to emphasize oral health importance to women during pregnancy. A very important factor leading to the success of this program is that the mobile dental staff is made up of four local, culturally competent dental health professionals who have been with the program since its inception and who continue to passionately carry out what they feel is missionary work in their own hometowns caring for their own people.

Innovative Ideas for a Multidisciplinary Team

Oral health has too often been perceived as the sole responsibility of dentists, and as such, opportunities for preventive counseling and care by physicians are frequently missed. Fluoride varnish application can be easily performed in a physician's office. The taste is tolerable and varnish application has been shown to prevent and even reverse the white spots characteristic of early demineralization.

Fluoride varnish comes in several varieties. The easiest to use are the single-use packets. The average cost of these materials is $1.00 to $2.00. Currently, Medicaid in Kentucky is reimbursing the application of varnish at $15.00 for two applications a year, at least ninety days apart for children up to four years of age. The code used is D1206 in conjunction with an office visit code. A fluoride varnish manual, entitled *Healthy Smile Happy Child* has been developed by the Kentucky Cabinet for Health and Family Service and Kentucky Department for Medicaid Services to guide physician's offices in providing this dental service to their child patients (Cabinet for Health and Family Service, 2007). Several other states are offering similar programs.

A full self-study module on childhood oral health and fluoride varnish application, complete with a video on the application itself can be found at www.smilesforlifeoralhealth.org. This is an American Academy of Family Physician and a Society of Teachers of Family Medicine–supported curriculum that provides comprehensive information on oral health from prenatal to geriatric patients. There are also links to other educational resources and materials (Douglass, 2008).

Physicians and other providers of health care for children have a unique opportunity to address the oral health needs of their patients. Applying fluoride varnish will help in reducing the burden of poor oral health to Kentuckians, particularly children, though it is only one part of the comprehensive management of patients that includes education and counseling on health behaviors, such as smoking and poor nutritional choices, that add to the severity of dental disease in this state. Because many children do not see a dentist, it is up to the clinicians in the child's medical home to initiate counseling about good oral health habits as well as providing treatments such as fluoride varnish, which can reduce early childhood caries (Wrightson & Stone, 2009).

Improving the oral health of Americans will take **multidisciplinary** partnerships (a team approach combining several disciplines to maximize expertise and optimize health outcomes) on all levels and out-of-the-box innovative models that bring care to those who have trouble accessing oral health care, especially for rural poor and underserved minorities.

This chapter focuses mostly on children's programs because it is necessary to start at the earliest age possible to affect significant change but much needs to be done for the adult and elderly populations as well. Pregnancy is now recognized as one of the most important times to access oral health care for the benefit of the mother and the child. The surgeon general's message is starting to be heard loud and clear across America: "You can't be healthy without oral health."

Conclusion

It is apparent from all available data sources, including the program described in this chapter, that school-based preventive dental outreach programs are effective at improving the oral health of communities. It is hoped, as this word gets out, that more and more programs of this type will develop across the nation.

As programs grow, they must keep in mind their overall goals. Primarily, such a program should provide the evidence-based preventive dental care needed to reverse the trend in rural and underserved areas toward poor dental health. Focusing efforts on the youngest age groups available should result in an increase in the proportion of preschool children who receive preventive dental care before age five.

Reaching parents will probably always be a challenge but it is a worthwhile part of an overall school-based program. Staff should make every attempt to contact parents of children enrolled in the program, informing them of the availability of affordable dental care at area safety-net providers, and then encouraging them to follow-up for comprehensive treatment.

Another big component of any dental program should be education. Seek to educate children and their families about the importance of dental care in overall health and well-being and begin a dialogue with family members to help them understand the importance of dental treatment. Educate families about the need to complete follow-up dental treatment by encouraging them to keep dental appointments and designate staff to help navigate any access issues such as transportation or finding a dental home where the family members feel comfortable.

Raising community awareness about oral health as a critical health issue is important. Be sure the community receives the message loud and clear that oral health is an integral part of overall health and well-being. Increasing the oral health literacy of families and community members, including the understanding that tooth decay is a chronic, transmissible, and preventable disease, will go a long way in improving the overall oral health of a community. Have staff work closely with school, daycare, and Head Start teachers and staff to educate them about the goals and objectives of the program, and the value of optimal oral health.

Summary

- Rural underserved populations with low socioeconomic status and low health literacy suffer a heavier burden of oral disease and are less likely to receive dental care.

- Tooth decay and dental caries have physical and emotional repercussions, ranging from pain and infection to impaired nutrition, impaired speech and growth and development, poor self-image and confidence, and inability to attend work or school.

- Expectant mothers and young children are important populations to reach when addressing oral health disparities. Pregnant mothers must be addressed for the benefit of the mother and child; young children should be targeted at the earliest possible age to affect significant change.

- A number of factors contribute to rural oral health disparities such as poor access to dental care, lifestyle choices (smoking and obesity), a cultural acceptance of poor oral and dental care, a lack of education and understanding about the consequences of untreated dental disease, a lack of dental preventive services for young children and expectant mothers, and an unfluoridated water supply.

- When targeting oral health disparities in rural communities, a multidisciplinary approach should be implemented with evidence-based preventive dental care, parental involvement, family education, and community awareness.

Key Terms

disease	oral health
disparities	preventive
multidisciplinary	underserved

For Practice and Discussion

1. Using the Internet as your data source, select one rural state and describe the oral health statistics for children. How can the lessons learned from Kentucky help the state you selected?

2. An emerging phrase in the dental profession is "put the mouth back in the body." Imagine that you have an opportunity to convince your state legislators that this should be a top priority for funding. Using the material from this chapter, please compose a fifteen-minute speech that would make the case crystal clear to even the most apathetic audience member.

References

ASTDD (Association of State and Territorial Dental Directors). (2010). *Best practice approach: Prevention and control of early childhood tooth decay.* Retrieved from http://www.astdd.org/prevention-and-control-of-early-childhood-tooth-decay -introduction/

Barnett, M. L. (2006). The oral-systemic disease connection: An update for the practicing dentist. *Journal of the American Dental Association, 137,* 5S–6S.

Beltran-Aguilar, E. D., et al. (2005). Surveillance for dental caries, dental sealants, tooth retention, edentulism, and enamel fluorosis: United States, 1988–1994 and 1999–2002. *MMWR Surveillance Summaries, 54*(03), 1–44.

Berkowitz, R. J. (2006). Mutans streptococci: Acquisition and transmission. *Pediatric Dentistry, 28*(2), 106–109.

Buerlein, J., Peabody, H., & Santoro, K. (2010). *Improving access to perinatal oral health care: Strategies and considerations for health plans.* Washington, DC: National Institute for Health Care Management. Retrieved from http://www.cdhp.org/resource/improving_access_perinatal_oral_health_care_strategies _considerations_health_plans

Cabinet for Health and Family Service and Kentucky Department for Medicaid Services. (2007). *Kentucky health choices, fluoride varnish manual: Healthy smile, happy child.* Frankfort: Author.

Casamassimo, P. S., Thikkurissy, S., Edelstein, B. L., & Maiorini, E. (2009). Beyond the dmft: The human and economic cost of early childhood caries. *Journal of the American Dental Association, 140,* 650–657.

Cecil, J. (2006). *Healthy Kentucky smiles: A lifetime of oral health.* Statewide oral health strategic plan, the Commonwealth of Kentucky. Retrieved from http://chfs.ky.gov/NR/rdonlyres/67ED0872-8504-43A0-8165-8739F320CAC9/0/ StrategicPlan.pdf

Centers for Disease Control (2003). Public health and aging: Retention of natural teeth among older adults—United States, 2002. *Mortality & Morbidity Weekly Report, 52*(50), 1226–1229.

Douglass, A. B., et al. (2008). *Smiles for life: A national oral health curriculum* (2nd ed.). Society of Teachers of Family Medicine. Retrieved from http://smilesforlifeoralhealth.org/default.aspx?tut = 555&pagekey = 62948&s1 = 1579471

Featherstone, J.D.B. (2008). Dental caries: A dynamic disease process. *Australian Dental Journal, 53,* 286–291.

Hardison, J. D., et al. (2003). *Final results: 2001 Kentucky children's oral health survey.* Lexington: Division of Dental Public Health, College of Dentistry, University of Kentucky.

Herbert, B. (2007, May 19). Young, ill and uninsured. *New York Times.* Retrieved from http://www.nytimes.com/2007/05/19/opinion/19herbert.html? _r = 1&scp = 6&sq = bob + herbert&st = nyt

KCHFS (Kentucky Cabinet for Health and Family Services). (2003, July). *Executive summary 2002: Kentucky adult oral health survey.* Frankfort: Author.

Kentucky Institute of Medicine. (2007). *The health of Kentucky: A county assessment.* Lexington: Author.

Kentucky KIDS COUNT County Data Book (KKCCDB). (2007). *Kentucky youth advocates*. Jeffersontown: Author.

NMCOHRC (National Maternal and Child Oral Health Resource Center). (2003). *Oral health and learning: When children's health suffers, so does their ability to learn* (2nd ed.). Washington, DC: Georgetown University.

Ruddy, G. (2007). *Health centers' role in addressing the oral health needs of the medically underserved*. Washington, DC: National Association of Community Health Centers.

Saman, D. M., Arevalo, O., & Johnson, A. O. (2010). The dental workforce in Kentucky: Current status and future needs. *Journal of Public Health Dentistry*, *70*(3),, 188–196.

Stone, D. N., Casey B., Skelton, J., Kovarik, R., Burch, S., Mullins, M. R., Arevalo, O., & Ebersole, J. L. (2007). *Early childhood caries disparities in rural communities of Kentucky*. Poster presentation at the 2007 International Association for Dental Research 85th General Session, New Orleans, LA.

Stone, D. N., Gross, D., Cornett, J., & Casey, B. (2010). *Partnering for pediatric oral health in rural Kentucky Head Starts*. Oral presentation at the 2010 National Rural Health Association Annual Conference. Savannah, GA.

Urbina, I. (2007, December 24). In Kentucky's teeth, toll of poverty and neglect. *New York Times*.

US Department of Health and Human Services. (2003). *Healthy people 2010 focus area 21 oral health* (2nd ed.). Washington, DC: Author.

US Department of Health and Human Services. (2000). *Oral health in America: A report of the surgeon general*. Rockville, MD: US Department of Health and Human Services, National Institute of Craniofacial Research, National Institute of Health.

US Department of Health and Human Services. (2003). *National call to action to promote oral health*. NIH Publication No. 03–5303. Rockville, MD: US Department of Health and Human Services, Public Health Service, National Institutes of Health, National Institute of Dental and Craniofacial Research.

Vos, S. (2008, November 9). State's dental disaster begins at an early age. Lexington Herald.

Weintraub, J. A., Ramos-Gomez, F., Jue, B., Shain, S., Hoover, C. I., Featherstone, J.D.B., & Gansky, S. A. (2006). Fluoride varnish efficacy in preventing childhood caries. *Journal of Dental Research*, *85*(2), 172–176.

WHO (World Health Organization). (2012). Definition of health. Retrieved from https://apps.who.int/aboutwho/en/definition.html

Wrightson, A. S., & Stone, N. (2009). Fluoride varnish: An effective method for family physicians to reduce childhood caries in their patients. *Kentucky Academy of Family Physicians Journal*, *65*, 20–22.

Chapter 16

Physical Activity Promotion in Rural America

Richard Kozoll
Sally M. Davis

Learning Objectives

- Be able to articulate the rationale for developing and implementing physical activity programs for rural communities.
- Identify unique issues and barriers to physical activity that may permeate rural communities.
- Understand the Step Into Cuba program and be able to describe how this could be adapted to other rural communities.
- Identify key aspects of the community guide that apply to the promotion of physical activity in communities.

• • •

America's recent attention to its epidemic of obesity has catapulted nutrition and physical activity intervention into the forefront of public health practice. Evidence supports national recommendations (CDC, 2005) for community-based physical activity promotion. Challenges arise, however, in adopting these recommendations for use in rural America. Few studies of effectiveness of physical activity interventions have considered the disparities experienced by rural populations.

This chapter will review what we know about the context of, need for, and implementation of physical activity promotion efforts in rural America.

It will begin with a review of changing lifestyle and health in our rural communities and discuss the benefits of physical activity and exposure to natural environments. The chapter will then present data on physical activity in modern American life with a focus on rural communities. The chapter will conclude with a review of the basis for current physical activity promotion recommendations and present an important case example of their adaptation for use in the rural and isolated community of Cuba, New Mexico.

Key Concepts

Early in the twentieth century, rural America was the center of American life. It was home to the majority of Americans and was the source of food and fiber for the nation's sustenance and commerce. Most rural people survived and earned wages through agriculture. The typical rural community in 1900 consisted of a small town or village with numerous small farms within a few miles. Most people lived their lives and fulfilled most of their needs, economic and otherwise, within this community. They had little contact outside their local community (US Department of Agriculture, Economic Research Service, 1995).

Rural America has changed dramatically since that time. The rural economy in particular has shifted from a dependence on farming, forestry, and mining to a striking diversity of economic activity. Roads and the automobile have created connection between rural areas and cities. Improvements in communication and transportation have reduced rural isolation and removed many cultural differences. Radio, television, phone service, and the Internet, along with improved transportation, have increasingly blurred the distinctions between urban and rural life.

As these changes were taking place, rural America became home to a smaller share of the US population. And although rural America continues to provide most of the nation's food and fiber, it has taken on additional roles such as providing labor for industry; land for agribusiness, natural resource extraction, and other industry; services for commercial and noncommercial through traffic; creating retirement communities; and providing natural settings for recreation and enjoyment.

Despite rural America's new roles, the loss of population has undermined economic opportunity and community infrastructure (Tarmann, 2003). A vigorous physical lifestyle, once central to rural America, has become a victim of the evolution as well.

Metabolic and Cardiovascular Health in Rural America

Persons living in rural areas have higher rates of mortality, chronic disease, and disability than those living in urban areas (Jones et al., 2009). According to the 2006 National Health Interview Survey (US Department of Health and Human Services, 2006), adults in nonmetro households reported higher rates of hypertension, heart disease, and stroke than those in metro (more than one million residents) areas.

Between 1980 and 2006, the number of Americans with diabetes has tripled (CDC, 2011) and has been called a national epidemic. The Hispanic and Native American populations, disproportionately represented in rural areas, have even higher rates of diabetes than the overall population (CDC, 2010; National Diabetes Education Program, 2009).

Obesity, a known precursor to cardiovascular disease and diabetes, is more prevalent among rural American adults (Jackson et al., 2005). Physical inactivity, a major contributor to unhealthy energy balance and consequent obesity, is also more common in rural America (Joens-Matre et al., 2008; Patterson et al., 2004). These statistics are even more striking when one considers the rise in overall childhood obesity rates since 1990. In 2007 to 2008, 17 percent of children and adolescents two to nineteen years of age were reported to be obese (Ogden et al., 2010). This report notes that child and adolescent obesity tracks to adulthood and in the short term leads to psychosocial problems and cardiovascular risk factors such as high blood pressure, high cholesterol, abnormal glucose tolerance, and diabetes. Obesity is more common in low-income populations such as those in 444 nonmetro counties with levels of poverty greater than 20 percent (Tarmann, 2003).

Obesity, a known precursor to cardiovascular disease and diabetes, is more prevalent among rural American adults.

Health Benefits of Physical Activity and Exposure to Nature

Healthy energy balance (defined by the type and quantity of food and amount of physical activity) improves indicators of metabolic and cardiovascular health. Physical activity alone, even without dietary change, has been demonstrated to improve many facets of health. A government report (US Department of Health and Human Services, (2008b) highlights the current evidence supporting the benefits of physical activity.

All-cause mortality (death rate from all causes) is 30 percent lower among most active compared with least active adults, with a clear dose-response (the greater the activity level, the lower the death rate) relationship. The most active adults have a 20 to 35 percent drop in risk of coronary heart disease, cerebrovascular disease, stroke, hypertension, and atherogenic dyslipidemia (cholesterol disorders causing arterial blockage), with similar effect among all ages and both sexes. Active adults have a 30 to 40 percent lower risk of developing diabetes when compared to sedentary peers, with a clear dose-response relationship and similar effect among all ages and both sexes.

There is strong evidence that physical activity maintains current weight, promotes weight loss when combined with a calorie-restricted diet, and prevents weight regain after loss. It also has been shown to reduce the quantity of abdominal and intra-abdominal fat. There are other demonstrated benefits of physical activity on musculoskeletal health, functional health, cancer incidence, and mental health, including cognitive function among elderly persons (Etgen et al., 2010).

There is also accumulating evidence that any activity performed outdoors or in view of a natural environment can have positive effects on one's quality of life. Cognitive function, particularly in children (including sustained attention and interest and improved problem solving), can be improved by having a nearby natural environment (McCurdy et al., 2010; Wells, 2000).

Mood and self-esteem have also been shown to improve as a result of exposure to the natural environment (Barton & Pretty, 2010). Men had the most dramatic improvement in mood, whereas youth and the mentally ill had the most improvement in measures of self-esteem.

Reduction in stress and anxiety, irritability and anger, accident rate, and employee illnesses as a result of natural exposure have also been demonstrated in various studies summarized by Barton and Pretty (2010).

Physical Activity by Americans: Recommendations and Reality

The preponderance of evidence for the positive health effects of physical activity has led to the formulation of guidelines for intensity, duration, and frequency of its use by Americans. Current guidance, the *2008 Physical Activity Guidelines for Americans* (US Department of Health and Human Services, 2008b), calls for unimpaired adults to engage in at least 2.5 hours of moderate intensity (3.0 to 5.9 units of energy expenditure or metabolic equivalent task [MET]; for example, walking at three miles per hour = 3.3 METs) or 1.25 hours of vigorous intensity (6.0 or more METs; for example, running a ten-minute mile = 10.0 METs) aerobic physical activity per week. Activity is beneficial, even if divided into intervals as small as ten minutes (US Department of Health and Human Services, 2008a, 2008b). The *Healthy People 2010* objectives (United States Department of Health and Human Services, 2000) call for thirty minutes of moderate activity at least five days per week or a vigorous twenty-minute workout three times weekly.

The American College of Sports Medicine recently issued similar guidelines for individuals with non-insulin dependent diabetes mellitus: 150 minutes per week of moderate or vigorous aerobic exercise spread out over at least three days per week with no more than two consecutive days between bouts of activity (American College of Sports Medicine and the American Diabetes Association, 2010).

Following issuance of the 2008 national recommendations, a CDC telephone survey (2008) showed only 64.5 percent of adults physically active by the new criteria and only 48.8 percent active by the *Healthy People 2010* criteria. The publication editors indicated a low response rate indicating that even these numbers may be an overestimate.

The rising proportions of rural people who are unable or unwilling to engage in recommended physical activity prompts several questions: what are the barriers to a return to a more active rural lifestyle? How can they be addressed? Who should address them?

What are the barriers to a return to a more active rural lifestyle? How can they be addressed? Who should address them?

A Rural Example

Sufficient evidence is available to recommend physical activity strategies for all Americans. This evidence has been translated into recommendations by the Task Force on Community Preventive Services and published as guidelines in the *Morbidity and Mortality Weekly Report* (Increasing physical activity, 2001) and the *American Journal of Preventive Medicine* (Kahn et al., 2002). Despite national dissemination of this guidance, there is little documentation of the implementation of these strategies in more remote and isolated communities, especially those with high rates of obesity and related chronic diseases. A project in Cuba, New Mexico, Step Into Cuba (the project), has been underway since 2008 and provides an important case example for adapting the guidelines for rural use. The project is operated by a 501(c)3 nonprofit organization, the Nacimiento Community Foundation, which offers a diverse array of health and community service programs. In addition to Step Into Cuba, the Foundation operates a farmer's market, community garden, food pantry, case management services, financial literacy training, and a program providing shelter, prescription medication, and utility assistance.

Evaluation of the project is underway by the University of New Mexico Prevention Research Center (UNM PRC). Together with the project's steering committee, the Step Into Cuba Alliance, the UNM PRC is prospectively evaluating the CDC recommendations adapted for use in the project. The UNM PRC has a particular interest in how to link research to practice and policy through the study of translation, dissemination, and implementation processes.

The primary site of the project is the Village of Cuba, New Mexico, and its surrounding, highly scenic natural environment. This community shares many of the same characteristics as other rural communities throughout the Southwest. In 2000, the Village and surrounding area had a total population of about 1,700. The population is tricultural (67 percent Hispanic, 17 percent Native American, and 16 percent Anglo), disproportionately low income, and is similar to many municipalities in New Mexico where, in 2000, a quarter of the population lived in villages of less than 2,500 (US Census Bureau, 2000). Eighty percent of the study area's residents ($n = 1,350$) live in a census block where, in 1999, 32 percent of the population lived below the poverty level compared to 18 percent of New Mexico residents (US Census Bureau, 2000, 2008). As in many small communities, people in Cuba experience limited transportation, long travel distances, limited access to recreational facilities and activities, language and cultural diversity, harsh climate, and high unemployment, all of which increase the need for services, compound the difficulty of providing services, and contribute to the known disparities in health status.

Lifestyle in Cuba, New Mexico, has changed dramatically in the last two generations, and outdoor activity, once central to subsistence, is now increasingly absent in people's lives. Disproportionately high rates of obesity and the related problems of metabolic syndrome, diabetes, hyperlipidemia, atherosclerotic cardiovascular disease, and osteoarthritis underscore the need for introduction or re-introduction of physical activity through the Step Into Cuba project.

Campaigns and Informational Approaches to Increase Physical Acivity

Community-wide Campaigns

The community guide review of ten published research studies that focused on communitywide campaigns identified sufficient evidence to support a "strongly recommended" designation. Specifically, communitywide campaigns are described as large-scale, high-intensity, communitywide campaigns with sustained high visibility that include messages regarding physical activity behavior that are promoted through television, radio, newspaper columns and inserts, and trailers in movie theaters.

Successful interventions were multicomponent and included support and self-help groups, physical activity counseling, risk factor screening and education, community events, and creation of walking trails. The task force evaluated these interventions as a combined package because separating out the incremental benefit of each component was impossible (Increasing physical activity, 2001).

The Step Into Cuba project included a community-wide campaign as one of the approaches to promoting physical activity. However, this rural community has no local television, radio stations, or movie theatres. *The Cuba News*, the local paper, is published once a month. Therefore, most of the activities included in the studies reviewed by the task force were thought to be inappropriate for the local community. Instead, the project has adapted the approach in several ways. Articles and inserts are included in the *Cuba News* along with photographs of local activities. Although the newspaper is published only once each month it has a wide readership reaching most of the local population. Additionally, the partnership with the UNM PRC provided access to the necessary resources to develop and maintain a website that features and promotes Step Into Cuba. The website is on the homepage of the computers at the Cuba library and is accessible at local schools, homes, and workplaces. The site was initiated in May 2009, and in 2010 experienced 66,303 requests for 28,663 of its pages. In the first year of the project the UNM Health Sciences Center produced a YouTube video on the new walking trails and walking groups in Cuba. The project implemented additional forms of promotional activities including posters, fliers, signs, walking maps, newsletters, informational kiosks promoting physical activity and use of the nearby Continental Divide National Scenic Trail, and planning meetings open to the community.

Behaviorial and Social Approaches to Increase Physical Activity

Social Support Interventions in Community Settings

The community guide review of nine published research studies regarding social support identified enough evidence to again support a "strongly recommended" category for this approach. The emphasis of recommended social support is to build, strengthen, and maintain social networks that provide participants supportive relationships to enhance and reinforce routine physical activity.

The project selected this intervention and has implemented it with independent funding obtained from the CDC and the New Mexico Department of Health. A contract supports a healthy communities coordinator who also serves as the local walking champion. The walking champion organizes, leads, and empowers walking groups and promotes group activity as part of the community campaign. She has found particular groups to be most receptive to walking together: Cuba Senior Center "regulars," employee groups (e.g., school staff, clinic staff, governmental office staffs), and student participants of a summer fitness camp organized by the champion. Physical activities other than walking are substituted when walking is not possible due to inclement weather. For example the walking group from the local senior center will participate in indoor games, yoga, and other activities when walking outside is impractical.

Individually Adapted Health Behavior Change Programs

The community guide review of eighteen published research studies of individually adapted health behavior changes identified sufficient evidence to support a "strongly recommended" category for this approach as well. Specifically, reviewed interventions included programs tailored to the person's readiness for change or specific interests. These interventions are designed to assist participants with incorporating physical activity into their daily routines by teaching them key behavioral skills, such as the following:

- Goal setting and self-monitoring
- Building social support
- Behavioral reinforcement through self-reward and positive self-talk
- Structured problem solving
- Relapse prevention

The interventions reviewed involved interaction in group settings or by mail, telephone, or directed media. The Step Into Cuba project selected this approach and chose as its primary focus a strategy of physical activity prescription or referrals by local practitioners, in part because of presence of a physician champion at Cuba's only health clinic. Prescription Trails, a program operated by several New Mexico municipalities, and promoted by the New Mexico Department of Health, was adapted for use in Cuba's rural setting. The Prescription Trails model focuses on making use of city parks and open spaces for physical activity. Because of the paucity of convenient walking venues and the time demands on the health care providers in the busy rural practice, the project chose to modify the program to include "referral trails." The principle is to encourage walking through motivational clinic counseling and follow up with a referral to the walking champion for additional counseling and individual planning and reinforcement of a walking program. Medical precautions and patient general goals are conveyed to the champion at the time of referral.

Environmental and Policy Approaches to Increase Physical Activity

Enhanced Access to Places for Physical Activity

The community guide review of twelve published research studies on the creation or enhancement of places for physical activity, combined with informational outreach, identified sufficient evidence to categorize this approach as "strongly recommended." This intervention is described as creating or enhancing access to places for physical activity by building trails or facilities or by reducing barriers to such places. Some of the programs reviewed also provide training in using equipment and incentives and health education.

In 2008 the Cuba area had very few attractive places to walk. The high school had an outdoor track that was fenced and not accessible after school hours. The school complex also has several miles of cross-country trails on adjacent public land that are partially fenced and have never been used for public recreation. The county fairgrounds had roadways that were fenced and unavailable to the public. City streets and state highways had no sidewalks. The five-lane highway (US Highway 550) that bisects the community has partial sidewalks but they are narrow and are not set back from the curb, making them hazardous and unpleasant for walking when large or speeding vehicles travel the two outer lanes. In the winter, US Highway 550 also has no location for cleared snow, leaving sidewalks blocked and impassable. The city park has a community center with a weight room, cardiovascular exercise room, and a gymnasium that can be accessed for a fee and have not been actively promoted. Given this selection of venues, it is not surprising that the Step Into Cuba Alliance saw much of Cuba's problem as the need for creating places to walk, including access points to its scenic surrounding federal lands.

The Village park has become a focal point of community efforts, which has spurred related activities such as support of a planning process for development of the park using community input and efforts of graduate students in landscape architecture from the University of New Mexico. A draft park plan is available for public review and comment on the Step Into Cuba website.

The county fairgrounds, one mile from the center of Cuba, has been another area of focus. A ten-year development plan is underway with leadership provided by the fairgrounds manager, a key Alliance member. Several miles of internal trails, campgrounds, RV parking, an indoor event arena, and a trailhead for the Continental Divide National Scenic Trail are among the current plans.

Another focal point has been the school campus where plans for more public use of the track, all-year use of an enclosed swimming pool, a safe-routes-to-school project, and use by the public of the cross-country trails are underway. A joint use policy is now in place.

In addition to improving existing places to walk, an impressive array of new trails has been constructed or is planned for construction. A one-mile walking path has been constructed by the Village of Cuba and Step Into Cuba volunteers and youth corps assignees around the perimeter of the city park. In order to make the path more attractive for walking, several hundred conservation seedlings, thirty-four transplanted conifers, eighty types of wildflowers, and one hundred deciduous trees, shrubs, and cacti have been planted and watered by volunteers, using a new drip irrigation system. Dozens of rocks and boulders have been relocated to the trail and two benches have been added for individuals who may need to rest while walking the path. Additional grant funds are being sought to construct an all-weather surface. A demonstration of various trail surface choices is on public display at the park in order to provide an opportunity for community members to give input as to their preferences.

A one-half-mile walking path has been constructed on village property adjacent to the city library, senior center, and low-income housing complex. The library trail has become a popular place for senior citizen and employer walking groups as well as residents of the housing units. Also, a one-quarter-mile path has been constructed by staff of the local health clinic and is used for brief activity during breaks and lunch hours.

A generous, private land donation to the Nacimiento Community Foundation has resulted in new public open space connecting the Village of Cuba to the nearest corner of the Santa Fe National Forest. A one mile trail has been constructed. This trail provides access to additional hiking opportunities on Cuba Mesa and the continental divide trail on national forest land and is becoming very popular with children and families (see Figure 16.1).

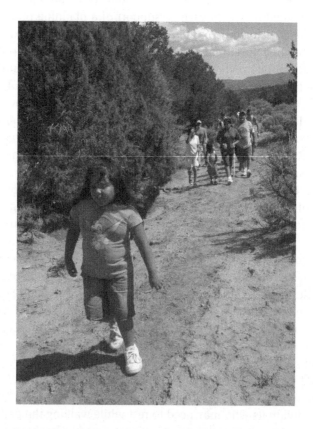

Figure 16.1. Hikers Follow the Fisher Trail Route Toward Cuba Mesa

Two potential new segments for the Continental Divide National Scenic Trail have been scouted, located by GPS readings, and mapped by the project volunteer coordinator with assistance from the Continental Divide Trail Alliance, a key Step Into Cuba Alliance partner, and the Santa Fe National Forest Cuba Ranger District. The proposed routes are undergoing environmental and cultural clearances during 2011. Completion of one or both of these segments should greatly enhance hiking by community members and visitors.

Street-Scale Design and Land Use Policies

The community guide review of six published research studies on street-scale urban design and land-use policies and practices to support physical activity identified sufficient evidence to support a recommendation for this approach. Reviewed interventions were multidisciplinary and involved planners, architects, engineers, developers, and public health professionals. Policy instruments used included building codes, roadway design standards, and environmental changes. Design components studied included street lighting, infrastructure projects to increase safety of street crossing, traffic-calming approaches (e.g. speed humps, traffic circles), and enhanced street landscaping.

The Step Into Cuba Alliance has promoted policy and environmental changes that would improve safe access to US Highway 550 as a venue for walking. A fortuitous development was selection of a Cuba sidewalk improvement project for funding by the New Mexico Department of Transportation in 2009. This decision, coupled with other efforts to improve Cuba's walkability, resulted in a half-day walkability workshop sponsored by the Step Into Cuba Alliance and supported by two critical Alliance partners: the UNM PRC and the US National Park Service Rivers, Trails, and Conservation Assistance program. As a result of the workshop and its walking audits, comprehensive recommendations for pedestrian enhancements were printed and distributed. Many of these recommendations related to the need to provide safe and attractive pedestrian connections between the emerging venues for physical activity previously described.

Alliance partners studied and participated in a regional planning process for pedestrian enhancements, including not only the funded sidewalk project but also five other proposed pedestrian walkway, crosswalk, and bikeway projects. Step Into Cuba developed all five proposals for the Village with the help of an external traffic planning consultant. The proposals have been submitted and accepted by the regional planning organization—the Mid-Region Council of Governments—and forwarded for consideration to the New Mexico Department of Transportation. The Alliance intends to remain an active player as these projects proceed through the administrative process and, if funded, their eventual development.

Point-of-Decision Prompts to Encourage Use of Stairs

The community guide review of six published research studies on point-of-decision prompts also identified sufficient evidence to support a "recommended" category for this approach. Point-of-decision prompts were limited to motivational signs placed close to elevators and escalators encouraging use of nearby stairs for health benefits or weight loss.

The Step Into Cuba project selected use of point-of-decision prompts as one of their interventions as well. However, there are no elevators or escalators and very few stairways in the Cuba area. This recommendation was adapted to include indoor and outdoor walking prompts that encourage people to walk for health or from one location (e.g., the post office) to another (e.g., the health clinic) instead of driving.

Conclusion

The health benefits of physical activity are well known and have become an important focus for health promotion in the United States. The increasing problem of overweight or obese Americans and their related chronic conditions underscores the need. **Evidence-based strategies** (approaches that have been shown effective by repeated scientific study) for increasing physical activity have been developed and recommended by the US Task Force on Community Preventive Services but much needs to be learned about their appropriateness and effectiveness in rural America. One comprehensive rural adaptation of the strategies is underway in Cuba, New Mexico, and under study by the University of New Mexico Prevention Research Center. It incorporates communitywide campaigns, point-of-decision prompts, social support, individually adapted health behavior change, enhanced access to places for physical activity combined with informational outreach, and street-scale urban design and land-use policies and practices. Additional studies of new and adapted strategies will be needed to guide future physical activity promotion in rural America.

Summary

- The transformation of the rural American lifestyle to one that requires less vigorous physical activity has compounded obesity, chronic disease, and disability rates of rural communities over time.

- Obesity and physical inactivity are more prevalent among rural American adults. Rural communities also report greater percentages of overweight and obese children, which are linked to a higher risk of adult obesity and related diseases.

- The obesity epidemic has prompted federal health guidelines for physical activity; however, few studies of effectiveness of physical activity interventions have been tailored to accommodate the disparities prevalent in a rural environment.

- The physical activity study conducted in Cuba, New Mexico, is a potential model of the adaptations necessary to foster a multifaceted approach in improving physical activity in a rural community.

For Practice and Discussion

1. Working with a colleague or two from your class, discuss how modernization has contributed to a decrease in physical activity in rural communities.

2. As a public health professional, how do you negotiate between evidence-based practice and tailoring an intervention to the needs and desires of a rural community?

Key Terms

evidence-based strategies

built environment

social support

individually adapted health behavior change

point-of-decision prompts

Acknowledgments

This publication was also supported by cooperative agreement (UNM PRC Grant) number 5U48DP001931 from the Centers for Disease Control and Prevention. The findings and conclusions in this article are those of the author(s) and do not necessarily represent the official position of the Centers for Disease Control and Prevention.

References

American College of Sports Medicine and the American Diabetes Association. (2010). Exercise and type 2 diabetes: American College of Sports Medicine and the American Diabetes Association: Joint position statement. *Medicine & Science in Sports & Exercise, 42*(12), 2282–2303.

Barton, J., & Pretty, J. (2010). What is the best dose of nature and green exercise for improving mental health? A multi-study analysis. *Environmental Science & Technology, 44*(10), 3947–3955.

CDC. (2005). *The guide to community preventive services: What works to promote health?* New York: Oxford University Press.

CDC. (2008). Prevalence of self-reported physically active adults—United States, 2007. *MMWR Morbidity and Mortality Weekly Report, 57*(48), 1297–1300.

CDC. (2010). *Trends in diabetes prevalence among American Indian and Alaska Native children, adolescents, and young Adults: 1990–1998.* Retrieved from http://www.cdc.gov/diabetes/pubs/factsheets/aian.htm

CDC. (2011). *Diabetes data and trends: Number (in millions) of civilian, non-institutionalized persons with diagnosed diabetes, United States, 1980–2009.* Retrieved from http://www.cdc.gov/diabetes/statistics/prev/national/figpersons.htm

Etgen, T., Sander, D., Huntgeburth, U., Poppert, H., Förstl, H., & Bickel, H. (2010). Physical activity and incident cognitive impairment in elderly persons: The INVADE study. *Archives of Internal Medicine, 170*(2), 186–193.

Increasing physical activity. A report on recommendations of the Task Force on Community Preventive Services. (2001). *MMWR Recommendations and Report, 50*(RR-18), 1–14.

Jackson, J. E., Doescher, M. P., Jerant, A. F., & Hart, L. G. (2005). A national study of obesity prevalence and trends by type of rural county. *Journal of Rural Health, 21*(2), 140–148.

Joens-Matre, R. R., Welk, G. J., Calabro, M. A., Russell, D. W., Nicklay, E., & Hensley, L. D. (2008). Rural-urban differences in physical activity, physical fitness, and overweight prevalence of children. *Journal of Rural Health, 24*(1), 49–54.

Jones, C. A., Parker, T. S., Ahearn, M., Mishra, A. K., & Variyam, J. N. (2009, August). *Health status and health care access of farm and rural populations* (ERS report summary). Washington, DC: US Department of Agriculture, Economic Research Service.

Kahn, E. B., Ramsey, L. T., Brownson, R. C., Heath, G. W., Howze, E. H., Powell, K. E., Stone, E. J., Rajab, M. W., & Corso, P. (2002). The effectiveness of interventions to increase physical activity. A systematic review. *American Journal of Preventive Medicine, 22*(4 Suppl.), 73–107.

McCurdy, L. E., Winterbottom, K. E., Mehta, S. S., & Roberts, J. R. (2010). Using nature and outdoor activity to improve children's health. *Pediatric and Adolescent Health Care, 40*(5), 102–117.

National Diabetes Education Program. (2009). *The diabetes epidemic among Hispanics/Latinos.* National Institute of Diabetes and Digestive and Kidney Diseases. Retrieved from http://www.diabetes.niddk.nih.gov/dm/pubs/statistics/

Ogden, C., Lamb, M., Carroll, M., & Flegal, K. (2010). Obesity and socioeconomic status in children and adolescents: United States, 2005–2008. *NCHS Data Brief, 51*, 1.

Patterson, P. D., Moore, C. G., Probst, J. C., & Shinogle, J. A. (2004). Obesity and physical inactivity in rural America. *Journal of Rural Health, 20*(2), 151–159.

Tarmann, A. (2003). *Fifty years of demographic change in rural America*. Retrieved from http://www.prb.org/Articles/2003/ FiftyYearsofDemographicChangeinRuralAmerica.aspx

US Census Bureau. (2000). *Urban/rural and metropolitan/nonmetropolitan population: 2000– state—urban/rural and inside/outside metropolitan area Census 2000 summary file 1 (SF 1) 100-percent data*. Retrieved from http://factfinder2 .census.gov/faces/tableservices/jsf/pages/productview.xhtml?pid = DEC_00_SF1 _GCTP1.US93&prodType = table

US Census Bureau. (2008). *US Census Bureau: State and county quick facts: New Mexico*. Retrieved from http://quickfacts.census.gov/qfd/states/35000.html

US Department of Agriculture, Economic Research Service. (1995). *Understanding rural America*. Washington, DC: Author.

US Department of Health and Human Services. (2000). *Healthy people 2010*. Washington, DC: Author.

US Department of Health and Human Services. (2006). *National health interview survey*. Retrieved from http://www.icpsr.umich.edu/icpsrweb/NACDA/ studies/20681/version/3

US Department of Health and Human Services. (2008a). *Physical activity guidelines Advisory Committee Report 2008*. Retrieved from http://www.health.gov/ paguidelines/committeereport.aspx

US Department of Health and Human Services. (2008b). *2008 physical activity guidelines for Americans*. Washington, DC: Author. Retrieved from http:// www.health.gov/paguidelines/pdf/paguide.pdf

Wells, N. M. (2000). At home with nature—effects of "greenness" on children's cognitive functioning. *Environment and Behavior, 32*(6), 775–795.

Chapter 17

Preventing Farm-Related Injuries
The Example of Tractor Overturns

Henry P. Cole
Susan C. Westneat

Learning Objectives

- Understand the significance of tractor overturns regarding injury and death.
- Articulate the value of forming community partnerships and community-based committees before planning and implementing intervention approaches for farmers.
- Describe the value of using theoretical approaches to achieving behavior change among farmers.
- Identify key attributes of effective intervention methods with farmers at risk of injury.

• • •

One unique aspect of rural life is the use of the land to grow crops or raise livestock, which provides families with incomes. Although farming is not a universal practice in rural America, it is done by millions of people. Unfortunately, farm accidents tend to be common thus creating a threat to rural public health that is quite special. A particularly deadly type of farm accident involves tractor overturns. This chapter describes a farm population at high risk for tractor overturn injuries and a collaborative partnership between farm community members and university researchers that resulted in a hazard reduction for these types of injury.

Farmers in Kentucky and five nearby states located in central Appalachia experience tractor overturn death rates greater than 9.8 per one hundred thousand workers per year, the highest in the nation. Farms in these six states account for only 8.4 percent of US farmland acres but for 19.0 percent of all US farms, 19.8 percent of all US farm tractors, 21.3 percent of US farms with less than 180 acres, 20.3 percent of US farms with annual value of sales less than $10,000, and 20.1 percent of US farms where the operator works an off-farm job more than two hundred days per year (Cole, McKnight, & Donovan, 2009). Many farm tractors in this six-state region lack a simple device called a rollover protective structure (ROPS) or roll bar that when installed is 98 percent effective in preventing operator deaths during tractor overturns (Murphy et al., 2010). Kentucky farmers' demographics make them particularly vulnerable to tractor overturn injuries. For example, 67.3 percent have annual sales of farm products less than $10,000 and 42.2 percent of principal farm operators work at off-farm jobs fewer than two hundred days per year. For 51.0 percent of Kentucky farms the combined value of their tractors and all other equipment is less than $20,000 (Cole et al., 2009).

Many farm tractors in this six-state region lack a simple device called a rollover protective structure (ROPS) or roll bar that when installed is 98 percent effective in preventing operator deaths during tractor overturns

Key Concepts

Leveraging behavior change is an extremely difficult task, one that may be compounded greatly when the target audience is composed of farmers (a traditional independent and isolated population in the United States). The intervention methods used in this study of tractor overturns are broadly applicable to other intervention challenges with US farmers, thus the expanded example may be quite useful to anyone working in the field of injury prevention in rural public health. Key features of this successful intervention directed toward rural farmers include (1) forming community partnerships and community committees, (2) developing replicable printed intervention materials, (3) predicating the program on surveillance findings, (4) using behavioral theory to guide intervention planning and design, (5) use of mass media in highly creative ways, (6) use of hands-on and highly interactive learning activities, and (7) use of motivational techniques such photos of overturned tractors.

The Community Partners ROPS Project

In October 1996, the researchers were awarded a three-year cooperative agreement as part of the National Institute for Occupational Safety and Health (NIOSH) Community Partners for Healthy Farming (CPHF) Initiative. The goal was to develop an intervention program to promote farmers retrofitting unprotected tractors with ROPS or replacing them with newer ROPS-equipped tractors. In April 1996, four counties were randomly selected from sixty central Kentucky farming counties. Two of the four were randomly assigned to the intervention condition and two to the control. Following funding in October 1996, a ROPS-promotion program was implemented in the two intervention counties across the three-year project period (Cole & Westneat, 2001).

The goal was to develop an intervention program to promote farmers retrofitting unprotected tractors with ROPS or replacing them with newer ROPS-equipped tractors.

The Community Partners

In November and December 1996, research team members identified and engaged key farm community leaders from forty local community groups and farm service agencies in the two intervention counties. These partners represented tractor equipment dealerships, banks, farm insurance agencies, farm producer organizations, the Farm Bureau, farm supply businesses, local and regional manufacturing plants that employed part-time farmers, hospitals and health care providers, local newspapers, locally owned AM radio stations, television stations, and rural electric cooperatives. Throughout the project, this array of community partners collaborated in developing, disseminating, revising, and evaluating the community intervention program. The partners suggested developing short and engaging messages that made good use of graphics and community stories accompanied by simple hands-on activities. They noted that equipping unprotected tractors with ROPS provides peace of mind and makes good business sense. The partners also suggested that incentive funds, even if relatively small, were needed to stimulate farmers' purchase of ROPS retrofit kits (Cole & Westneat, 2001).

The Workshops

Community-partner committees (small groups of key leaders) were established in each intervention county. Thereafter, the two intervention county committees, located 184 miles apart, worked separately. Public health nurses Brandt and Muehlbauer, each of whom resided adjacent to one of the two intervention counties, arranged monthly meetings between University of

Kentucky (UK) research team members and community partners. In each intervention county, the UK public health nurse and community partner leaders met on a weekly basis. Over the three-year period a series of two-hour workshops also were conducted, occasionally on the UK campus but more often at the Farm Bureau and agricultural extension offices in the two intervention counties. Typically four to eight community partners, three or four UK researchers, and occasionally one or two of the National Institute for Occupational Safety and Health (NIOSH) program officers attended the workshops.

The Kentucky ROPS Notebook

Over the project period, ten sets of easy-to-use community education messages and activities were collaboratively produced. The collection became known as the *Kentucky ROPS notebook* (Cole et al., 2004). Early and incomplete versions of the notebook were produced in hard copy and CD formats in 1997, 1998, and 1999. Multiple copies were distributed to community partners in the two intervention counties. Each notebook activity included a tips page that described the intended learning outcomes and suggestions for engaging participants in active dialogue and hands-on learning as opposed to lecturing or making formal presentations. The notebook was updated again in 2001 and became available online via the NIOSH National Agricultural Safety Database (NASD, 2011).

The program materials were based on injury surveillance data for fatal, nonfatal injury, and noninjury tractor overturn events for non-ROPS and ROPS-equipped tractors. The case materials were drawn from four sources:

- Statewide Kentucky tractor-overturn fatality investigations conducted by the UK Injury Prevention and Research Center (KIPRC) as part of the NIOSH national Fatality Assessment and Control Evaluation (FACE) project
- Tractor overturn stories in the two intervention counties as reported by local and regional equipment dealers, emergency medical staff, newspapers, radio, and television media
- Similar tractor overturn stories from a ten-year compilation of national press clipping
- Personal tractor overturn stories told by the farmers who attended the intervention county meetings and workshops

Theoretical Approach

Development of the ROPS notebook messages and activities was guided by three theories. The first is the conceptual model shown in Figure 17.1 that

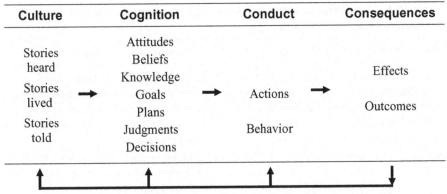

Culture	Cognition	Conduct	Consequences
Stories heard	Attitudes		
	Beliefs		Effects
	Knowledge		
Stories lived →	Goals →	Actions →	
	Plans		Outcomes
Stories told	Judgments	Behavior	
	Decisions		

Feedback loops by which consequences of individuals' actions modify conduct, cognition, and socio-cultural norms

Figure 17.1. A Sociocultural, Cognitive, and Behavioral Psychology Model of How Health Beliefs and Behaviors Are Learned
Source: Adapted from Cole (1997, 2002).

integrates behavioral, cognitive, sociocultural, and narrative psychology explanations of human behavior (Bruner, 1990; Cole, 1997, 2002; Sarbin, 1986). The second a set of well-known behavioral theories and principles, includes the **theory of reasoned action** and its adaptation by Witte's (1992) **extended parallel process model,** which combines fear appeals with personal **self-efficacy** messages and **response efficacy** messages, in this case the injury prevention effectiveness of ROPS. This combination produces public health campaign messages that promote individuals' reasoned (logical) actions to prevent a potential injury (Morgan et al., 2002; Witte, 1992; Witte & Allen, 2000). The third is Pavio's (1971) **dual-coding theory,** the idea that human brains have two primary modes for processing information, one by language and the other by images. Simple images and short narratives that simultaneously convey congruent information promote rapid processing, deeper understanding, and better retention of message content.

The project community education messages and activities that compose the ROPS notebook are summarized in Table 17.1.

Mass Communication Messages

Each of the one hundred public service announcements (PSAs) is a six- to eight-line story that can be read aloud in thirty seconds. Some PSAs are stories told by individuals who overturned a ROPS tractor and survived and others

Table 17.1. The Kentucky ROPS Notebook Mass Communication Messages and Interactive Learning Activities

Mass Communication Messages	Community Meeting Activities
• Radio public service announcements (PSAs) about tractor overturn injuries and the injury protection provided by ROPS and seatbelts (one hundred each of thirty seconds duration)	• Mr. Good Egg Farmer scale model tractor overturn demonstration using a hen's raw eggs as simulated operators on non-ROPS and ROPS-equipped scale model tractors
• Newspaper stories about tractor overturns each about a half-page in length (twenty published in local papers)	• Examination and discussion of seven 8 × 10-inch color photos of fatal and nonfatal tractor overturns
• Charts, posters, and photographs about the injury outcomes from tractor overturns with and without ROPS (fifteen sets widely duplicated and displayed)	• Skits role-played by community partner farmers that re-created authentic dialogues about tractor overturn close call events and decisions related to obtaining ROPS
• A trifold flier that listed tractor equipment dealers' contact information and tractor features needed by the dealer to order a ROPS (ten thousand copies distributed)	• Facts and figures about tractor overturn injuries and their prevention by ROPS; a series of simple graphs and illustrations were widely displayed as posters and also used in presentations at community meetings
• Envelope stuffer messages; each combined a graphic illustration and a short narrative about overturns of non-ROPS and ROPS-equipped tractors and the injury outcomes and consequences—fifteen stuffers with local sponsors' bylines listed at the bottom (one hundred thousand copies distributed)	• Five interactive simulation exercises about non-ROPS and ROPS-equipped tractor overturns wherein as the story progressed the participants made decisions about the story characters' actions and then learned the consequences of those decisions

are shared by family members of farmers who were injured or died in overturns. Stories also were contributed by individuals involved in the rescue and treatment of farmers injured in tractor overturns as well as by those involved in the recovery of fatally injured farmers. Many of the stories describe the profound grief and economic consequences following a disabling injury or death that resulted in a broken family and loss of a farm and way of life. Other PSAs described the circumstances that motivated farmers to equip their tractors with ROPS, often following an overturn by a spouse or other family member who narrowly escaped injury or was injured or killed. Some PSAs promoted the relative low cost of a ROPS retrofit kit, for example, by comparing the $780 total cost associated with a $3.00 purchase of a soft drink and snack at a local convenience store, five days a week for a year.

Intervention county AM radio station computer logs revealed that the one hundred thirty-second PSAs were broadcast multiple times a day in conjunction with daily farm market and weather reports. New PSAs were mixed with older messages as they were developed throughout the project. Individual PSAs also were included as print messages in local newsletters and similar publications. Sometimes a few PSAs were selected, printed, and distributed to individuals who attended community meetings. At intervals during the meeting those individuals stood and read aloud their PSAs.

Reporters in the two intervention counties wrote twenty-six stories that were published in the farm sections of local newspapers. The stories described cases in which farmers debated retrofitting a tractor with a ROPS, their reasons for obtaining a ROPS, and the process of finding and installing a ROPS. Other stories described overturns in which a ROPS prevented an injury. Some stories described the peace of mind achieved by installing ROPS because of the injury protection provided for family members who drive tractors.

Twelve other stories are first-person accounts about non-ROPS tractor overturns that resulted in severely disabling injuries or death. These stories often were read aloud at community gatherings by the severely injured survivor or by a family member of the deceased. The individuals involved provided written permission for inclusion of their verbatim stories in the notebook.

Other notebook stories were pre-scripted skits developed from authentic farmer dialogues about tractor overturn close calls, injuries, and decisions related to obtaining ROPS. Dyads of individuals attending community meetings were each given different skits. Each pair of actors read aloud the skit dialogue and role-played their skit's characters.

A trifold pocket pamphlet titled "How to Get a ROPS and Seatbelt on Your Tractor" was developed for each county by intervention county equipment dealers, insurance agents, and bankers and widely disseminated. Each pamphlet listed the contact information for all the farm tractor dealers in that county as well as the local banks that offered low-interest loans for ROPS purchases. A three-panel worksheet prompted the farmer to gather and write down the tractor information needed prior to meeting with an equipment dealer. Another panel listed reasons for obtaining ROPS (e.g., one-third of all fatal or disabling injuries from non-ROPS tractor overturns result in loss of the farm; a ROPS is like a life insurance policy with a one-time payment that protects all who drive the tractor). Approximately ten thousand copies of the pamphlet were duplicated and widely distributed in both counties by many farm businesses, service agencies, and also by manufacturing plants that

If this happened to your son. . .

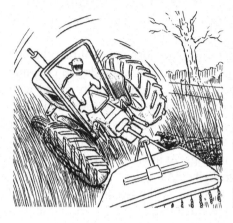

Wouldn't you want him on a ROPS-equipped tractor?

Wouldn't you hope he was wearing the seat belt?

Set a good example! Protect your loved ones and yourself. Get a ROPS and buckle up!

ROPS are available for most tractors at local equipment dealers, usually for less than $1000 including shipping and installation.

A message from _____ [Name of organization] _____

and the Community Partners for Healthy Farming Project

Figure 17.2. Example of a Graphic and Narrative Stuffer Message

printed and distributed copies to their employees, many of whom were part-time farmers.

Approximately one hundred thousand copies of the fifteen envelope-stuffer messages that paired a simple graphic image with a short narrative were distributed throughout the intervention counties by agencies and companies that routinely sent mail to farmers (see Figure 17.2). The stuffers also were distributed as countertop handouts by those same groups. A line at the bottom of each stuffer message included the statement, "A message from___," followed by the name of a local farm business or service provider (Morgan et al., 2002).

Hands-on Activities

The Mr. Good Egg Farmer activity used two scale model tractors, one with a ROPS and seatbelt and the other with no ROPS and no seatbelt. Participants were placed in small groups. Each group was given a hen's raw egg, asked to draw a face on the egg, and then to name their Mr. Good Egg. Each group then drew straws. Groups that drew long straws placed and secured their Mr. Good Egg farmers on a ROPS-equipped model tractor. Groups that drew short straws placed their unbelted Mr. Good Eggs on a non-ROPS model tractor. In turn, the model tractors were run up a ramp onto a simulated stream bank that collapsed resulting in an overturn. The belted eggs on the ROPS tractor

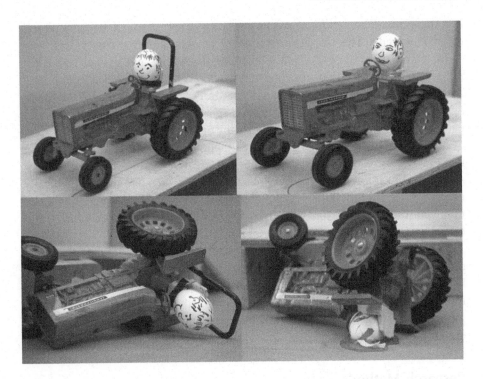

Figure 17.3. The Mr. Good Egg Farmer Demonstration of ROPS and non-ROPS Model Tractor Overturns

were not damaged. The unbelted eggs on the non-ROPS tractors were crushed (see Figure 17.3). Farmers found the demonstration to be sobering and convincing that ROPS and seatbelts avert overturn injuries.

Photos of fatal and nonfatal tractor overturns were another widely used hands-on activity. Groups of three to five individuals were given one 8 × 10-inch color photo of an overturned tractor. Some photos were of overturns where a ROPS had stopped a lateral overturn at approximately 90 to 115 degrees with the tractor on its side. Other photos showed rear overturns of ROPS tractors where the ROPS had stopped the overturn at approximately 90 degrees with the tractor's front end pointing straight up in the air. In both cases the tractor steering wheels, seats, and operator compartments were undamaged. Other photos of non-ROPS tractors overturns showed tractors that were completely upside down with their wheels facing upward following either a 180-degree lateral roll or backward flip. In these cases the operator's compartment, seat, and steering wheel were crushed beneath the tractor. No bodies were shown. The fatal overturn photos were selected from Kentucky FACE investigations. The nonfatal overturn photos were supplied by agricultural extension agents, farmers, farm equipment dealers, and first responders.

Each small group was asked to examine one photo and answer two questions; "What do you think happened here?" and "What were the consequences?" After a five-minute examination and discussion each group displayed the photo and shared their conjectures with the whole group. After all groups had reported, each individual small group was given a copy of the fifty- to sixty-word summary of the formal field investigation for the photo they had examined. Group members then read and discussed the investigative report. The groups then shared and examined all seven photos and the investigative reports. Typically every farmer present knew personally multiple individuals who had been involved in tractor overturns, many that resulted in no or minor injuries and others that resulted in serious injury or death.

The photos and their accompanying short investigative reports also were duplicated and displayed as posters at the nine tractor equipment dealerships in the two intervention counties and elsewhere as well. The dealers reported that the photos and investigative reports grabbed farmers' attention and promoted discussions about obtaining ROPS for unprotected tractors (Struttmann et al., 2001).

Research Methods

The Kentucky farm tractor telephone survey was cooperatively designed and administered under a contractual agreement with the National Agricultural Statistics Service, Kentucky field office (KY-NASS). Four counties were randomly selected from among sixty central Kentucky counties. Two were assigned to the intervention condition and two as controls. KY-NASS statisticians then constructed a sampling frame of 4,422 farms stratified by farm acres and annual value of sales that included 79.3 percent of the total farms in the four counties. In January 1997 the preintervention survey was administered and completed by 1,648 randomly sampled farm operators. In January 2000 following the intervention 1,227 of the original farmers surveyed completed the postintervention survey, a 74.5 percent response rate. Both surveys gathered information about the number of ROPS and non-ROPS tractors on each farm. Additional items on the second survey asked farmers if they had obtained ROPS retrofit kits and ROPS-equipped tractors since January 1997 and if so from what source or sources. Table 17.2 provides the sampling frame details.

Just prior to the intervention activities that began in February 1997 we visited each of the equipment dealers in the two intervention counties and inquired about the number of ROPS retrofit kits they had sold in 1996, the year prior to the project. The nine dealers reported they had sold a combined total of only four ROPS. They also agreed to meet with us at their sales

Table 17.2. Number (1,227) and Percent of Farms Included in the 1997 Pre- and 2000 Postintervention Surveys by County with Respect to the 1997 Census of Agriculture 5,577 Total Farms and the KY-NASS Sampling Frame of 4,422 Farms

Data Source	01 Barren	02 Fleming	03 Hardin	04 Nelson	Total farms
Farms 1997 USDA census	1,818	1,063	1,480	1,216	5,577
Tractors 1997 USDA census	3,443	2,005	3,056	2,521	11,025
Mean tractors per farm	1.89	1.89	2.06	2.07	1.98
Farms included in the KY-NASS sampling frame	1,444	765	1,264	949	4,422
Total farms surveyed pre and post	301	283	322	321	1,227
Percent of farms included within the KY-KASS sampling frame	20.8	37.0	25.5	33.8	27.7
Percent of farms included within the 1997 USDA Census of Agriculture	16.6	26.7	23.0	26.4	22.0

Source: USDA (1997).

offices every two months to provide an ongoing record of their ROPS retrofit kit sales throughout the three-year project. Control county dealers were not contacted.

Additional program impact and evaluation methods used within the two intervention counties throughout the intervention period included the following:

- Interviews of nine manufacturing companies' employers who through their human resource and safety programs delivered the ROPS project campaign messages to their employees, many of whom were part-time farmers (Brandt et al., 2001)
- Collection of local newspaper articles about ROPS
- Radio station logs of PSA broadcasts
- Recording the numbers of graphic stuffers distributed
- Data compiled from a one-page, eighteen-item outreach and event and activity reporting form that was completed on a weekly basis by the community partners (the two UK public health nurses and the UK researchers)

The event categories on the outreach form included presentations, group activities, community meetings, displays and posters, and news articles. The form documented the date and location of the event, its purpose, number of individuals attending, the number and affiliations of the community partner leaders involved in planning and hosting the event, as well as estimates of their time to prepare and conduct the event, plus additional costs related to duplicating and distributing materials (Cole & Westneat, 2001).

Results

Results are reported in two sections. The first section describes the increase in ROPS-equipped tractors in intervention counties 01 and 02 compared to county 03, the one true control county. County 04, although planned as a control, became an intervention county after the John Deere dealer in that county mounted his own ROPS promotion effort following the non-ROPS tractor overturn death of one of his customers in early 1997 (Myers, Cole, & Westneat, 2005). The second section describes intervention counties' 01 and 02 use of the CPHF ROPS project messages and activities. The data reported in both sections are summarized from the Kentucky ROPS project final report (Cole & Westneat, 2001). Three different data sources were used to estimate the increase in ROPS-equipped tractors in intervention and control counties.

Postintervention Interviews

The data in Table 17.3 were derived from the postintervention interviews of the sample of 1,227 farmers in the intervention and control counties. Rows one through three of this table list each individual county's pre- to postintervention increase in ROPS-equipped tractors including ROPS retrofits and newer ROPS-equipped tractors that were purchased for the protection provided by the ROPS. Rows four and five reveal that counties 02 and 04 had respectively a 20.8 percent and 20.6 percent increase in ROPS tractors acquired for the protective value of the ROPS. The 95 percent confidence intervals in row five indicate that these two counties had a significant increase in ROPS ($p < .05$) compared to the true control county 03 and to intervention county 01. Row six lists the newer ROPS-equipped tractors acquired for features other than the ROPS. The 95 percent confidence intervals in row seven reveal no significant difference across the four counties. Row eight lists the total number of ROPS tractors acquired by each county and row nine the respective 95 percent confidence intervals. Only county 04, where a John Deere dealer mounted his own ROPS campaign, had a statistically significant ($p < .05$) increase in total ROPS tractors acquired.

Table 17.3. Number of Farms Surveyed (1,227) Across Counties Pre- and Postintervention by Percent of ROPS Retrofits and ROPS Replacement Tractors Purchased for the ROPS and Percent of ROPS Tractors Purchased for Features Other Than the ROPS

Kentucky County	01 Barren	02 Fleming	03 Hardin	04 Nelson
Number of farms surveyed	301	283	322	321
• Number of ROPS retrofits	15 (5.0%)	27 (9.5%)	8 (2.5%)	33 (10.3%)
• Number of ROPS tractors acquired for the ROPS	10 (3.3%)	15 (5.3%)	8 (2.5%)	7 (2.2%)
• Number of ROPS tractors acquired for the ROPS plus other features	18 (6.0%)	17 (6.0%)	19 (5.9%)	26 (8.1%)
• Total tractors acquired for the ROPS	43 (14.3%)	59 (20.8%)	35 (10.9%)	66 (20.6%)
• 95% confidence interval	(10.3–14.3)	(16.1–25.6)	(7.5–10.9)	(16.1–25.0)
• ROPS tractors acquired for features other than the ROPS	84 (27.9%)	65 (23.0%)	99 (30.8%)	91 (28.3%)
• 95% confidence interval	(22.8–33.0)	(18.1–27.9)	(25.7–35.8)	(23.4–33.3)
• Total ROPS tractors acquired	127 (42.2%)	124 (43.8%)	134 (41.6%)	157 (48.9%)
• 95% confidence interval	(33.6–47.8)	(38.0–49.7)	(36.2–47.0)	(43.4–54.4)

Tractor Dealers' ROPS Sales

The second independent data source was the Barren and Fleming county tractor equipment dealers ROPS retrofit kit sale records. By the end of the project a total of eighty-one ROPS retrofit kits were sold to seventy-nine farmers. The eighty-one tractors had a mean age of 22.6 years (SD = 8.7). Barren County dealers reported that 63.5 percent of their ROPS sales were within their county with the remainder to farmers in nearby counties. Fleming County dealers reported that only 34.7 percent of their ROPS sales were within the county and the remainder in nearby counties. Overall 39.5 percent of total

ROPS retrofits sales by dealers in the two counties were to farmers in nearby counties. Kentucky's 120 counties are relatively small. The number of farm equipment dealers decreased markedly during the decade prior to the study. Dealers that remained served farmers from multiple counties.

SAF-T-CAB Sales Records

SAF-T-CAB was the primary after-market ROPS supplier at that time of the study. It sold a total of eight ROPS kits in the two control counties and fifty in the two intervention counties during the first two and a half years of the project. Records after this period were not available. The proportion of sales to equipment dealers versus individual farmers was unknown.

Impact of Intervention Messages and Activities

During March and April 2001, fifty-nine (74.5 percent) of the seventy-nine farmers whose equipment dealers reported had retrofitted eighty-one ROPS were interviewed by telephone. Fourteen could not be reached despite repeated attempts. Six declined the interview because they were too busy. Of the fifty-nine interviewed, 85 percent reported having seen or heard the campaign messages, and 80 percent reported the messages influenced them to equip their tractors with a ROPS. The most frequently stated motives for ROPS retrofits were the following:

- The injury protection provided to family members
- Increased awareness of overturn risks and injuries
- Knowing someone who had been injured or killed in a non-ROPS tractor overturn
- The risk of collisions posed by drivers who become angry and aggressive when encountering slow-moving farm equipment
- The financial costs related to tractor overturn injuries
- Fear of civil suits from injuries to nonfamily workers
- The protection from skin cancer by installing a sun shade on the ROPS

The radio PSAs, graphic stuffers, newspaper stories, and the "How to Get a ROPS" pamphlet were widely disseminated within the two intervention counties but also spread to counties adjacent to or near the intervention counties, in large part because Barren and Fleming county agencies and businesses also serve farmers in adjacent and nearby counties. The Mr. Good Egg farmer and the photos of fatal and nonfatal overturns activities were very popular. As a result individuals in the two intervention counties shared these and other materials with colleagues, family, and friends in other counties. As one farmer in Meade County said, "Mr. Good Egg was soon running wild throughout Kentucky."

Community Partners' Contributions

The outreach and event and activity reporting form data that were used to calculate the in-kind dollar contribution of the community partners in the two intervention counties. Over the three-year project period the estimated in-kind dollar contributions from Barren and Fleming counties totaled $174,724, a value that exceeded the $130,884 CDC-NIOSH grant that supported the UK researchers' three-year effort to design, develop, implement, disseminate, and evaluate the project methods and materials (Myers et al., 2005). The community partners' dollar contributions were estimated from community partner volunteers' labor hours, donated radio and TV preparation and broadcast costs, newspaper ROPS promotion ads and ROPS story preparation, local duplication costs for the stuffer messages, the "How to Get a ROPS" pamphlet, photos of fatal and nonfatal overturns chart displays, and locally raised cash funds of $5,450 of which $3,750 was used as incentive fund awards for farmers' purchase of ROPS retrofit kits. In both counties the incentive awards were widely advertised and then awarded three times a year by random drawings held at public community gatherings. Barren County raised a total of $750 and made five incentive awards of $100 each and one award of $250. Fleming County raised $4,700 of which $3,000 was used for twelve ROPS incentive awards of $250 each. The remaining $1,700 was used for advertising the drawings and duplicating and distributing selected notebook posters, charts, and other materials to beef, dairy, pork, tobacco, and other farm producer groups (Cole & Westneat, 2001).

Discussion

Examination of rows one through four in Table 17.3 reveals that for three counties the number of ROPS retrofit kits were a small proportion of the total ROPS tractors acquired for the protection provided by the ROPS. The respective values were Barren, 34.9 percent; Fleming, 16.9 percent; Hardin, 22.9 percent; and Nelson 50.0 percent. Nelson County was an exception because the dealer was part of a national John Deere program. Unlike many other tractor brands, John Deere continued to stock ROPS for its older tractors. It supplied ROPS retrofit kits to its dealers at cost and with no shipping charges. The Nelson County dealer in turn provided farmers with ROPS at cost and no shipping costs plus a modest installation charge. ROPS retrofit kits for John Deere tractors are generally less expensive than for other tractor brands.

ROPS typically are not available for tractors manufactured prior to 1966. Most tractors manufactured from 1970 to 1985 were designed to accept ROPS but were not include as original equipment. The NIOSH-funded New York Center for Agricultural and Occupational Health (NEC) found that the average cost of a ROPS retrofit including shipping and installation was $935. In addition 23 percent of farmers who inquired about ROPS retrofits had older tractors for which no ROPS was available (Murphy et al., 2010). Many farmers have difficulty finding and purchasing ROPS for older tractors. This problem is more acute in Kentucky where 67.3 percent of farmers have annual value of farm product sales less than $10,000, and 51 percent have tractors plus all other equipment valued at less than $20,000.

The study had a number of limitations. The number of ROPS retrofits and ROPS-protected tractors reported in Table 17.3 are from the interviews of the 1,227 farmers in the four counties. Yet, Nelson county equipment dealers reported 65.3 percent of their ROPS kit sales were to farmers in other counties. For Barren county dealers 36.5 percent of ROPS kits were out of county. This suggests that the ROPS-promotion program may have been more effective than the values in Table 17.3 indicate. In addition, the in-county dealer records were accurate but incomplete. The 1,227 farmers in the intervention and control counties obtained ROPS kits and ROPS-equipped tractors from many sources other than their county equipment dealers. These included used equipment dealers in their counties and other counties, ROPS purchased from other farmers located in their and other counties, and thirteen ROPS that were fabricated by farmers or by local machine shops, a dangerous practice because the ROPS may not meet design standards and fail during an overturn.

The lack of incentive funds to assist farmers' purchase of ROPS retrofit kits was a major limitation. Fleming County, with its twelve incentive fund awards of $250 each, was more effective in promoting ROPS retrofits than Barren County's one $250 and five $100 incentive awards.

Effectiveness of incentive awards was demonstrated by the New York Center. Over a three-year period it initiated a ROPS social marketing campaign. In addition, NEC obtained $200,000 from the New York State legislature to provide farmers with rebates for ROPS retrofits up of up to 70 percent of the cost of a ROPS or a maximum of $600. Within the first twelve months 268 tractors were retrofitted. Thirty-four months into the project and with incentive funds of up to $700, a total of seven hundred tractors had been retrofitted (Murphy et al., 2010). An earlier NEC study found that the social marketing messages alone without incentive fund rebates were ineffective for promoting ROPS retrofits (Sorensen et al., 2008).

The NEC used a small array of social marketing messages developed in partnership with a professional marketing firm and then consistently disseminated these messages to their intervention counties. The Kentucky project used a wide array of messages and activities developed by the UK researchers in collaboration with many community partners. From an experimental design perspective the Kentucky study would have been stronger if it had produced and evaluated a smaller and more consistent array of intervention materials and messages. However, the wide array of materials, activities, and methods in the Kentucky ROPS notebook attracted a wide range of individuals and organizations in the intervention counties who used different combinations of the materials. Following the project many farm safety organizations and individuals sought out, adopted, adapted, and used the Kentucky ROPS notebook materials and methods with a wide range of individuals in other states. Beginning in 2000 Bruce Stone and his colleagues at the Virginia Farm Bureau adopted, adapted, and incorporated many of the notebook materials and messages into their statewide ROPS promotion and incentive fund program (personal communication, B. Stone, January 9, 2011). Charles Privette at Clemson University worked with safety extension specialists at Clemson and South Carolina State University to create a shortened version of the notebook tailored for use with South Carolina's limited resource farmers in fourteen counties (Privette & Cole, 2003). The agricultural extension program at Kentucky State University used selected notebook materials to mount a ROPS promotion effort in nineteen northern counties with a high prevalence of limited resource and minority farmers (personal communication, M. Simon, May 7, 2005). In 2008 and 2009 the Penn State Lancaster County Extension Service adapted five of the simulation exercise stories in the notebook for use with Old Order Amish and Mennonite teachers, parents, and children. The simulations were used by twenty-three teachers and adult family members in fifteen Lancaster, Pennsylvania, schools, as well as by two additional large Amish families. The simulations also were used by two Old Order Mennonite schools and two large Mennonite families in Canada. The simulations were well received and rated highly by children, teachers, and family members (Moyer, undated). As demonstrated by numerous requests for the materials addressed to the Southeast Center (located in Lexington, Kentucky) and searches and downloads of notebook materials from the NASD website, the notebook methods and materials continue to be used by a wide range of individuals and organizations.

Conclusion

Tractor rollovers are a common form of farm-related injury. Thus, this threat to health and well-being is largely unique to rural America. Fortunately, the innovation of ROPS offers substantial protection against morbidity and mortality caused by rollovers. The adoption of ROPS, however, has been problematic. Findings from this Kentucky-based study suggest that community-based intervention programs may be a vital method of ROPS promotion to farmers. Farmers may indeed be reluctant to spend money on this form of protection yet study results suggests that a carefully planned set of educational approaches may change their thinking and eventually lead to the adoption of ROPS.

Summary

- Tractor rollover is a common problem in rural America yet these death- and injury-producing events can be largely avoided through installation of a simple innovation.

- As an innovation, ROPS may not be universally adopted by farmers. Therefore, it is imperative that rural public health efforts include educational programs and promotion efforts designed to foster improved implementation.

- A theory-based intervention program that uses mass media and other social marketing techniques as well as educational materials may be an effective approach to the problem of low uptake of ROPS among rural farmers.

For Practice and Discussion

1. Please consider the Kentucky ROPS notebook that was referred to throughout this chapter. How might this notebook be different in communities located other parts of the country such as the Pacific Northwest or the northeastern United States? To what degree is local culture a determining factor in materials such as this notebook?

2. Working with a colleague from class, design an added component to the notebook and the social marketing approach that you each agree would greatly magnify the effect of rural public health efforts to reduce tractor rollover–related morbidity and mortality. Describe your added component in detail and justify how it improves on the existing approach described in this chapter.

Key Terms

community-partner committees

dual-coding theory

extended parallel process model

response efficacy

self-efficacy

theory of reasoned action

Acknowledgments

The work reported in this chapter was completed under CDC/NIOSH cooperative agreement numbers U06/CCU412900–01, 02, and 03 awarded to the University of Kentucky Southeast Center for Agricultural Health and Injury Prevention, under human subjects protocol IRB number 01–0499-P2b. The authors gratefully acknowledge the assistance of research team members Larry Piercy, Tim Struttmann, Vickie Brandt, Joan Muehlbauer, and Susan Morgan; NIOSH project officers Janet Ehlers, Terri Palermo, and Ted Scharf; and the many farmers and farm community service and business organizations and individuals who made this project possible.

References

Brandt, V.A., Struttmann, T. W., Cole, H. P., & Piercy L. R. (2001). Delivering health and safety education messages for part-time farmers through local businesses and employers. *Journal of Agromedicine, 7,* 23–30.

Bruner, J. S. (1990). *Acts of meaning.* Cambridge, MA: Harvard University Press.

Cole, H. P. (1997). Stories to live by. A narrative approach to health behavior research and injury prevention. In D. S. Gochman (Ed.), *Handbook of health behavior research IV. Relevance for professionals and issues for the future.* New York: Plenum Press.

Cole, H. P. (2002). Cognitive-behavioral approaches to farm community safety education: A conceptual analysis. *Journal of Agricultural Safety and Health, 8,* 145–159.

Cole, H. P., McKnight, R. H., & Donovan, T. A. (2009). Epidemiology, surveillance and prevention of farm tractor overturn fatalities. *Journal of Agromedicine, 14,* 164–171.

Cole, H. P., & Westneat, S. C. (2001). *The Kentucky ROPS project. Final technical report for partners in prevention: Promoting ROPS and seatbelts on family farm tractors.* Lexington: University of Kentucky, Southeast Center for Agricultural Health and Injury Prevention.

Cole, H. P., Westneat, S., Piercy, L. R., Brandt, V., Muehlbauer, J., & Morgan, S. (2004). *The Kentucky ROPS project notebook.* Retrieved from http://nasdonline.org/document/1014/2/d000997/the-kentucky-community-partners-for-healthy-farming-rops-project.html

Morgan, S. E., Cole, H. P., Struttmann, T., & Piercy, L. (2002). Stories or statistics? Farmers' attitudes toward messages in an agricultural safety campaign. *Journal of Agricultural Safety and Health, 8,* 225–239.

Moyer, K. (undated). *Farm safety stories.* Lancaster: Pennsylvania State University, College of Agricultural Sciences, Lancaster County Cooperative Extension.

Murphy, D. J., Myers, J., McKenzie, E. A., Cavaletto, R., May, J., & Sorensen, J. (2010). Tractors and rollover protection in the United States. *Journal of Agromedicine, 15,* 249–263.

Myers, M. L., Cole, H. P., & Westneat, S. C. (2005). Cost effectiveness of a dealer's intervention in retrofitting rollover protective structures. *Injury Prevention, 11,* 169–173.

NASD. (2011). *The Kentucky community partners for healthy farming ROPS project.* Retrieved from http://nasdonline.org/document/1014/2/d000997/the-kentucky -community-partners-for-healthy-farming-rops-project.html

Pavio, A. (1971). A dual coding approach to perception and cognition. In J. Pick, H. L. Pick, & E. Saltzman (Eds.), *Modes of perceiving and processing information* (pp. 39–51). Hillsdale, NJ: Erlbaum.

Privette III, C. V., & Cole, H. P. (2003). Tractor safety using the SC ROPS Program. *Journal of Extension, 41*(6), 1–14.

Sarbin, T. R. (Ed.). (1986). *Narrative psychology: The storied nature of human conduct.* New York: Prager.

Sorensen, J. A., May, J., O'Hara, P., Ostby-Malling, R., Lehman, T., Strand, J., Stenland, H., Weinehall, L., & Emmelin, M. (2008). Encouraging the installation of rollover protective structures in New York State: The design of a social marketing intervention. *Scandinavian Journal of Public Health, 36,* 859–869.

Struttmann, T. W., Brandt, V. A., Morgan, S. E., Piercy, L. R., & Cole, H. P. (2001). Equipment dealers' perceptions of a community based ROPS campaign. *Journal of Rural Health, 17,* 131–140.

USDA. (1997). *Machinery and equipment on place: 1997 and 1992 [for Barren, Fleming, Hardin, and Nelson Counties].* Table 9. Retrieved from http:// www.agcensus.usda.gov/Publications/1997/Vol_1_Chapter_2_County_Tables/ Kentucky/ky2_09.pdf

Witte, K. (1992). Putting fear back into fear appeals: The extended parallel process model. *Communication Monographs, 59,* 329–349.

Witte, K., & Allen, M. (2000). A meta-analysis for fear appeals: Implications for effective public health campaigns. *Health Education and Behavior, 27,* 591–615.

Chapter 18

Addressing Mental Health Issues in Rural Areas

Carly E. McCord
Timothy R. Elliott
Daniel F. Brossart
Linda G. Castillo

Learning Objectives

- Gain an understanding of the contextual, ethical, and diversity issues facing rural citizens with mental health needs.
- Gain knowledge of the unique models to address community needs for primary and mental health services.
- Understand the use of technology to provide mental health services to rural areas.
- Understand the critical role of nondoctoral-level providers within the community to promote healing and health adaptation.

• • •

Glaring disparities in access and availability of **mental health** (services like counseling, therapy, assessment and consultation) care in rural areas necessitates the interdisciplinary collaboration of students, researchers, clinicians, stakeholders, and policy makers in developing realistic, sustainable solutions relevant to particular communities. In this chapter, we will provide an overview of the mental health issues that face rural citizens and present perspectives on the contextual and ethical issues that characterize these problems. We will address empirically supported interventions and conclude with directions for future work that are informed by a broader perspective of community-based programs and capacity building.

Almost 20 percent (fifty-five million people) of the total US population live in rural areas and are faced with the barriers of low accessibility, availability, and perceived acceptability of mental health services (Health Resources and Services Administration, 2005). Accessibility to mental health services is hindered by higher rates of poverty, inadequate housing and transportation, lower rates of insurance, and poorer health (Stamm et al., 2003; Wagenfeld, 2003). In many cases, mental health care remains scarce or unavailable because more than 85 percent of MHPSAs are in rural areas (Bird, Dempsey, & Hartley, 2001). An estimated one-third of rural counties in the United States lack *any* health professionals equipped to address mental health issues, with a much larger ratio of rural counties lacking any kind of specialty mental health services (Gamm, Stone, & Pittman, 2003).

An estimated one-third of rural counties in the United States lack any health professionals equipped to address mental health issues.

When mental health services are present in rural communities, individuals often receive disjointed care across stages of treatment (Fox et al., 1994). And if services are available, people in rural areas who have mental health concerns are more likely to receive pharmacology and less likely to receive psychotherapy (Fortney et al., 2010). Men and women in rural areas are less likely to receive mental health treatment of any sort than their urban counterparts (Hauenstein et al., 2006), and if they do they will likely find a mental health provider with less advanced training than their urban peers (Wagenfeld et al., 1994) or they opt for informal counseling provided by ministers, local self-help groups, family, or friends (Fox, Merwin, & Blank, 1995). Greater travel distances required to obtain expert mental health services (including treatment for substance abuse) are associated with fewer outpatient visits and an increased probability of hospitalization (Fortney et al., 1995; Fortney, Owen, & Clothier, 1999).

Key Concepts

Rural populations often face unique hardships related to mental health and require consideration of several, characteristic ethical concerns. The structure and availability of mental health care services in rural areas are frequently inadequate but multiple, viable alternatives are emerging.

Disparities in Mental Health

We know the prevalence of behavioral disorders and mental health problems are at least as high in rural areas as in metropolitan areas, yet mental health issues in rural communities are exacerbated by the lack of mental health services and highly trained mental health service providers. There is evidence, however, to suggest that some behavioral problems may be disproportionately higher in rural areas than in their urban counterparts (Hauenstein et al. 2006; Smalley et al., 2010; Stamm et al., 2007). For example, several studies have reported higher rates of depression, substance abuse, and domestic violence in rural areas (Bushy, 1998; Cellucci & Vik, 2001; Murty et al., 2003).

The prevalence of depression among rural women is higher (35.5 percent of those seen in a primary care clinic (Sears, Danda, & Evans, 1999) than those for the general population of women (8.6 percent in the National Comorbidity Survey, http://www.hcp.med.harvard.edu/ncs/publications.php). Women in rural areas experience unique problems that increase their risk for depression and abuse including social isolation, limited occupational options (which contribute to financial instability and poverty), and lack of childcare (Annan, 2006; Hauenstein & Peddada, 2007; Thurston, Patten, & Lagendyk, 2006).

Rates of suicide and suicide attempts are higher in rural areas, particularly among men (Eberhardt & Pamuk, 2004, Singh & Siahpush, 2002). Higher rates of depression and substance abuse (including alcohol, tobacco, cocaine, methamphetamine, inhalants, and marijuana) are found among rural youth (National Center on Addiction and Substance Abuse, 2000; Substance Abuse and Mental Health Services Administration, 2001). Alcohol use is often implicated in the high rates of suicide in rural areas (Johnson, Gruenewald, & Remer, 2009). These complex characteristics and disparities of rural residence provide an important context for understanding rural mental health issues.

Issues of Diversity

Diversity is more than just ethnic variation. All factors that make an individual unique, including gender, age, and rurality in general, affect accessibility, service delivery, and outcomes. Individuals in rural areas vary greatly in their degree of acculturation to modern society (think Amish elder versus small town teenager) and the population density across rural areas can be quite disparate. Furthermore, the value systems and customs of rural areas may have commonalities but generalizing all rural residents as self-sustaining, religious, family folk certainly ignores the reality of a diverse rural culture.

In the past, rural areas have been less ethnically diverse than urban areas, but the percentages of minority residents are rising. Rural communities are on average composed of about 15.9 percent Hispanics and 16.5 percent African Americans (US Census Bureau, 2006).Individuals from ethnic and minority backgrounds often encounter more overdiagnosis and misdiagnosis and poorer treatment outcomes across mental health settings generally (Ridley, 2005), and the health disparities they encounter in rural areas are greater than those experienced by their urban counterparts (Probst et al., 2004). African Americans and Hispanics underuse mental health services, even among those who have insurance (Padgett et al., 1994) and perceived racial discrimination is associated with depression among both groups (Brown, Brody, & Stoneman, 2000; Kogan et al., 2007; Torres & Ong, 2010). The lack of bilingual mental health providers, language and cultural barriers, and the geographic isolation of rural communities place a hardship on rural Hispanics to receive treatment for depression.

Age is another important diversity consideration relevant to mental health in rural communities. In most rural areas, the elderly constitute a large percentage of rural residents due to the influx of retired individuals and the exodus of young adults to suburban and metropolitan areas (Crowther, Scogin, & Norton, 2010). In fact, in 2004, the National Advisory Committee on Rural Health and Human Services reported that a quarter of the older adult population of America lives in rural areas. What qualifies someone as an "older adult" varies greatly and often ranges from fifty to eighty-five years of age, with sixty-five being a commonly used cutpoint because the Social Security Administration uses this as the designated age for retirement.

Many of the same barriers to mental health care that exist for rural residents are exacerbated for older adults. For example, older adults in rural areas experience higher rates of depression and dementia, less social support and greater isolation, and poorer overall physical health. Care for the mental health of older adults in rural areas must be carefully designed to meet the unique needs of this population. For example, when using technology to increase accessibility, socially acceptable and user-friendly set-ups should be considered. Or when using a psychoeducational approach (such as cognitive behavioral therapy), providers can adjust their approach appropriately to accommodate an older adult's decreased rate of learning and increased difficulty with memory tasks (Crowther et al., 2010).

On the other end of the age spectrum, the mental health of rural adolescents is often overlooked. Studies have shown the incidence of illegal drug and alcohol use, suicide, and depression surpasses their urban counterparts (Biddle, Sekula, & Puskar, 2010; Sloboda, 2002). Of the few national studies that have examined rural-urban differences in children's mental health needs and use of services, prevalence of mental health problems are at a similar rate for rural (36 percent) and urban (37 percent) children (Ziller et al., 2003). However, after controlling for insurance status and accessibility to mental health services, rural children are 20 percent less likely to use mental health services than urban children (Ziller et al., 2003). Rural schools are often placed in the position of identifying and handling students with mental health problems. However, rural schools lack the resources and personnel to address many of the mental health concerns seen in the classroom.

Rural areas are also characterized by a large percentage of military veterans in the population. Rural individuals serve at a disproportionately higher rate in the military than those in urban areas; over 44 percent of current military recruits are from rural areas (Rogers, 2009). Rural-residing veterans tend to be older, less likely to be employed, and report a lower health-related quality of life (physical and mental) than their urban counterparts (Weeks et al., 2004). Rural communities will bear a significant burden with the influx of veterans from Operation Iraqi Freedom and Operation Enduring Freedom with the chronic "signature wounds" of these conflicts—posttraumatic stress disorder and traumatically acquired brain injuries. Our soldiers will encounter "particularly poor access to mental health care" in rural and frontier regions of the country (Tanielian & Jaycox, 2008, p. 302).

Ethical Issues

Several ethical concerns characterize the provision of mental health services in rural areas. Dual relationships are often inescapable, boundaries of competence can be unclear, confidentiality can be difficult to maintain, and clientele may be less educated about the role and scope of the professional. Not surprisingly, professionals are less inclined to provide psychological services to those living in rural areas where they are subject to greater ethical risk, less compensation, higher burnout rates due to lack of referral sources, increased isolation, and infringement of their personal privacy by the scrutinizing eyes of the community.

Professionals are less inclined to provide psychological services to those living in rural areas where they are subject to greater ethical risk.

Rural residents often surrender their anonymity when visiting a mental health professional whose office and parking lot are visible to anyone driving by. Also, rural residents are quite familiar with the speed and breadth of communication coverage attained by the town's "grapevine." Often an individual's participation in counseling quickly becomes known within the community resulting in stigmatization of the individual seeking help. Professionals must strive to address issues of stigma by facilitating greater trust in the therapeutic relationship and within the community at large. Without the assurance of anonymity and confidentiality, treatment outcomes are unpredictable and malfeasance is likely. Professionals should take extra steps to provide anonymity outside the building by providing parking not visible from the street and inside the building so that clients feel safe even in the waiting room. Additionally, office staff and professionals must take extreme caution with any information related to a client's involvement in treatment (Werth, Hastings, & Riding-Malon, 2010).

Creating buy-in with community stakeholders must be done thoughtfully to reduce future occurrences of dual relationships. Individuals helping increase access to mental health services may be a consumer of the service in the future. The American Psychological Association (APA) ethical code explains that not all dual relationships are unethical but that professionals should carefully evaluate each dual relationship and assess whether the dual relationship may impair the professional's objectivity, thereby creating the potential for harming the client (APA, 2002).

Unfortunately, most training programs operate from an urban model and do not emphasize or teach about the specific treatment concerns of rural residents. The APA ethics code states, "Psychologists provide services, teach, and conduct research with populations and in areas only within the boundaries of their competence, based on their education, training, supervised experience, consultation, study, or professional experience" (APA, 2002, p.1063). This ethical standard, paired with the current urban training models, creates a recipe for ethical dilemmas. Moreover, no one clinician can possibly be competent in treating all problems presented in his or her office. Due to the lack of health resources available in rural communities, practitioners are likely to run into issues that are outside the scope of their expertise. It could be tempting to treat the individual because the other options may be limited, nonexistent, or located hours away.

Mental Health Services

Currently, mental health services in rural areas rely on a patchwork of de facto providers composed of formal (primary care clinics, federally qualified health centers [FQHCs], etc.) and informal (churches, law enforcement, etc.) entities in a region (Fox et al., 1995). Provision and care coordination is initiated by "gateway providers" (e.g., ministers, law enforcement officers, primary care and emergency room physicians) who have an understandable unfamiliarity with the complexity of mental health diagnoses and treatment options. Law enforcement is often responsible for handling mental health emergencies. The outcomes of this loose-knit and highly variable system are predictably poor (Hauenstein, 2007).

Alternative systems are distinguished by strategic coordination and integration of available services. For example, FQHCs—particularly community health centers and migrant health centers—are well positioned to provide an array of primary and mental health services. One such program was initiated in a series of state policies in Hawaii to provide behavioral health services to reach medically underserved populations throughout the islands (Oliveira et al., 2006). The program provides behavioral health expertise throughout all primary and mental health care services, ensuring care to individuals with mental health diagnoses and to those who have mental issues comorbid with chronic and acute health conditions.

The Department of Veterans Affairs (VA) has responded to rural military veterans with integrated clinics that address the needs of the chronically mentally ill and those who present in primary care. A network of mental health–intensive case management programs serves veterans in rural and urban areas, employing an assertive community treatment approach to service provision and coordination. Evaluation data indicate that military veterans in smaller and remote rural areas receive less-intensive and fewer recovery services than urban veterans (Mohamed, Neale, & Rosenheck, 2009). To address mental health care needs often seen in primary care, the VA has developed community-based outpatient clinics— satellite facilities to provide primary and ambulatory care—with almost one hundred in areas designated as rural or highly rural (Elder & Quillen, 2007). These clinics are staffed primarily with doctoral-level service providers.

Access to and provision of specific mental health services in rural areas may be best remedied with the use of long-distance **technologies**. Long-distance technologies and telecommunications for health care purposes (commonly referred to as *telehealth*) includes the use of telephone, videoconferencing, or Internet transmissions to provide an array of mental health services (e.g., screening, assessment, consultation, education, counseling, psychotherapy).Telephone use is less expensive, allows for greater anonymity, and greater sense of control and convenience than other methods(Reese, Conoley, & Brossart, 2006).Other work clearly indicates that recipients of telephone counseling are satisfied with the experience and believe it "helped them improve their lives" (Reese, Conoley, & Brossart, 2002, p. 239).

There is considerable evidence supporting the use of telephone counseling for a variety of mental health problems. In a study of depressed patients from a rural primary care clinic, Mohr, Hart, and Marmar (2006) found that providing cognitive behavioral therapy (CBT) in telephone sessions significantly reduced symptoms assessed on two separate depression inventories. Data from relevant randomized control trials (RCTs) indicate similar effects for standardized CBT in reducing depression symptoms among family caregivers of stroke survivors (Grant et al., 2002) and traumatic brain injury (Rivera et al., 2008). Telephone counseling has been found effective for specific problems such as anxiety disorders among children (Lynehan, & Rapee, 2006).

Telephone counseling can also be effectively implemented in treatment and in follow-up programs for behavioral health problems often encountered in primary care. Cupertino et al. (2007) used telephone counseling in a smoking cessation program with rural participants and reported a high rate of satisfaction across the two years of treatment. Participants rated their counseling as a highly important part of the tobacco dependence treatment program. Perri et al. (2008) found that extended care telephone counseling of obese women from rural communities who had completed an initial weight loss program was an effective option for long-term weight management compared to receiving education alone.

Other technologies, such as videoconferencing, e-mail, and Internet contacts, have considerable promise for providing a variety of mental health services. For example, instant messaging has been used to provide real-time group counseling with rural Latina adolescents (Archuleta, Castillo, & King, 2006). The counseling services were provided in collaboration with three rural school districts and school counseling students at a Texas university located over two hundred miles away. Additional technologies have yet to be implemented in any systematic fashion (e.g., remote monitors, wearable sensors, texting).

Videoconferencing has been used effectively to conduct assessments, consultation, clinical supervision, training, counseling, and psychotherapy in rural settings (McCord et al., 2011; Richardson et al., 2009; Schopp, Demeris, & Glueckauf, 2006). Videoconferencing has increased in usage with favorable Medicare reimbursement policies, and services can be provided in a culturally competent manner to the satisfaction of individuals from ethnic and minority groups (e.g., Native Americans, Shore et al., 2008; Native Hawaiians, Oliveira et al., 2006; Hispanics, Nelson & Bui, 2010). The use of videoconferencing, however, is often limited by the quality of the infrastructure in rural areas for computer transmissions through existing telephone lines or satellite coverage.

Current Issues and Future Directions

To a certain extent, many are aware of the impact rural culture can have on initiating and developing therapeutic rapport, obtaining consent, and providing clinical services to rural clientele. Missing from this equation is the perspective and potential buy-in of stakeholders in the rural community (Sears, Evans, & Kuper, 2003). This kind of community engagement is often time-consuming, and it requires interdisciplinary collaboration to successfully cultivate a long-term investment in, as well as leverage available resources for, the provision of mental health services. These matters are necessary for ensuring adequate use of services, cultivating a positive presence in the community, and defining commitments for local stakeholders—all of which are crucial for sustainability.

Yet many solutions to mental health service delivery issues in rural areas are made in a manner that seems more "linear" (i.e., what is the best way to provide a service?) than systemic (how can the community work together to provide services to its residents?). A systemic perspective requires the involvement and buy-in of stakeholders in the rural community. It requires a realization of the need to build community capacity to identify needs, potential solutions, and possible collaborations to implement those solutions (Iscoe & Harris, 1984; Trickett, 2009).

This time-intensive process is necessary to develop realistic solutions relevant to a particular community and that are sustainable over time. For example, a recent project in the Brazos Valley region of Texas developed after a series of community surveys of the health status and needs of the residents resulted in the creation of a health resource commission (composed of elected and informal community leaders and representatives from various nonprofit and for-profit service providers and from various state and local agencies including law enforcement), and a series of meetings convened to prioritize needs and identify potential resources to address them (Wendel et al., 2011). As a result of this process, a "town and gown" partnership emerged in which the telehealth capacity of a regional FQHC was expanded to offer counseling and assessment services to a health resource clinic located an hour away in a rural county. The therapeutic services are provided by trainees in an accredited doctoral program in counseling psychology (who gain valuable clinical experiences that count toward their training requirements), supervised by faculty members of the program.

This arrangement illustrates the value of collaborative problem solving and capacity building among constituents in rural communities. But it also reflects the need to identify innovative solutions that maximize the use of nondoctoral-level providers and long-distance technologies in rural areas. It is becoming quite clear that doctoral-level service providers will not relocate to rural areas in numbers that will support sustained activity; therefore, the reliance on doctoral-level providers and third-party payers is unreasonable and unsustainable (Hauenstein, 2007). Despite several policy initiatives (and incentives) for service personnel to work in rural areas, and the recent expansion of Veterans Affairs health care systems, rural communities have not experienced a significant increase in available doctoral-level providers. Current budget constraints throughout the states will undermine the reimbursement of doctoral-level service provision in rural communities. It is also likely that the lack of evidence from well-controlled RCTs of mental health interventions in rural areas will be used by third-party payers to deny coverage (despite the recognized inappropriate reliance on RCTs to determine evidence for the treatment of chronic, complex conditions, particularly with understudied populations in underserved areas).

In order to improve the quality and cost-effective delivery of mental services in rural communities, nondoctoral-level service providers must be strategically implemented. This will involve the use of master's-level counselors to provide counseling and a greater use of physician extenders and other qualified personnel to administer and monitor prescriptions. In New Mexico and Louisiana, for example, psychologists who have obtained approved training in psychopharmacology can be licensed to have prescription privileges (Jameson & Blank, 2007; Norfleet, 2002). To a great extent, mental health nurses have already played a major role in providing the bulk of mental health services in rural areas (Hauenstein, 2007).

The provision of mental health services by doctoral- and master's-level practitioners is often limited to empirically established psychotherapy treatments. However, psychotherapy is a uniquely Western phenomenon that excludes indigenous methods of healing. Although psychotherapy may be an effective form of mental health treatment for many individuals the number of trained mental health professionals in rural areas limits its capacity. One suggested solution to resolve this issue and at the same time have buy-in of stakeholders in the rural community is to use an ecological approach to addressing mental health issues in a community. The Hawaiian model discussed previously, for example, integrated feedback from Native Hawaiians in developing various treatment options and included native healers as part of the program (Oliveira et al., 2006).

An ecological model—one that emphasizes the relationships between people and settings in which they live (Trickett, 1984)—may be required for developing sustainable services tailored for a specific community. This perspective emphasizes the identification of naturally occurring resources and solutions within communities to promote well-being, healing, and healthy adaptation. Furthermore, it promotes the enhancement of coping and adaptational strategies that enable individuals and communities to respond effectively to stressful situations.

One ecological approach to mental health work involves the training of community-based mental health workers. This approach has its roots in the health-promoter model (Werner & Bower, 1990). In the southwestern border of the United States, community-based health workers are known as *promotoras*. Promotoras are fundamental to prevention efforts aimed at improving the health of disadvantaged populations in southern New Mexico and west Texas. Because promotoras tend to be individuals from the local community and have similar backgrounds to patients, they are more likely to facilitate trust with patients (Castillo & Caver, 2009). In one study, promotoras were trained in mental health screening, recognizing depression and other mental health disorders, ethics, patient privacy and confidentiality, professional behaviors in medical settings, fundamentals of interview, and mobilizing local resources for patients (Getrich et al., 2007). Results of the study found that the use of promotoras was associated with patient empowerment.

Innovative initiatives will necessitate changes in reimbursement policies and collaborations within and between state licensing boards so that services can be expanded without being circumscribed by guild interests that conflict with the health and well-being of rural residents. Furthermore, private, state, and nonprofit health care systems will have to find ways to collaborate effectively to address the issues that an aging populace and returning veterans will place on rural communities. Many of the mental health problems that will accompany older age will present in primary and emergency care. The demands and needs of rural veterans necessitate a coordinated effort between federal and state community mental health services (Wallace et al., 2006) because the complex nature of the signature wounds from the current conflicts will have chronic, long-lasting, and disruptive effects that will tax health care and legal systems.

Conclusion

Rural communities face dilemmas in mental health care delivery and accessibility that require awareness and purposeful interventions. In this chapter we provided an overview of the contextual, ethical, and diversity issues facing rural citizens and also gave examples of creative ways researchers, clinicians, and policy makers are attempting to meet community needs to provide an array of primary and mental health services. The most effective and sustainable mental health services may be achieved with increased community capacity that facilitates cooperation among various stakeholders to realize strategic solutions. Furthermore, the use of long-distance technology and nondoctoral-level providers may be one of the best ways to provide mental health services for rural areas, and the existing literature is encouraging regarding consumer satisfaction and positive treatment outcomes. Systemic solutions are needed that go beyond linear, single services to helping community stakeholders and invested policymakers to collaboratively develop ecological and sustainable services that respect the unique relationships between the people and the setting in which they live.

Summary

- The prevalence of mental health problems are at least as high in rural areas as in metropolitan areas; however, there is evidence to suggest that some behavioral problems may be disproportionately higher in rural areas. These complex characteristics and disparities provide an important context for understanding rural mental health issues.
- All factors that make an individual unique including gender, age, degree of rurality, ethnicity, veteran status, and so on affect accessibility, service delivery, and treatment outcomes.

- Mental health professionals in rural areas are subject to greater ethical risks related to competence and confidentiality, have higher burnout rates, and must typically work for less compensation.
- Technologies such as telephone, videoconferencing, e-mail, and the Internet have considerable promise for increasing access to mental health care.
- The ecological model for health care provision emphasizes the identification of naturally occurring resources (such as FQHCs, promotoras, and natural healers) within communities to promote healing and health adaptation.

Key Terms

diverse(ity)   technology(ies)

mental health

For Practice and Discussion

1. Working with one or two colleagues from class, discuss the impact of diversity (gender, age, veteran status, etc.) on the accessibility, availability, and acceptability of mental health services.

2. Create your own ecological model to meet a specific community need (refer to Chapter One for an example).

3. Working with one or two colleagues from class, discuss how a broader perspective of community-based programs and capacity programs can improve mental health service delivery in rural areas.

Acknowledgments

This research was supported in part by grant number D06RH07934 from the Office of Rural Health Policy, Health Resources and Services Administration. The findings and conclusions presented are the authors' and do not necessarily represent the official position of the Office of Rural Health Policy.

References

APA. (2002). Ethical principles of psychologists and code of conduct. *American Psychologist, 47,* 1597–1611.

Annan, S. L. (2006).Sexual violence in rural areas: A review of the literature. *Family & Community Health, 29,* 164–168.

Archuleta, D. J., Castillo, L. G., & King, J. J. (2006). Working with Latina adolescents in online support groups. *Journal of School Counseling, 4*, 3–16.

Biddle, V. S., Sekula, L. K., & Puskar, K. R. (2010). Identification of suicide risk among rural youth: Implications for the use of heads. *Journal of Pediatric Health Care, 24*, 152–167. doi:10.1016/j.pedhc.2009.03.003.

Bird, D.C., Dempsey, P., & Hartley, D. (2001). *Addressing mental health workforce needs in underserved rural areas: Accomplishments and challenges* (Working Paper No. 23). Portland: Maine Rural Health Research Center.

Brown, A. C., Brody, G. H., & Stoneman, Z. (2000).Rural black women and depression: A contextual analysis. *Journal of Marriage and the Family, 62*,187–192.

Bushy, A. (1998). Health issues of women in rural environments: An overview. *Journal of the American Medical Women's Association, 53*(2), 53–56.

Castillo, L. G., & Caver, K. (2009). Expanding the concept of acculturation in Mexican American rehabilitation psychology research and practice. *Rehabilitation Psychology, 54*, 351–362. doi:10.1037/a0017801.

Cellucci, T., & Vik, P. (2001).Training for substance abuse treatment among psychologists in a rural state. *Professional Psychology: Research and Practice, 32*, 248–252.

Crowther, M.R., Scogin, F., & Norton, M. J. (2010). Treating the aged in rural communities: The application of cognitive-behavioral therapy for depression. *Journal of Clinical Psychology, 66*, 502–512.

Cupertino, A. P., Mahnken, J. D., Richter, K., Cox, L., Casey, G., Resnicow, K., et al. (2007). Long term engagement in smoking cessation. *Journal of Health Care for the Poor and Underserved, 18*, 39–51.

Eberhardt, M. S., & Pamuk, E. R. (2004). The importance of place of residence: Examining health in rural and nonrural areas. *American Journal of Public Health, 94*, 1682–1686.

Elder, M., & Quillen, J. H. (2007). A reason for optimism in rural mental health care: Emerging solutions and models of service delivery. *Clinical Psychology: Science and Practice, 14*, 299–303.

Fortney, J. C., Booth, B. M., Blow, F. C., Bunn, J. Y., & Cook, C. A. (1995).The effects of travel barriers and age on the utilization of alcoholism treatment aftercare. *American Journal of Drug and Alcohol Abuse, 21*, 391–406.

Fortney, J. C., Harman, J. S., Xu, S., & Dong, F. (2010). The association between rural residence and the use, type, and quality of depression care. *The Journal of Rural Health, 26*, 205–213. doi:10.1111/j.1748-0361.2010.00290.

Fortney, J. C., Owen, R., & Clothier, J. (1999).Impact of travel distance on the disposition of patients presenting for emergency psychiatric care. *Journal of Behavioral Health Services and Research, 26*, 104–109.

Fox, J. C., Blank, M. B., Kane, C. F., & Hargrove, D. S. (1994). Balance theory as a model for coordinating delivery of rural mental health services. *Applied and Preventative Psychology, 3*, 121–129.

Fox, J., Merwin, E., & Blank, M. (1995). De facto mental health services in the rural South. *Journal of Health Care for the Poor and Underserved, 6*, 434–467.

Gamm, L., Stone, S., & Pittman, S. (2003). Mental health and mental disorders—a rural challenge: A literature review. In L. D. Gamm, L. L. Hutchison, B. J. Dabney, & A. M. Dorsey (Eds.), *Rural healthy people 2010: A companion document to Rural Healthy People 2010*. College Station: The Texas A&M University System Health Science Center, School of Rural Public Health, Southwest Rural Health Research Center.

Getrich, C., Heying, S., Willging, C., & Waitzkin, H. (2007). An ethnography of clinic "noise" in a community-based, promotora-centered mental health intervention. *Social Science and Medicine, 65,* 319–330.

Grant, J. S., Elliott, T. R., Weaver, M., Bartolucci, A. A., & Giger, J. N. (2002). Telephone intervention with family caregivers of stroke survivors after rehabilitation. *Stroke, 33,* 2060–2065.

Hauenstein, E. J. (2007). Building the rural mental health system: From de facto system to quality care. *Annual Review of Nursing Research, 26,* 143–173.

Hauenstein, E. J., & Peddada, S. (2007). Women and primary care: Prevalence of major depressive disorder. *Journal of Health Care for the Poor and Underserved, 18,* 185–202.

Hauenstein, E. J., Petterson, S., Merwin, E., Rovnyak, V., Heise, B., & Wagner, D. (2006). Rurality, gender, and mental health treatment. *Family & Community Health, 29,* 169–185.

Health Resources and Services Administration. (2005). *Mental health and rural America: 1994–2005.* Rockville, MD: Author.

Iscoe, I., & Harris, L. C. (1984). Social and community interventions. *Annual Review of Psychology, 35,* 333–360.

Jameson, J. P., & Blank, M. B. (2007). The role of clinical psychology in mental health services: Defining problems and developing solutions. *Clinical Psychology: Science and Practice, 14,* 283–298.

Johnson, F. W., Gruenewald, P. J., & Remer, L. G. (2009). Suicide and alcohol: Do outlets play a role? *Alcohol: Clinical and Experimental Research, 33,* 2124–2133.

Kogan, S. M., Brody, G. H., Crawley, C., Logan, P., & Murry, V. M. (2007). Correlates of elevated depressive symptoms among rural African American adults with type 2 diabetes. *Ethnicity and Disease, 17,* 106–112.

Lynehan, H. J., & Rapee, R.M. (2006). Evaluation of therapist-supported parent-implemented CBT for anxiety disorders in rural children. *Behavior Research and Therapy, 44,* 1287–1300.

McCord, C. E., Elliott, T. R., Wendel, M. L., Brossart, D. F., Cano, M., Gonzalez, G., & Burdine, J. N. (2011). Community capacity and teleconference counseling in rural Texas. *Professional Psychology: Research and Practice, 42,* 521–527.

Mohamed, S., Neale, M., & Rosenheck, R. A. (2009). VA intensive mental health case management in urban and rural areas: Veteran characteristics and service delivery. *Psychiatric Services, 60,* 914–921.

Mohr, D. C., Hart, S. L., & Marmar, C. (2006). Telephone administered cognitive-behavioral therapy for the treatment of depression in a rural primary care clinic. *Cognitive Therapy and Research, 30,* 29–39.

Murty, S. A., Peek-Asa, C., Zwerlong, C., Stromquist, A. M., Burmeister, L. F., & Merchant, J. A. (2003). Physical and emotional partner abuse reported by men and women in a rural area. *American Journal of Public Health, 93*, 1073–1075.

National Center on Addiction and Substance Abuse. (2000). *No place to hide: Substance abuse in mid-size cities and rural America.* New York: Author.

Nelson, E. L., & Bui, T. (2010). Rural telepsychology services for children and adolescents. *Journal of Clinical Psychology, 66*, 490–501.

Norfleet, M. A. (2002). Responding to society's needs: Prescription privileges for psychologists. *Journal of Clinical Psychology, 58*, 599–610.

Oliveira, J. M., Austin, A. A., Miyamoto, R.E.S., Kaholokula, J. K., Yano, K. B., & Lunasco, T. (2006). The rural Hawai'i behavioral health program: Increasing access to primary care behavioral health for native Hawaiians in rural settings. *Professional Psychology: Research and Practice, 37*, 174–182.

Padgett, D. K., Patrick, C., Burns, B. J., & Schlesinger, H. J. (1994). Ethnic differences in use of inpatient mental health services by blacks, whites, and Hispanics in a national insured population. *Health Services Research, 29*, 135–153.

Perri, M. G., Limacher, M. C., Durning, P. E., Janicke, D. M., Lutes, L. D., Bobroff, L. B., et al. (2008). Extended-care programs for weight management in rural communities. *Archives of Internal Medicine, 168*, 2347–2354.

Probst, J. C., Moore, C. G., Glover, S., & Samuels, M. (2004). Person and place: The compounding effects of race/ethnicity and rurality on health. *American Journal of Public Health, 94*, 1695–1703.

Reese, R. J., Conoley, C. W., & Brossart, D. F. (2002). Effectiveness of telephone counseling: A field based investigation. *Journal of Counseling Psychology, 49*, 233–242.

Reese, R. J., Conoley, C. W., & Brossart, D. F. (2006). The attractiveness of telephone counseling: An empirical investigation of client perceptions. *Journal of Counseling & Development, 84*, 54–60.

Richardson, L. K., Frueh, B. C., Grubaugh, A., Egede, L., & Elhai, J. D. (2009). Current directions in videoconferencing tele-mental health research. *Clinical Psychology: Science and Practice, 16*, 323–338.

Ridley, C. R. (2005).*Overcoming unintentional racism in counseling and therapy: A practitioner's guide to intentional intervention.* Newbury Park, CA: Sage.

Rivera, P., Elliott, T., Berry, J., & Grant, J. (2008). Problem-solving training for family caregivers of persons with traumatic brain injuries: A randomized controlled trial. *Archives of Physical Medicine and Rehabilitation, 89*, 931–941.

Rogers, I. P. (2009). *TRVA's rural veteran study.* Texas Rural Area Veterans Association. Retrieved from http://www.ruraltx.com/ruralstudy.pdf

Schopp, L., Demeris, G., & Glueckauf, R. L. (2006).Rural backwaters or front-runners? Rural telehealth in the vanguard of psychology practice. *Professional Psychology: Research and Practice, 37*, 165–173.

Sears, S. F., Danda, C. E., & Evans, G. D. (1999). PRIME-MD and rural primary care: Detecting depression in a low-income rural population. *Professional Psychology: Research and Practice, 30*, 357–360.

Sears, S. F., Evans, G. D., & Kuper, B. D. (2003). Rural social services systems as behavioral health delivery systems. In B. Stamm (Ed.), *Rural behavioral health care: An interdisciplinary guide*. Washington, DC: American Psychological Association.

Shore, J. H., Brooks, E., Savin, D., Orton, H., Grigsby, J., & Manson, S. M. (2008). Acceptance of telepsychiatry in American Indians. *Telemedicine and e-Health, 14,* 461–466.

Singh, G. K., & Siahpush, M. (2002). Increasing rural-urban gradients in US suicide mortality, 1970–1997. *American Journal of Public Health, 92,* 1161–1167.

Sloboda, Z. (2002). Drug abuse in rural America: A growing problem. *Counselor, 3*(6), 16–21.

Smalley, K. B., Yancey, C. T., Warren, J. C., Naufel, K., Ryan, R., & Pugh, J. L. (2010). Rural mental health and psychological treatment: A review for practitioners. *Journal of Clinical Psychology, 66,* 479–489.

Stamm, B. H., Lambert, D., Piland, N. F., & Speck, N. C. (2007). A rural perspective on health care for the whole person. *Professional Psychology: Research and Practice, 38,* 298–304.

Stamm, B. H., Piland, N. F., Crouse, B., Boulger, J., Davis, G., Ide, B. A., Buchner, M. S., Galliher, R. V., & Tidwell, K. (2003). Essays from the field. In B. Stamm (Ed.), *Rural behavioral health care: An interdisciplinary guide* (pp. 11–20). Washington, DC: American Psychological Association.

Substance Abuse and Mental Health Services Administration. (2001). *Summary of findings from the 2001 National Household Survey on Drug Abuse*. Rockville, MD: Office of Applied Studies.

Tanielian, T. L., & Jaycox, L. H. (2008). *Invisible wounds of war: Psychological and cognitive injuries, their consequences, and services to assist recovery*. Santa Monica, CA: RAND Corporation.

Thurston, W. E., Patten, S., & Lagendyk, L. E. (2006). Prevalence of violence against women reported in a rural health region. *Canadian Journal of Rural Medicine, 11,* 259–267.

Torres, L., & Ong, A. D. (2010). A daily diary investigation of Latino ethnic identity, discrimination, and depression. *Cultural Diversity and Ethnic Minority Psychology, 16,* 561–568.

Trickett, E. (1984). Toward a distinctive community psychology: An ecological metaphor for the conduct of community research and the nature of training. *American Journal of Community Psychology, 12,* 264–279.

Trickett, E. J. (2009). Community psychology: Individuals and interventions in community context. *Annual Review of Psychology, 60,* 395–419.

United States Census Bureau. (2006). *USA quickfacts*. Retrieved from http://quickfacts.census.gov/qfd/states/00000.html

Wagenfeld, M. O. (2003). A snapshot of rural and frontier America. In B. Stamm (Ed.), *Rural behavioral health care: An interdisciplinary guide*. Washington, DC: American Psychological Association.

Wagenfeld, M. O., Murray, J. D., Mohatt, D. F., & DeBruyn, J. (Eds.). (1994). *Mental health and rural America: An overview and annotated bibliography 1978–1993*. Washington, DC: US Government Printing Office.

Wallace, A. E., Weeks, W. B., Wang, S., Lee, A. F., & Kazis, L. E. (2006). Rural and urban disparities in health-related quality of life among veterans with psychiatric disorders. *Psychiatric Services, 57*, 851–856.

Weeks, W. B., Kazis, L. E., Shen, Y., Cong, Z., Ren, X., Miller, D., Lee, A., & Perlin, J. (2004). Differences in health-related quality of life in rural and urban veterans. *American Journal of Public Health, 94*, 1762–1767.

Wendel, M., Brossart, D., Elliott, T., McCord, C., & Diaz, M. (2011).Use of technology to increase access to mental health services in a rural Texas community. *Family and Community Health, 34*, 134–140.

Werner, D., & Bower, B. (1990). *Aprendiendo a Promover la Salud*. Palo Alto, CA: Hesperian Foundation.

Werth, J. L., Hastings, S. L., & Riding-Malon, R. (2010). Ethical challenges of practicing in rural areas. *Journal of Clinical Psychology, 65*, 537–548.

Ziller, E. C., Coburn, A. F., Loux, S. L., Hoffman, C., & McBride, T. D. (2003). *Health insurance coverage in rural America* (No. 4093). Washington, DC: The Kaiser Commission on Medicaid and the Uninsured; University of Southern Maine, Edmund S. Muskie School of Public Service, Institute for Health Policy.

Chapter 19

Cancer Prevention and Control in Rural Communities

Robin C. Vanderpool
Laurel A. Mills

Learning Objectives

- Recognize cancer disparities that are present in rural and minority populations.
- Learn about barriers to cancer screening and prevention among rural residents.
- Learn about evidence-based programs that have proven successful in increasing cancer screening among rural communities.
- Understand how community partners and organizations can be an efficient and effective tool in reducing cancer disparities in rural populations.

• • •

As the second leading cause of death and disease in the United States, cancer is a significant focus for public health practitioners working in rural and urban communities alike. However, rural communities carry a disproportionate burden of cancer due to the higher prevalence of **risk factors** related to cancer development such as cigarette smoking, sun exposure, poor diet, physical inactivity, alcohol consumption, and human papillomavirus (HPV) infection (Eberhardt & Pamuk, 2004; Gosschalk & Carozza, 2003; Haynes & Smedley,

1999). Further compounding these elevated risk factors for cancer is the demographic makeup of rural communities. Typically, rural communities have an aging population, increased concentrations of minority populations and poor whites, higher rates of unemployment and poverty, lower rates of education, and are geographically isolated (Hartley, 2004; Institute of Medicine, 2005; Phillips & McLeroy, 2004; Probst et al., 2004; Ricketts, Johnson-Webb, & Randolph, 1999). Furthermore, rural populations are recognized for lower rates of cancer screening (e.g., mammography, Pap testing, and colonoscopy) (Bennett, Probst, & Bellinger, 2011; Coughlin, Thompson, Hall, et al., 2002; Gosschalk & Carozza, 2003) and limited access to cancer-related health care, including screening services, health insurance, clinical trials, and oncology specialists (Baldwin et al., 2008; Gosschalk & Carozza, 2003; Institute of Medicine, 2005; Sateren et al., 2002; Schur & Franco, 1999). Lack of or delayed screening may predicate later-stage diagnoses with poorer clinical prognosis and aggressive treatment regimens. Evidence suggests that rural residents are at risk for later-stage cancer diagnoses compared to their urban counterparts (Howe et al., 1992; Liff, Chow, & Greenberg, 1991; Monroe et al., 1992). Cancer is an obvious area of concern for rural public health practitioners; based on survey results from *Rural Healthy People 2010,* cancer tied with nutrition and overweight (tenth and eleventh rankings) as a priority area for rural public health (Gosschalk & Carozza, 2003).

Although there are many types of cancer and cancer care is a continuum from prevention through the end of life, this chapter will focus specifically on prevention and screening efforts for breast, cervical, and colorectal cancer in rural communities. For each of these three cancers, the chapter will provide basic statistics, including rural-specific data; discuss related prevention and screening measures, statistics, and barriers to care for rural residents; and highlight successful examples of awareness campaigns, educational programs, and intervention studies focused on rural populations. Examples will draw from recent studies and the research of the Centers for Disease Control and Prevention (CDC)-funded University of Kentucky (UK) Rural Cancer Prevention Center (RCPC).

Key Concepts

Decreasing cancer disparities in rural and minority populations is important in cancer-control efforts because these populations suffer from undue cancer burden. The barriers faced by these populations make primary and secondary prevention efforts challenging for public health practitioners; however, using community assets, such as churches, health care providers, and community leaders, is an effective way to decrease rural cancer disparities.

Breast Cancer

Among women, breast cancer is the leading cause of cancer and the second leading cause of related mortality behind lung cancer (ACS, 2011a). More than 207,000 women are diagnosed with breast cancer annually and approximately 40,000 women die from the disease each year (ACS, 2010a). Increased breast cancer mortality, often due to a later-stage diagnosis, has been reported among specific rural populations such as African American women in the Deep South (Coughlin, Thompson, Seeff, et al., 2002; Friedell et al., 2003).

Primary prevention of breast cancer, preventing the disease before it starts, is difficult considering scientists do not exactly know what causes breast cancer. For example, there are no distinct risk factors for breast cancer as there are for lung cancer and its significant link to cigarette smoking. Modifiable risk factors for breast cancer may include alcohol consumption, weight, physical activity, use of postmenopausal hormone replacement therapy, use of birth control pills, having children, and breastfeeding (ACS, 2011a; NCI, 2011a). Risk factors for breast cancer that are not modifiable include age, gender, personal or family history of breast cancer, race and ethnicity, dense breast tissue, and young age at first menstruation (ACS, 2011a).

Although focused breast cancer prevention efforts are lacking due to causative uncertainties, research suggests that **screening** for breast cancer using clinical breast exams and mammography can significantly affect related morbidity and mortality (ACS, 2011a). In public health terms, this is recognized as **secondary prevention,** in other words, detecting the disease before symptoms are present. National mammography rates among women age forty and over now approach 62 percent (2008 data) (ACS, 2010b). However, certain segments of women, including minorities and those residing in rural America, have substantially lower screening rates, putting themselves at risk for a later-stage breast cancer diagnosis (Bennett et al., 2011; Coughlin, Thompson, Hall, et al., 2002; Friedell et al., 2003). For example, Hall and colleagues report that mammography screening rates (mammograms in the past two years) for Appalachian women are 69 percent compared to their non-Appalachian counterparts at 72 percent (Hall et al., 2002). Similarly, rural African American women in the southern Black Belt (eleven southern states) also have lower breast cancer screening rates compared to white women in the same region (66 percent versus 69 percent, respectively) (Coughlin, Thompson, Hall, et al., 2002). In addition, Cummings and colleagues examined mammography screening rates in rural North Carolina and found that African Americans (sixty-five years and older) reported the lowest screening rates (42 percent), whereas white women aged fifty to sixty-four reported the highest rates (58 percent) (Cummings et al., 2002). Lower rates of mammography screening may be due in part to a variety of behavioral, psychosocial, and socioeconomic **barriers,** which prevent women from obtaining needed breast cancer screening. These barriers include cost, limited access to screening services, lack of transportation, distance to medical services, lack of child care, fear of the mammography procedure, initiation of first mammography, fear of a cancer diagnosis, fewer qualified providers, and cultural beliefs (Coughlin, Thompson, Hall, et al., 2002; Coughlin, Thompson, Seeff, et al., 2002; Rauscher, Hawley, & Earp, 2005).

In an effort to address these barriers faced by rural women, public health practitioners and researchers have designed various awareness campaigns, educational programs, and intervention studies targeted to rural women. These programs, interventions, and community collaborations are done in hopes of increasing breast cancer screening rates and decreasing subsequent morbidity and mortality. For example, the Indiana County Cancer Coalition (ICCC) in rural southwest Pennsylvania adapted an evidence-based intervention to increase breast cancer screening in low-income rural women (Bencivenga et al., 2008). The ICCC chose the Tell A Friend program from the American Cancer Society. This program is based on peer counseling and incorporates the use of media, small incentives, and reminders to encourage women to make appointments for mammograms. The ICCC implemented this program through a partnering organization, the Indiana County Community Action Program, which is an association of eighteen food pantries. In collaboration with these food pantries, posters about breast cancer were displayed and female customers were sent to a screening recruitment area to speak with a staff member where screening eligibility was determined. Women forty and older with no history of screening were scheduled for a mammogram (Bencivenga et al., 2008). Subsequently, women were reminded by providers' offices to ensure completion of screening. A total of 158 women were identified as eligible for screening; 138 (87 percent) women were screened. For thirteen of these women, this was their first screening mammogram. The success of this evidence-based program helped disadvantaged Appalachian women receive mammograms and shows the impact local coalitions and community collaborations can have on cancer control in rural communities.

Additionally, the Delta Project was implemented to increase breast cancer screening among minority rural women in the Arkansas Delta. This intervention targeted health care providers and sought to increase their knowledge of screening guidelines, how to correctly perform a clinical breast exam, and to give appropriate counsel for breast cancer screening (Coleman et al., 2003). This project used in-office intervention methods such as pocket cards, prompts (posters), and short newsletters to reach rural physicians. Thirty-five percent of eligible African American women were screened in the intervention counties compared to 21 percent in the comparison group. This project demonstrated that rural health care providers are critical in cancer control and play a vital role in increasing their patients' screening behaviors.

As evidenced by the Tell A Friend program and the Delta Project, there are successful programs that public health practitioners and community organizations can adapt and implement in their own rural communities to affect breast cancer.

Cervical Cancer

The American Cancer Society reports approximately 12,000 women are diagnosed with cervical cancer each year and 4,200 women will die from the disease annually (ACS, 2010a). Cervical cancer is preventable through primary and secondary prevention measures. Increased cervical cancer incidence and mortality rates are observed among specific rural female populations such as Appalachians, Hispanics, and African Americans (Coughlin, Thompson, Hall, et al., 2002; Coughlin, Thompson, Seeff, et al., 2002; Huang et al., 2002; Wingo et al., 2008; Yabroff et al., 2005). The Papanicolaou (Pap) test has been an established cervical cancer screening exam since the 1950s and has been made widely available through private clinicians, federally qualified health centers, rural health centers, and local health departments. One noteworthy program is the federally funded National Breast and Cervical Cancer Early Detection Program (NBCCEDP), which provides free and low-cost screening services to women in need (see Box 19.1). Using the Pap test procedure, clinicians can identify and remove precancerous lesions as well as detect cervical cancer.

More recently, two pharmaceutical companies (GlaxoSmithKline and Merck & Co.) have developed an HPV vaccine to prevent infections from virus types 16 and 18, the two virus types responsible for 70 percent of all cervical cancer cases (NCI, 2009). Clinical evidence strongly suggests HPV vaccination among girls nine to twenty-six years old helps prevent the development of precancerous and cancerous cervical lesions (ACIP, 2010; Markowitz et al., 2007).

Despite the advent of these effective public health measures, rural women carry an undue burden of increased cervical cancer incidence and mortality primarily due to lower rates of screening and HPV vaccination, limited access to cervical cancer–related health care services, and lower socioeconomic status (Yabroff et al., 2005). Nationally, 83 percent of women eighteen years and older have had a Pap test within the past three years (2008 data) (ACS, 2010b). In examining specific rural populations, screening rates for Appalachian women are 81 percent compared to their non-Appalachian counterparts at 84 percent (Hall et al., 2002). Thompson and colleagues examined rural Hispanic cancer screening behaviors in Yukima County, Washington, and found that Hispanic women had lower cervical cancer screening rates

---

Box 19.1. National Breast and Cervical Cancer Early Detection Program (NBCCEDP)

In 1990, Congress passed the Breast and Cervical Cancer Mortality Prevention Act. The NBCCEDP provides funding to all fifty states and offers the following services to women who are economically disadvantaged or are uninsured: clinical breast exams, mammograms, Pap smears, pelvic exams, diagnostics, and treatment referral. Between 8 and 11 percent of US women are thought to be eligible for the NBCCEDP. To date, the NBCCEDP has served nearly four million women and provided nine million breast and cervical cancer screenings. This program has helped decrease mortality from breast and cervical cancer in underserved women.

The NBCCEDP serves as an example and a resource for rural public health practitioners. Partnering with local health departments can help ensure that underserved women can be served by the NBCCEDP and increase breast and cervical cancer screening in rural areas.

Source: CDC (2010b).

---

compared to non-Hispanic whites (90 percent Hispanic versus 98 percent white) (Thompson et al., 2002). Similar to breast cancer, rural women experience noted barriers to cervical cancer screening, which include modesty, fear of a cancer diagnosis, cultural beliefs such as fatalism, not wanting a male health care provider to perform the screening, daily family and job responsibilities, financial concerns, limited access to screening services, lack of transportation, and the invasive nature of the Pap test procedure (Freeman & Wingrove, 2005).

Rural women carry an undue burden of increased cervical cancer incidence and mortality primarily due to lower rates of screening and HPV vaccination, limited access to cervical cancer–related health care services, and lower socioeconomic status.

Despite the promise of a vaccine that can prevent cervical cancer, enthusiasm for the HPV vaccine has been limited because of its tie to a sexually transmitted disease, three-dose regimen, lack of promotion by health care providers, controversy about the incorporation into school-based vaccination requirements, and parental safety concerns (Gollust et al., 2010). Katz and colleagues report that Appalachian Ohio women, health care providers, and community members have significant concerns about the HPV vaccine, specifically with vaccine safety, the adolescent vaccination age recommendation, and the fact the vaccine prevents a sexually transmitted disease (Katz et al., 2009).

Nationally, HPV vaccine uptake and adherence rates are marginal at best. Among thirteen- to seventeen-year-old females in 2009, only 44 percent had at least dose one of the HPV vaccine and among women nineteen to twenty-six years old only 17 percent had at least dose one of the HPV vaccine (CDC, 2010a; Dorell et al., 2010). Even with documented interest in HPV vaccination by rural women (Fazekas, Brewer, & Smith, 2008; Hopenhayn et al., 2007), recent research suggests some rural adolescent girls and young adult women have lower HPV vaccination uptake and adherence rates. Crosby and colleagues compared HPV vaccination uptake between a rural sample of women and an urban sample in Kentucky and discovered that rural women were less likely to initiate dose one of the HPV vaccine (even though it was offered for free) and almost seven times less likely to return for subsequent doses compared to their urban counterparts (Crosby et al., 2011).

Fortunately, there are awareness campaigns, educational programs, and intervention studies that public health practitioners can identify in the literature and in practice to help increase cervical cancer screening and HPV vaccination rates in rural communities. Related specifically to Pap testing, Faith Moves Mountains (FMM) is a community-based participatory research (CBPR) project conducted in the heart of Appalachia Kentucky (see Chapter One). This program aims to increase Pap testing among rarely and never screened Appalachian women by the use of lay health advisors (LHAs) and also involves faith-based organizations in this multiphase program (Schoenberg et al., 2009). This program was highly tailored to the community and used local assets and collaborations to deliver the program. For example, the development of this program took eighteen months and used formative techniques such as ethnographic, survey, and focus group research (Schoenberg et al., 2009). This level of intense preparation was used to increase community buy-in and to ensure that the program truly reflected the central role religion plays in these rural communities. Although intervention results are pending, over four hundred Appalachian women and their families have interacted with the FMM program and its staff. FMM is an excellent example of a successful collaboration between community members and academic researchers to affect cancer in a medically underserved, rural area of the United States.

Regarding HPV vaccination, the UK RCPC has initiated a randomized-control study that uses a DVD-based counseling intervention to promote return for doses two and three of the HPV vaccine and routine Pap testing among women nineteen to twenty-six years old in Appalachia Kentucky. The campaign is entitled, "1–2–3 Pap"; women in the intervention group receive usual care (i.e., a telephone reminder from a nurse) and the DVD counseling program

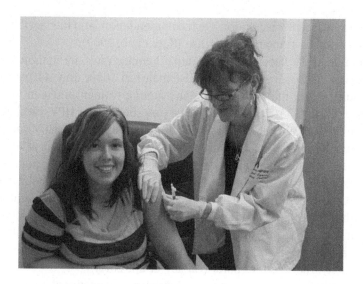

Figure 19.1. Young Woman Receiving the HPV Vaccine

and women in the control group receive only usual care. Research from a previous pilot study revealed that uptake and adherence of the HPV vaccine among young adult women in an eight-county region of Appalachia Kentucky was quite low, despite the vaccine series being offered free of charge (Crosby et al., 2011). Return rates for dose two of the vaccine were 32.0 percent and rates for dose three were 11.7 percent. As a result of these findings, RCPC researchers solicited feedback from its community advisory board members who suggested a communitywide social marketing campaign with billboard, radio, and television public service announcements, community hog roasts, and partnerships with the local health departments to encourage women to receive dose one of the HPV vaccine. Figure 19.1 shows a young Appalachian woman receiving dose one of the HPV vaccine from the RCPC research nurse.

In order to promote return for doses two and three, community members suggested a visual- and audio-based educational program with local "actors" to increase the salience of the health messages. Based on message testing with young adult women from eastern Kentucky, the RCPC partnered with the University of Kentucky Department of Communication to develop a twelve-minute DVD starring three young women from eastern Kentucky, two local female health care providers (a nurse practitioner and a physician), and a female television reporter from the regional news station. The primary messages of the DVD, entitled *1–2–3 Pap*, include increasing self-efficacy, increasing young women's understanding of the value of the HPV vaccine and Pap testing,

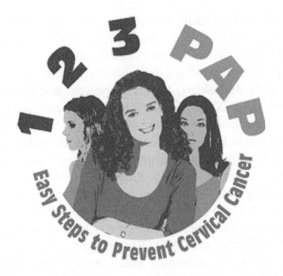

Figure 19.2. 1, 2, 3 Pap Logo

stressing the importance of receiving all three doses, and addressing barriers to the vaccination series (see Figure 19.2) (Cohen et al., in press).

Nine months after starting the study, 170 young women had received dose one of the HPV vaccine as a result of outreach and social marketing efforts. At that time, preliminary results from the randomized controlled trial intervention study suggested that the DVD intervention may have created a significantly ($P = .04$) greater return rate for all three doses (81.8 percent) compared to the rate observed for women randomized to the control condition (47.6 percent). Although these findings are only preliminary, they do suggest potential efficacy of this easy-to-deliver strategy for effectively protecting young rural women against cervical cancer via HPV vaccination.

As evidenced from the Faith Moves Mountains and the Rural Cancer Prevention Center's "1-2-3 Pap" campaign, there are a variety of ways communities and researchers alike can affect cervical cancer in rural areas.

Colorectal Cancer

Colorectal cancer (CRC, cancer of the colon and rectum) is the second leading cause of cancer and related mortality among men and women combined in the United States (ACS, 2011b). According to the American Cancer Society, 142,000 cases of colorectal cancer are diagnosed annually and 51,000 individuals die from the disease each year (ACS, 2011b). Increased colorectal cancer incidence and mortality rates have been observed among specific rural populations such as Appalachians (Huang et al., 2002; Wingo et al., 2008), African Americans (Bennett et al., 2011; Campbell et al., 2004), and Hispanics (Bennett et al., 2011; Thompson et al., 2002). Colorectal cancer risk factors include diet, physical inactivity, family history of colorectal cancer, cigarette smoking, age (fifty and older), history of polyps, and history of prolonged ulcerative colitis (NCI, 2011b). Similar to cervical cancer screening, screening for colorectal cancer can also prevent the development of cancer through the removal of precancerous polyps. Clinical research strongly suggests sigmoidoscopy and colonoscopy can significantly reduce incidence and mortality from colorectal cancer (Atkin et al., 2010; Kahi et al., 2009). However, nationally, both screening procedures are provided at rates that are suboptimal, at approximately 60 percent for men and women over age fifty (2008 data) (ACS, 2010b). Moreover, in rural communities the rates are even lower (Tarasenko & Schoenberg, 2011; Thompson et al., 2005). For example, Tarasenko and colleagues examined colorectal cancer screening among Appalachian residents and found that less than half (44 percent) of participants had a CRC screening in the past two years (Tarasenko & Schoenberg, 2011). Similarly, Thompson and colleagues found that rural Hispanics had lower rates of ever having a CRC screening (sigmoidoscopy or colonoscopy) than non-Hispanic rural whites (26 percent and 44 percent, respectively) (Thompson et al., 2005). In order to improve CRC screening rates in rural communities, the following barriers must be addressed: limited physician recommendation, limited access to endoscopy services, lack of transportation, being underinsured or uninsured, limited knowledge about CRC screening, invasive nature of screening procedures, embarrassment, fear of a cancer diagnosis, fatalistic views of cancer, and a lack of a personal physician. Further, only a limited number of gastroenterology specialists are available for referrals from rural family physicians (ACS, 2011c; Baldwin et al., 2008; Greiner et al., 2004).

Efforts to decrease barriers to colorectal cancer screening and increase uptake of the actual clinical procedure(s) are greatly needed in rural communities. Several exemplars of awareness campaigns, educational programs, and intervention studies have been previously conducted in rural communities. As an example, researchers in rural Colorado implemented an awareness campaign that involved items such as posters, community talks, advertisements, personal stories, news articles, and small incentives to bolster CRC screening rates (Zittleman et al., 2009). The High Plains Research Network in eastern Colorado used CBPR and was able to increase the regional populations' intentions to get screened for CRC and intentions to speak with a doctor about CRC screening.

In North Carolina, the Wellness for African Americans Through Churches (WATCH) program was conducted in twelve rural churches. The program aimed to promote behaviors such as increasing physical activity, improving diet (i.e., increasing fruit and vegetable consumption and monitoring fat intake), and increasing colorectal cancer screening through promotion of fecal occult blood testing (FOBT). Researchers compared two interventions: (1) a print and video component tailored to church members and (2) LHAs (Campbell et al., 2004). The print and video intervention was personalized and tailored to each individual from baseline survey data; videotapes and newsletters were sent periodically throughout the intervention time frame to participants. The LHAs provided diet, physical activity, and screening-related educational and awareness activities within the churches. Notably, the tailored print and video intervention was more successful than the LHA intervention. Among the tailored print and video intervention group, the screening rate for FOBT increased by 15 percentage points compared to the LHA group (10 percent) (Campbell et al., 2004). As evidenced by this research, rural churches can be a community asset when conducting colorectal cancer–related prevention and screening interventions.

Rural churches can be a community asset when conducting colorectal cancer–related prevention and screening interventions.

As demonstrated by the High Plains Research Network and the WATCH program, there are successful initiatives that public health practitioners and community organizations can adapt and implement in their own rural communities to affect colorectal cancer.

Conclusion

As evidenced by the disparities in disease rates and screening for breast, cervical, and colorectal cancer in rural populations, cancer control in rural communities is necessary. Reducing barriers to care, emphasizing community assets, building collaborations, and increasing capacity all play a role in how successful community members and researchers can be in implementing cancer control programs in rural locales. Although cancer is just one of many health disparities in rural communities, it is an important one that can indeed be rectified through carefully constructed public health programs.

Summary

- Rural communities have higher rates of cancer because of the prevalence of cancer-related risk factors such as alcohol consumption, cigarette smoking, sun exposure, poor diet, and physical inactivity.

- Rural populations are associated with lower rates of cancer screening, which may predicate later-stage diagnoses with poorer clinical prognosis and more aggressive treatment regimens.

- Common barriers to receiving breast, cervical, and colorectal cancer screenings in rural communities are financial constraints, limited access to screening services, lack of transportation, fear of the screening procedure, fear of a cancer diagnosis, and cultural norms.

- Successful, evidence-based programs promoting cancer screenings in rural communities are available for public health practitioners and community organizations to adapt, implement, and evaluate in their own rural communities.

Key Terms

barriers

primary prevention

risk factors

screening

secondary prevention

For Practice and Discussion

1. Working with a classmate, discuss why rural communities experience higher rates of cancer and lower rates of screening. Consider the top three barriers to cancer screening articulated by rural residents and formulate a related intervention(s) to alleviate those barriers. Could you design one intervention to address all three cancer situations or do you need three individual programs? Please be prepared to explain your answer.

2. Consider the University of Kentucky Rural Cancer Prevention project focused on increasing adherence to doses two and three of the HPV vaccine. If you were designing a similar campaign in your rural community, what key questions would you ask your community advisory board? How would you balance your ideas for an intervention project with the community's ideas? How would you continue to solicit feedback from the community members throughout the development and implementation of the project?

3. For all three cancers discussed in this chapter, it is clear that increasing cancer screening rates would make a substantial impact on disease rates. Working with a classmate, design a social marketing

campaign that would resonate with your rural community focused on either breast, cervical, or colorectal cancer screening. What would be your campaign's call to action? What community resources would you use? Which local "celebrities" would you call on?

Acknowledgments

This publication was also supported by cooperative agreement number 1U48DP001932–01 from the Centers for Disease Control and Prevention. The findings and conclusions in this article are those of the author(s) and do not necessarily represent the official position of the Centers for Disease Control and Prevention.

References

ACIP. (2010). Recommended adult immunization schedule: United States, 2010. *Annals of Internal Medicine, 152*(1), 36–39.

ACS. (2010a). *Cancer facts & figures 2010.* Retrieved from http://www.cancer.org/ Research/CancerFactsFigures/CancerFactsFigures/cancer-facts-and-figures-2010

ACS. (2010b). *Cancer prevention and early detection.* Retrieved from http:// www.cancer.org/acs/groups/content/@epidemiologysurveilance/documents/ document/acspc-027876.pdf

ACS. (2011a). *Breast cancer.* Retrieved from http://www.cancer.org/acs/groups/cid/ documents/webcontent/003090-pdf.pdf

ACS. (2011b). *Colorectal cancer.* Retrieved from http://www.cancer.org/acs/groups/ cid/documents/webcontent/003096-pdf.pdf

ACS. (2011c). *Colorectal cancer facts and figures 2011–2013.* Retrieved from http:// www.cancer.org/acs/groups/content/@epidemiologysurveilance/documents/ document/acspc-028323.pdf

Atkin, W. S., Edwards, R., Kralj-Hans, I., Wooldrage, K., Hart, A. R., Northover, J.M.A., et al. (2010). Once-only flexible sigmoidoscopy screening in prevention of colorectal cancer: A multicentre randomised controlled trial. *The Lancet, 375*(9726), 1624–1633.

Baldwin, L. M., Cai, Y., Larson, E. H., Dobie, S. A., Wright, G. E., Goodman, D. C., et al. (2008). Access to cancer services for rural colorectal cancer patients. *Journal of Rural Health, 24*(4), 390–399.

Bencivenga, M., DeRubis, S., Leach, P., Lotito, L., Shoemaker, C., & Lengerich, E. J. (2008). Community partnerships, food pantries, and an evidence-based intervention to increase mammography among rural women. *The Journal of Rural Health, 24*(1), 91–95.

Bennett, K. J., Probst, J. C., & Bellinger, J. D. (2011). Receipt of cancer screening services: Surprising results for some rural minorities. *The Journal of Rural Health, 28*(1), 63–72.

Campbell, M. K., James, A., Hudson, M. A., Carr, C., Jackson, E., Oates, V., et al. (2004). Improving multiple behaviors for colorectal cancer prevention among African American church members. *Health Psychology, 23*(5), 492–502.

CDC. (2010a). *2009 adult vaccination coverage, NHIS.* Retrieved from http://www.cdc.gov/vaccines/stats-surv/nhis/2009-nhis.htm

CDC. (2010b). *National breast and cervical cancer early detection program (NBCCEDP): About the program.* Retrieved from http://www.cdc.gov/cancer/nbccedp/about.htm

Cohen, E. L., Vanderpool, R. C., Crosby, R. A., Noar, S. M., Bates, W., Collins, T., et al. (in press). 1–2–3 Pap: A campaign to prevent cervical cancer in eastern Kentucky. In M. J. Dutta & G. L. Kreps (Eds.), *Communication and health disparities.* Cresskill, NJ: Hampton Press.

Coleman, E. A., Lord, J., Heard, J., Coon, S., Cantrell, M., & Mohrmann, C., et al. (2003). The Delta project: Increasing breast cancer screening among rural minority and older women by targeting rural healthcare providers. *Oncology Nursing Forum, 30*(4), 669–677.

Coughlin, S. S., Thompson, T. D., Hall, H. I., Logan, P., & Uhler, R. J. (2002). Breast and cervical carcinoma screening practices among women in rural and nonrural areas of the United States, 1998–1999. *Cancer, 94*(11), 2801–2812.

Coughlin, S. S., Thompson, T. D., Seeff, L., Richards, T., & Stallings, F. (2002). Breast, cervical, and colorectal carcinoma screening in a demographically defined region of the southern U.S. *Cancer, 95*(10), 2211–2222.

Crosby, R. A., Casey, B. R., Vanderpool, R., Collins, T., & Moore, G. R. (2011). Uptake of free HPV vaccination among young women: A comparison of rural versus urban rates. *The Journal of Rural Health, 27,* 380–384.

Cummings, D. M., Whetstone, L. M., Earp, J. A., & Mayne, L. (2002). Disparities in mammography screening in rural areas: Analysis of county differences in North Carolina. *The Journal of Rural Health, 18*(1), 77–83.

Dorell, C., Stokley, S., Yankey, D., & Cohn, A. (2010). National, state, and local area vaccination coverage among adolescents aged 13–17 years—United States, 2009. *Morbidity and Mortality Weekly Report, 59*(32), 1018–1023.

Eberhardt, M. S., & Pamuk, E. R. (2004). The importance of place of residence: Examining health in rural and nonrural areas. *American Journal of Public Health, 94*(10), 1682–1686.

Fazekas, K. I., Brewer, N. T., & Smith, J. S. (2008). HPV vaccine acceptability in a rural southern area. *Journal of Women's Health, 17*(4), 539–548.

Freeman, H. P., & Wingrove, B. K. (2005). *Excess cervical cancer mortality: A marker for low access to health care in poor communities.* Rockville, MD: National Cancer Institute, Center to Reduce Cancer Health Disparities.

Friedell, G. H., Linville, L. H., Sorrell, C. L., & Huang, B. (2003). Kentucky breast cancer report card. *Journal of the Kentucky Medical Association, 101*(10), 449–454.

Gollust, S. E., Dempsey, A. F., Lantz, P. M., Ubel, P. A., & Fowler, E. F. (2010). Controversy undermines support for state mandates on the human papillomavirus vaccine. *Health Affairs, 29*(11), 2041–2046.

Gosschalk, A., & Carozza, S. (2003). Cancer in rural areas: A literature review. *Rural healthy people 2010: A companion document to Healthy People 2010* (Vol. 2). College Station: The Texas A&M University System Health Science Center, School of Rural Public Health, Southwest Rural Health Research Center.

Greiner, K. A., Engelman, K. K., Hall, M. A., & Ellerbeck, E. F. (2004). Barriers to colorectal cancer screening in rural primary care. *Preventive Medicine, 38*(3), 269–275.

Hall, H. I., Uhler, R. J., Coughlin, S. S., & Miller, D. S. (2002). Breast and cervical cancer screening among Appalachian women. *Cancer Epidemiology Biomarkers & Prevention, 11*, 137–142.

Hartley, D. (2004). Rural health disparities, population health, and rural culture. *American Journal of Public Health, 94*(10), 1675–1678.

Haynes, M., & Smedley, B. (Eds.). (1999). *The unequal burden of cancer: An assessment of NIH research and programs for ethnic minorities and the medically underserved.* Washington, DC: National Academies Press.

Hopenhayn, C. R., Christian, A., Christian, W. J., & Schoenberg, N. E. (2007). Human papillomavirus vaccine: Knowledge and attitudes in two Appalachian Kentucky counties. *Cancer Causes Control, 16*(6), 627–634.

Howe, H. L., Katterhagen, J. G., Yates, J., & Lehnherr, M. (1992). Urban-rural differences in the management of breast cancer. *Cancer Causes and Control, 3*(6), 533–539.

Huang, B., Wyatt, S., Tucker, T., Bottorff, D., Lengerich, E., & Hall, H. (2002). Cancer death rates—Appalachia, 1994–1998. *Morbidity and Mortality Weekly Report, 51*(24), 527–529.

Institute of Medicine. (2005). *Quality through collaboration: The future of rural health.* Washington, DC: National Academies Press.

Kahi, C. J., Imperiale, T. F., Juliar, B. E., & Rex, D. K. (2009). Effect of screening colonoscopy on colorectal cancer incidence and mortality. *Clinical Gastroenterology and Hepatology, 7*(7), 770–775.

Katz, M. L., Reiter, P. L., Heaner, S., Ruffin, M. T., Post, D. M., & Paskett, E. D. (2009). Acceptance of the HPV vaccine among women, parents, community leaders, and healthcare providers in Ohio Appalachia. *Vaccine, 27*, 3945–3952.

Liff, J. M., Chow, W.-H., & Greenberg, R. S. (1991). Rural-urban differences in stage at diagnosis. Possible relationship to cancer screening. *Cancer, 67*(5), 1454–1459.

Markowitz, L., Dunne, E. F., Saraiya, M., Lawson, H., Chesson, H., & Unger, E. (2007). Quadrivalent human papillomavirus vaccine: Recommendations of the ACIP. *Morbidity and Mortality Weekly Report, 56*(RR02), 1–24.

Monroe, A. C., Ricketts, T. C., & Savitz, L. A. (1992). Cancer in rural versus urban populations: A review. *The Journal of Rural Health, 8*(3), 212–220.

NCI. (2009). *Human papillomavirus (HPV) vaccines.* Retrieved from http://www.cancer.gov/cancertopics/factsheet/Prevention/HPV-vaccine

NCI. (2011a). *What you need to know about breast cancer: About this booklet.* Retrieved from http://www.cancer.gov/cancertopics/wyntk/breast

NCI. (2011b). *What you need to know about cancer of the colon and rectum: Risk factors.* Retrieved from http://www.cancer.gov/cancertopics/wyntk/colon-and-rectal/page4

Phillips, C. D., & McLeroy, K. R. (2004). Health in rural America: Remembering the importance of place. *American Journal of Public Health, 94*(10), 1661–1663.

Probst, J. C., Moore, C. G., Glover, S. H., & Samuels, M. E. (2004). Person and place: The compounding effects of race/ethnicity and rurality on health. *American Journal of Public Health, 94*(10), 1695–1703.

Rauscher, G. H., Hawley, S. T., & Earp, J. A. (2005). Baseline predictors of initiation vs. maintenance of regular mammography use among rural women. *Preventive Medicine, 40*(6), 822–830.

Ricketts, T. C., Johnson-Webb, K. D., & Randolph, R. K. (1999). Populations and places in rural America. In T. C. Ricketts (Ed.), *Rural health in the United States.* New York: Oxford University Press.

Sateren, W. B., Trimble, E. L., Abrams, J., Brawley, O., Breen, N., Ford, L., et al. (2002). How sociodemographics, presence of oncology specialists, and hospital cancer programs affect accrual to cancer treatment trials. *Journal of Clinical Oncology, 20*(8), 2109–2117.

Schoenberg, N. E., Hatcher, J., Dignan, M. B., Shelton, B., Wright, S., & Dollarhide, K. F. (2009). Faith moves mountains: A cervical cancer prevention program in Appalachia. *American Journal of Health Behavior, 33*(6), 627–638.

Schur, C. L., & Franco, S. J. (1999). Access to health care. In T. C. Ricketts (Ed.), *Rural health in the United States.* New York: Oxford University Press.

Tarasenko, Y. N., & Schoenberg, N. E. (2011). Colorectal cancer screening among rural Appalachian residents with multiple morbidities. *Rural and Remote Health Journal, 11,* 1553.

Thompson, B., Coronado, G., Neuhouser, M., & Chen, L. (2005). Colorectal carcinoma screening among Hispanics and non-Hispanic whites in a rural setting. *Cancer, 103*(12), 2491–2498.

Thompson, B., Coronado, G. D., Solomon, C. C., McClerran, D. F., Neuhouser, M. L., & Feng, Z. (2002). Cancer prevention behaviors and socioeconomic status among Hispanics and non-Hispanic whites in a rural population in the United States. *Cancer Causes and Control, 13*(8), 719–728.

Wingo, P. A., Tucker, T. C., Jamison, P. M., Martin, H., McLaughlin, C., Bayakly, R., et al. (2008). Cancer in Appalachia, 2001–2003. *Cancer, 112*(1), 181–192.

Yabroff, K., Lawrence, W., King, J., Mangan, P., Washington, K., Yi, B., et al. (2005). Geographic disparities in cervical cancer mortality: What are the roles of risk factor prevalence, screening, and use of recommended treatment? *The Journal of Rural Health, 21*(2), 149–157.

Zittleman, L., Emsermann, C., Dickinson, M., Norman, N., Winkelman, K., Linn, G., et al. (2009). Increasing colon cancer testing in rural Colorado: Evaluation of the exposure to a community-based awareness campaign. *BMC Public Health, 9*(1), 288.

Chapter 20

Tobacco Use in Rural Populations

Geri A. Dino
Rose M. Pignataro
Kimberly A. Horn
Andrew Anesetti-Rothermel

Learning Objectives

- Identify differences between rural and urban residents' use of and addiction to tobacco products.
- Understand the primary challenges facing rural Americans regarding tobacco addiction.
- Describe programs and strategies that may be highly effective for the primary prevention of tobacco use among people in rural areas.
- Describe programs and strategies that may be highly effective for the cessation of tobacco use among people in rural areas.

•••

The evidence is indisputable that tobacco use is a national and worldwide problem. By the year 2020, it is projected that 8.4 million lives will be lost annually as a result of cigarette smoking (Bernhard et al., 2007), and the direct effects of smoking and related comorbidities will comprise the greatest global health problems (Csordas et al., 2008). Within the United States, tobacco use is the most pervasive cause of premature morbidity and mortality, accounting for more than 443,000 deaths per year, and results in $193 billion dollars annually in health care costs and lost productivity (Cokkinidies et al., 2009).

Smoking is the most prevalent form of tobacco use (Yanbaeva et al., 2007), creating health risks for smokers (active smoking) as well as others through environmental tobacco smoke (ETS) exposure (passive smoking) (Stampfli & Anderson, 2009; Yanbaeva et al., 2007). Smoking is a primary risk factor for multiple cancers (Hecht, 2006), coronary artery disease and stroke (Swan & Lessov-Schlaggar, 2007), peripheral vascular disease, lung diseases (Stampfli & Anderson, 2009), autoimmune diseases (Costenbader & Karlson, 2006; Harel-Meir, Sherer, & Shoenfeld, 2007), and adverse pregnancy outcomes (Salihu & Wilson, 2007). Smokeless tobacco use is also associated with health problems including cancer, coronary artery disease, peptic ulcers, and neuromuscular disease (Campbell-Grossman, Hudson, & Fleck, 2003).

Key Concepts

Rural populations are at increased risk for tobacco-related health disparities, including higher rates of initiation, current use, intensity of use, exposure to secondhand smoke, and cessation failure (Fagan et al., 2007; Weg et al., 2010). Rural youths and adults also experience more ETS exposure than do those living in urban areas (Weg et al., 2010; York et al., 2010). Use of smokeless tobacco is also highest in US rural areas (Nelson et al., 2006; Weg et al., 2010). This chapter presents rural tobacco use prevalence rates and associated chronic disease risks as well as tobacco-control strategies, including specific recommendations for reducing tobacco-related health disparities in rural populations.

Tobacco Use Prevalence

Whereas tobacco prevalence declined slightly in US urban areas, rural residents show increasing rates (Doescher et al., 2006; Weg et al., 2010). Underscoring the importance of this chapter, there is significant disparity in tobacco use between youth and adults living in rural versus urban areas. For example, approximately twelve million adult smokers live in rural communities (Hutcheson et al., 2008), representing the highest self-reported rates of adult tobacco use in the nation (Northridge et al., 2008).

Smoking

The prevalence of current smoking is 24.2 percent in Appalachia versus 21.9 percent in non-Appalachia America (Meyer et al., 2008). In Ohio, 30.0 percent of the state's Appalachian residents smoke compared to the statewide prevalence of 25.1 percent (Ahijevyyk et al., 2003). Rural smokers also tend to smoke more cigarettes per day than do nonrural smokers (Hutcheson et al., 2008).

To illustrate, 2007 BRFSS data show that the three states with the highest smoking prevalence are Kentucky (28.3 percent), West Virginia (27.0 percent), and Oklahoma (25.8 percent) (Davis et al., 2009).

We conducted an exploratory spatial (e.g., geographical) **data analysis** (Anselin, 1994) to examine the geographic distribution of cigarette smoking rates in the contiguous United States using county-level data from the forty-eight states and the District of Columbia, highlighting counties in Appalachia. Figure 20.1 shows the spatial distribution of county-level smoking rates in the United States from 2000 to 2009. The average US county rate was 21.46 percent (SD = 4.28). The lowest rate was found in Madison, Idaho (3.54 percent), and the highest in Shannon, South Dakota (44.07 percent). We also found that the average Appalachian county smoking rate (24.31 percent; SD = 4.40) was noticeably higher than the national average. The minimum Appalachian county smoking rate (13.53 percent) was found for Forsyth, Georgia, and the maximum (39.30 percent) was found in Lewis, Kentucky. Further examination of Figure 20.1 shows that most Appalachian counties are in the top two quintiles of smoking rates.

Figure 20.2 illustrates the spatial association between rurality and cigarette smoking rates based on 2000 to 2009 BRFSS data (CDC, 2010). Rurality was categorized into a nine-part classification scheme using 2003 RUCCs (US Department of Agriculture, 2004). Metro counties were subdivided into three classes based on the population size of their metro areas; nonmetro (rural) counties were subdivided into six classes based on their degree of urbanization and adjacency to a metro area(s). Cigarette smoking rates were calculated based on the total number of smokers per county and used respondent-weighted smoking rates and spatial empirical Bayes smoothed raw smoking rates in its construction. Counties without smokers were given their state's mean imputed rate.

We found a spatial association between rurality and cigarette smoking rates (Moran's I = 0.06; SD = .01; pseudo p = .001) after randomization (999 permutations). A total of 227 counties were clustered as having high rurality and high smoking, whereas 225 counties were clustered as having low rurality and low smoking (P < .05). Spatial outliers are identified as areas atypical to this causal association, for example, low rurality–high smoking (157 counties) or high rurality–low smoking (162 counties). As seen in Figure 20.2, central Appalachia is a geographic region of concern with significantly higher rates of smoking and rurality. In contrast, other rural areas such as in the Northwest have much lower rates of smoking than expected based on their rural nature. Future research is needed to understand the factors associated with these spatial outliers.

Rural smoking disparities exist with young people as well. Youths in tobacco-growing areas start smoking at an earlier age and smoke more

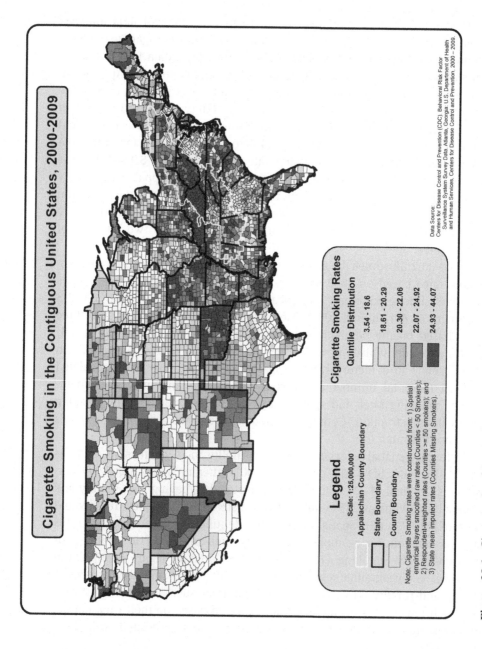

Figure 20.1. Cigarette Smoking in the Contiguous United States, 2000–2009

Note: Cigarette smoking rates were constructed from (1) spatial empirical Bayes smoothed raw rates (counties < 50 smokers); (2) respondent-weighted rates (counties ≥ 50 smokers); and (3) state mean imputed rates (counties missing smokers).

Source: CDC (2010).

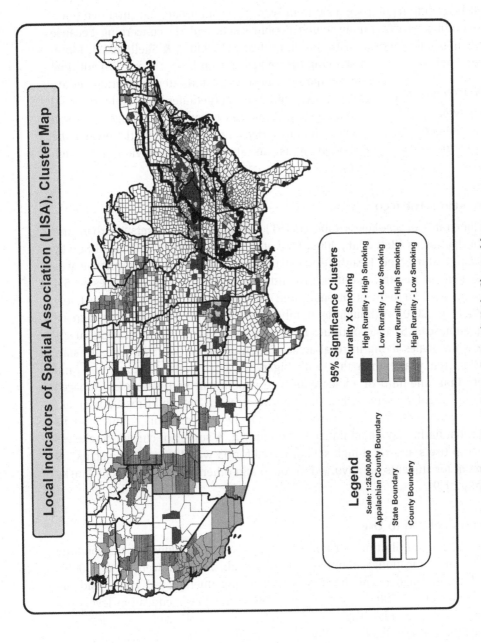

Figure 20.2. Local Indicators of Spatial Association (LISA), Cluster Map

Note: Cigarette smoking rates were constructed from (1) spatial empirical Bayes smoothed raw rates (counties < 50 smokers); (2) respondent-weighted rates (counties ≥ 50 smokers); and (3) state mean imputed rates (counties missing smokers).

Source: CDC (2010); US Department of Agriculture (2004).

frequently than do their nonrural peers (Denham, Meyer, & Toborg, 2004). Lutfiyya and colleagues (2008) merged YRBS data from 1997 to 2003 and found that rural high school students were at greater risk for using tobacco products and becoming regular smokers than were their suburban and urban counterparts. Tobacco use among young people is particularly concerning because addiction rates increase with duration of use (Newman & Shell, 2005). Moreover, youths who begin smoking before age sixteen have a more difficult time quitting than do those who start later (Northridge et al., 2008). Early initiation perpetuates the cycle of rural tobacco-related disparities because the younger a person is when she or he begins to use tobacco, the greater the likelihood of use as an adult (Hu, Davies, & Kandel, 2006).

Youths in tobacco-growing areas start smoking at an earlier age and smoke more frequently than their nonrural peers.

Smokeless Tobacco

Higher rates of smokeless tobacco (ST) use exist in rural versus urban and suburban areas (Bell et al., 2009; Weg et al., 2010). The 2008 National Survey on Drug Abuse and Health revealed that adult past-year ST prevalence was 10.0 percent in rural counties in contrast to county prevalence rates of 5.4 percent and 3.1 percent in small and large metropolitan areas, respectively (Weg et al., 2010). Although the number of adults using ST is stable or decreasing, adolescent ST use continues to be a problem. The majority of young users are white males living in rural areas. Experimentation with ST tends to start earlier (ten years) than that with cigarettes (age twelve to fourteen), and more than one-third of adolescents who experiment with smokeless tobacco become regular users within one to two years (Campbell-Grossman et al., 2003). Smokeless tobacco use is often deeply embedded in culture and its potential harm may be minimized or unknown. A survey of current smokeless tobacco users at a rural high school in California was 49.1 percent versus 5.9 percent for students not involved in rodeo and other organized sports (Gansky et al., 2009).

Factors Related to Use

Two factors contributing to rural tobacco disparities are lower socioeconomic status and educational attainment (Fagan et al., 2007; Wewers et al., 2000). To illustrate, higher smoking rates exist among unemployed rural residents (Doescher et al., 2006), children of parents with lower education levels are more likely to smoke (Fagan et al., 2007), and people with lower levels of education are less likely to achieve successful cessation (Fagan et al., 2007; Wewers et al., 2000). Other factors associated with rural tobacco disparities include low levels of medical coverage (Hutcheson et al., 2008), geographic isolation with reduced access to medical services (Hutcheson et al., 2008; Northridge et al., 2008), reduced availability of resources that promote cessation (Hutcheson et al., 2008), cultural attitudes that foster greater acceptance of tobacco use, and a regional economy that relies on tobacco production (Northridge et al., 2008). Ease of access to tobacco products facilitated early initiation and use (Denham et al., 2004; Smith et al., 2008), especially for youths living in tobacco-producing regions (Denham et al., 2004).

Tobacco advertising is a consistent predictor of tobacco use. Impact of tobacco advertising may be magnified in adolescents in that it contributes to a distorted perspective of widespread use (Smith et al., 2008). In rural communities, manufacturers may seek to capitalize on the cultural uniqueness to increase sales, for example, through sponsorship of sporting events such as local rodeos (American Legacy Foundation, 2009).

Exposure to Environmental Tobacco Smoke

ETS ranks third among preventable risk factors for premature mortality in the United States, accounting for fifty-three thousand annual deaths among non-smokers (Hahn et al., 2009). ETS includes sidestream smoke, the smoke that is released from the burning end of combustible tobacco products, and mainstream smoke, the exhaled smoke from smokers. Given the higher smoking prevalence rates in rural compared to nonrural areas, it is perhaps not surprising that rural children and adults are also more likely to be exposed to ETS than are those living in urban areas (York et al., 2010).

In addition to heightened ETS exposure in the home, rural communities are less likely than urban communities to have smoke-free restrictions (York et al., 2010). For instance, McMillen, Breen, and Cosby (2004) found that smoking bans in homes, cars, and public places, except outdoor parks, were less common in rural areas than they were in other locations. A recent study by Weg and colleagues (2010) used BRFSS data from 2006 and 2008 to examine geographic differences in self-reported tobacco use, ETS exposure in homes and public places, as well as policies regarding smoking at home and in workplaces. Study findings revealed that compared to suburban and urban residents, rural residents were more likely to have smoked and used ST in their lifetimes and to be current smokers, less likely to have quit, and more likely to experience ETS in the home and workplace. Rural residents also reported less restrictive smoking policies in homes and workplaces than their nonrural counterparts.

Racial and Ethnic Diversity in Tobacco Use Prevalence

Diversity exists throughout rural America. The racial and ethnic mix within US rural communities varies widely, and racial and ethnic differences in tobacco use may contribute to tobacco-related health disparities. Among racial and ethnic groups living in rural areas, Asians have the lowest prevalence and Native Americans have the highest prevalence of current smoking (Doescher et al., 2006). There is also a very low smoking prevalence among Amish communities living in Appalachia (Ferketich et al., 2008). Native Americans and Alaskan Natives have the highest rates of tobacco use in the United States (Fagan et al., 2007). Tobacco use among rural Native Americans is particularly high (Fagan et al., 2007)—20 percent higher than among other ethnic and racial groups living in similar areas (Doescher et al., 2006). Sale of tobacco products through Native American smoke shops helps stimulate the tribal economy and may contribute to increased prevalence of smoking within this population (Eichner et al., 2005). Influence of ceremonial tobacco use among Native Americans on rates of nontraditional smoking remains under investigation (Forster, Widome, & Bernat, 2007).

Tobacco Use and Chronic Disease

Tobacco use remains the leading preventable cause of many chronic diseases. The negative health consequences are extensive and varied, and compared to their urban counterparts, rural populations experience a disproportionate burden of health disparities causing tobacco-related diseases.

Diseases from Smoking

Cardiovascular disease is the leading cause of death in the United States but is particularly prominent in certain rural areas (Eberhardt & Pamuk, 2004). High rates of coronary heart disease have been observed in the Mississippi Delta, Ohio River Valley, and Appalachia, as well as the Piedmont areas of North and South Carolina and Georgia (Cooper et al., 2000). As a primary risk factor (Csordas et al., 2008; Leone et al., 2008; Tanriverdi et al., 2006), smoking contributes to heart disease through a number of mechanisms including chronic hypoxia and direct damage to the heart muscle, as well as thickening and calcification of the small coronary blood vessels (Leone et al., 2008), inflammation and oxidative stress (Csordas et al., 2008), and impaired antioxidant defense (Tanriverdi et al., 2006). Rural residence is also a risk factor for cerebrovascular disease (Cooper et al., 2000). Smoking is a significant risk factor for ischemic stroke (Bhat et al., 2008) and the prevalence of silent cerebral infarction was 1.8 times higher in current smokers versus nonsmokers (Swan & Lessov-Schlaggar, 2007).

A significant cardiovascular risk factor is diabetes. Of significance, rural areas experience a 17 percent higher diabetes prevalence rate compared to urban areas (Keppel, Pearcy, & Klein, 2004) and rural communities emphasize diabetes as a top health priority (Gamm & Hutchison, 2004). Research demonstrates a dose-dependent relationship between active smoking and the risk of type 2 diabetes (Willi, Bodenmann, & Ghali, 2007). Tobacco use may contribute to reduced glucose tolerance (Rafalson et al., 2009) by affecting glucose metabolism and insulin resistance (Willi et al., 2007). In people with diabetes, smoking accelerates renal failure (Jaimes, Tian, & Raij, 2007) and increases the incidence of peripheral neuropathy (Tamer et al., 2006; Tesfaye et al., 2005).

Cancer is the second leading cause of death in the United States. Smoking is well established as a risk factor for many cancers including lung, kidney, bladder, oral, esophageal, stomach, liver, and cervical cancer, and risk is correlated to duration and intensity of smoking (Gandini et al., 2008; Hecht, 2006). Lung cancer is the leading cause of cancer mortality nationally and worldwide. Smoking is the primary risk factor for lung cancer (Cornfield et al., 2009) and is responsible for 85 to 90 percent of lung cancers in the United States (Freedman et al., 2008). Smoking has also been implicated as a causal factor for higher rates of lung cancer for women residing in rural areas (Jemal et al., 2008).

Smoking is the primary risk factor for chronic obstructive pulmonary disease (Mannino & Buist, 2007), a leading cause of morbidity and mortality worldwide and in the United States, with a higher prevalence in rural areas versus other locations (Eberhardt & Pamuk, 2004). Smokers with asthma have more severe symptoms, accelerated decline in respiratory function, greater rates of hospitalization, and an impaired response to corticosteroids compared to nonsmokers. Cessation mitigates or reverses these symptoms (Chaudhuri et al., 2006).

Smoking can also lead to suppression of the immune system (Harel-Meir et al., 2007), impaired wound healing (Costenbader & Karlson, 2006; Martin et al., 2009), and is a risk factor for rheumatoid arthritis, lupus (Costenbader & Karlson, 2006; Harel-Meir et al., 2007), Graves' hyperthyroidism, Crohn's disease, and cirrhosis (Costenbader & Karlson, 2006).

Smokeless Tobacco

The amount of nicotine in a single dose of chewing tobacco is the same as or greater than the amount obtained from smoking a cigarette (Campbell-Grossman et al., 2003). There are a wide variety of negative health outcomes associated with ST, including oral and pancreatic cancers and cardiovascular disease (Boffetta & Straif, 2009; Campbell-Grossman et al., 2003; Nelson et al., 2006). In a twenty-year follow-up of people who had switched from cigarettes to ST, rates of all-cause mortality, lung cancer, coronary artery disease, and stroke were still significantly higher than among people who had ceased using tobacco entirely (Henley et al., 2007).

Environmental Tobacco Smoke

ETS exposure increases the risk for cardiovascular disease and stroke (Jefferis et al., 2010) by reducing circulating levels of antioxidants resulting in endothelial damage (Kosecik et al., 2005) and increasing inflammatory markers related to endothelial dysfunction (Jefferis et al., 2010). Even exposure to ETS for short time periods, for example, less than thirty minutes, can result in heightened cardiovascular risk in nonsmokers (Flouris et al., 2010; Hahn et al., 2009; Sullivan & Glantz, 2010). ETS exposure is also associated with heightened cancer risk and immune suppression (Stampfli & Anderson, 2009).

Harmful ETS exposure begins before birth due to smoking during pregnancy (Song & Fish, 2006). Smoking during pregnancy increases the likelihood of infertility, preterm delivery, low birth weight, and sudden infant death syndrome (Salihu & Wilson, 2007). Tobacco use has also been implicated in later pregnancy miscarriage (Dorfman, 2008). The CDC's state-specific **Pregnancy Risk Assessment Monitoring System** (PRAMS) gathers information on maternal attitudes and experiences before, during, and briefly after pregnancy. PRAMS data between 2000 and 2005 indicate that West Virginia, the only state fully encompassed by Appalachia, had the highest rate of smoking before, during, and after pregnancy, as well as the lowest rate of cessation during pregnancy (Tong et al., 2005). Nicotine readily crosses the placenta, has toxic effects on the fetus, and can reduce blood flow to the fetus and uterus through vasoconstriction (Swan & Lessov-Schlaggar, 2007). Exposure to cigarette smoke in utero has lasting implications including an increased life-long risk of cancer (Stampfli & Anderson, 2009) and heightened risk of behavioral disorders such as personality disorder, attention deficit disorder, and lower cognitive abilities (Julvez et al., 2007). Prenatal exposure to smoking and tobacco toxins has also been associated with decreased temporal lobe function and deficits in visuo-spatial memory (Swan & Lessov-Schlaggar, 2007).

More than 30 percent of children in the United States live in homes with at least one smoker (Poole-DiSalvo et al., 2010). ETS in childhood results in increased rates of lower respiratory and middle ear infections, increased severity of asthma, and also may be associated with increased risk of metabolic syndrome (Poole-DiSalvo et al., 2010). Tobacco smoke also increases risk of dental caries and may be associated with childhood obesity (Winickoff, Van Cleave, & Oreskovic, 2010). ETS exposure contributes to oxidative stress in children and can lead to early atherosclerosis (Kosecik et al., 2005).

Tobacco-Control Strategies in Rural America

The most effective way to address the burden of tobacco use is evidence-based, comprehensive, integrated, and sustained programs that affect social norms, networks, and systems (CDC, 2007; Institute of Medicine, 2007; World Health

Organization, 2008). Critical components include smoke-free policies; cessation assistance; prevention education; restrictions on tobacco advertising, promotion, and sponsorship; and increases in tobacco taxes.

Rural environments can present challenges for tobacco control because of, for example, favorable attitudes regarding tobacco use, highlighting the need for targeted strategies for rural populations. However, rural communities do have varying cultural, geographic, and population characteristics. Effective strategies must consider this variation rather than applying blanket strategies to all rural areas; a one-size-fits-all approach is destined for failure (Phillips & McLeroy, 2004).

Rural environments can present challenges for tobacco control because of, for example, favorable attitudes regarding tobacco use.

Rural communities also possess characteristics that can enable health promotion, especially if those strategies are tailored to capitalize on rural assets (Phillips & McLeroy, 2004). For example, public health researchers encountered strong family ties that served as channels of communication within parts of rural Appalachia (Denham et al., 2004; Meyer et al., 2008; Northridge et al., 2008). In such environments, efforts could focus on existing family networks as an advantageous means of disseminating information and implementing interventions. Other potential assets include the strong religious ties in many rural communities (Denham et al., 2004), making faith-based organizations a possible avenue for tobacco control (Hutcheson et al., 2008). For example, African Americans in some rural areas were more likely than whites to quit smoking, attributed partly to involvement of local African American churches in cessation efforts (Northridge et al., 2008).

Prevention

Research indicates that effective prevention efforts in rural communities should start in elementary school (Sarvela et al., 1999; Smith et al., 2008) because the peak age for experimental use of tobacco was predicted to occur as early as the fifth and sixth grades (Sarvela et al., 1999). However, population size may be an impediment to implementation of rural prevention efforts. Larger rural communities with greater population size had an improved capacity and better resources for tobacco-control efforts than did smaller rural areas (York et al., 2010). Resources include higher numbers of volunteers as well as dedicated staff to promote public health measures, and better access to nonprofit organizations that can assist in these efforts (York et al., 2010).

Cessation

Weg and colleagues (2010) suggested that access to **cessation services** (assistance with quitting tobacco use) constitute an important element in rural tobacco control. Compared to their suburban and urban counterparts, rural residents have more limited access to health care providers, including medical and mental health specialists, and worse levels of insurance coverage. Coupled with the higher tobacco use prevalence rates, these findings highlight the need for targeted tobacco cessation services (Cupertino et al., 2007). Rural residents will participate in pharmacological and behavioral cessation programs, especially when cost containment is incorporated (Cupertino et al., 2007; Weg et al., 2010). For example, tobacco cessation efforts tailored to meet the unique needs of a rural population can be found at the US-Mexico border region, home to a grassroots program named Campesinos Sin Fronteras. This program was designed to target and meet the needs of transient farm workers who are mostly Hispanic and who experience high poverty with low literacy rates. Educational interventions and strategies to promote prevention and cessation took place aboard the buses that provided transportation to and from the work fields (2009).

Historically, much of the focus on smoking cessation has been with adults, yet most smoking begins in adolescence (Curry, Mermelstein, & Sporer, 2009; Dino et al., 2004). In one study, quit rates among rural youths were lower than rates found in other equivalent studies of nonrural youths, suggesting that the former represent a recalcitrant smoking subgroup (Horn et al., 2004). This, coupled with rural teen smoking rates (Denham et al., 2004; Lutfiyya et al., 2008), underscores the need for cessation services directed at rural teens.

Population-Based Strategies

Years of research demonstrate that population-based approaches are the most effective for reducing ETS exposure (Cokkinidies et al., 2009; Jemal et al., 2008). Clean-air ordinances are particularly effective tobacco-control strategies. Smoking is less prevalent in areas with stronger restrictions on indoor smoking (Dinno & Glantz, 2009). Studies have also found positive health effects from enactment of clean indoor air legislation. Rayens and colleagues (2008) found that emergency department visits for asthma in Kentucky were reduced following passage of smoke-free legislation. Similarly, Sargent, Shepard, and Glantz (2004) found that admissions for myocardial infarction dropped significantly during the implementation of a smoke-free law that applied to public places and workplaces in Helena, Montana. Unfortunately, such policies are less common in rural areas (Weg et al., 2010; York et al., 2010), especially in those that produce tobacco (Ferketich et al., 2010). Lower education levels also reduced the likelihood of public support (York et al., 2010). Ferketich and colleagues (2010) conducted a policy analysis for Alabama, Georgia, Kentucky, Mississippi, South Carolina, North Carolina, Virginia, and West Virginia that showed weak statewide legislation that did not prohibit smoking in bars, restaurants, and many other workplaces. Regulations in Tennessee banned smoking in restaurants but not in bars. In some cases, policies can be set by local governments to regulate indoor exposure to ST. In Tennessee, state law precluded this by preventing local jurisdictions from passing laws attempting to limit sale or distribution of tobacco products.

Hahn and colleagues (2009) examined the relationships among tobacco-control capacity, efforts, and resources in rural communities with sociodemographic, political, and health-ranking variables. Only population size showed a significant association with tobacco control. Larger communities had stronger tobacco-control programs than did smaller ones, leading the authors to recommend that smaller communities be targeted for training, technical assistance, and resource allocation.

Pricing is also a strategy for reducing tobacco consumption. Increase in cost been shown to be an effective deterrent, especially among adolescent users (Rahilly & Farwell, 2007), and leads to a reduction in the number of cigarettes smoked as well as increasing overall cessation rates (Dinno & Glantz, 2009). Retrospective studies on local cigarette pricing and state excise taxes show a decrease in cardiovascular mortality for states with higher pricing (Polendak, 2009), demonstrating the long-range benefits of these types of strategies.

Conclusion

Empirical evidence confirms that tobacco use in rural populations presents unique risks, challenges, and, conversely, opportunities for public health intervention. The high prevalence of all types of tobacco use, as well as secondary exposure, necessitate innovative and culturally tailored tobacco-control policy and practice strategies. Careful consideration of the issues presented in this chapter may lead us one step closer to reducing tobacco-related health disparities in rural populations.

Summary

- Rural populations are at increased risk for tobacco-related health disparities, including higher rates of initiation, current use, intensity of use, exposure to secondhand smoke, and cessation failure.
- Rural populations experience health disparities in tobacco-linked diseases such as cardiovascular disease, cerebrovascular disease,

ischemic stroke, coronary heart disease, diabetes, and various cancers such as lung, kidney, bladder, oral, esophageal, stomach, liver, and cervical.

• Factors contributing to rural tobacco disparities are lower socioeconomic status and educational attainment, low levels of medical coverage, geographic isolation with reduced access to medical services, reduced availability of resources that promote cessation, cultural attitudes that foster greater acceptance of tobacco use, and a regional economy that relies on tobacco production.

• Youths in rural communities are at a greater risk for using tobacco products, smoking at an earlier age, and becoming regular smokers. Early initiation of tobacco product use is linked to increased addiction rates, increased chances of adult use, and more difficulty quitting.

• Although rural communities may have barriers to smoking prevention and cessation efforts, they also possess characteristics that can enable health promotion, such as strong community support networks for implementing interventions. Capitalizing on these assets of rural communities is essential toward initiating effective tobacco-control strategies.

For Practice and Discussion

1. Investigate the CDC website to determine the availability of programs that work for the prevention of tobacco use among youths. Compare these programs to the needs of rural American youths and determine which of the options would potentially be the best for use in a rural community in your state.

2. Using the Internet determine the amount of state taxes collected for each pack of cigarettes sold in your state. If possible, determine the annual statewide revenue generated by these taxes. Then, create a budget and prevention program that would use about 50 percent of this revenue to reduce rates of tobacco use. Be sure that the program you create has a strong potential to influence tobacco use declines in rural communities.

Key Terms

cessation services

pregnancy risk assessment monitoring system

References

Ahijevyyk, K., Kuun, P., Christman, S., Wood, T., Browning, K., & Wewers, M. (2003). Beliefs about tobacco among Appalachian current and former users. *Applied Nursing Research, 16*(2), 93–102.

American Legacy Foundation. (2009). *Tobacco control in rural America.* Retrieved from http://www.legacyforhealth.org/PDF/Tobacco_Control_in_Rural_America.pdf

Anselin, L. (1994). Exploratory Spatial Data Analysis and Geographic Information Systems. Paper presented at the New Tools for Spatial Analysis, Luxembourg.

Bell, R., Arcury, T., Chen, H., Anderson, A., Savoca, M., Kohrman, T., et al. (2009). Use of tobacco products among rural older adults: Prevalence of ever use and cumulative lifetime use. *Addictive Behavior, 34*, 662–667.

Bernhard, D., Moser, C., Backovic, A., & Wick, G. (2007). Cigarette smoke—an aging accelerator? *Experimental Gerontology, 42*, 160–165.

Bhat, V., Cole, J., Sorkin, J., Wozniak, M., Malarcher, A., Giles, W., et al. (2008). Dose-response relationship between cigarette smoking and risk of ischemic stroke in young women. *Stroke, 39*, 2439–2443.

Boffetta, P., & Straif, K. (2009). Use of smokeless tobacco and risk of myocardial infarction and stroke: Systematic review with meta-analysis. *BMJ, 339*(b3060).

Campbell-Grossman, C., Hudson, D., & Fleck, M. (2003). Chewing tobacco use: Perceptions and knowledge in rural adolescent youth. *Issues in Comprehensive Pediatric Nursing, 26*, 13–21.

CDC. (2007). *Best practices for comprehensive tobacco control programs.* Retrieved from http://www.cdc.gov/tobacco/stateandcommunity/best_practices/pdfs/2007/BestPractices_Complete.pdf

CDC. (2010). *BRFSS annual survey data.* Retrieved from http://www.cdc.gov/BRFSS/technical_infodata/surveydata.htm

Chaudhuri, R., Livingston, E., McMahon, M., Lafferty, J., Fraser, I., Spears, M., et al. (2006). Effects of smoking cessation on lung function and airway inflammation in smokers with asthma. *American Journal of Respiratory and Critical Care Medicine, 174*, 127–133.

Cokkinidies, V., Bandi, P., McMahon, C., Jemal, A., Glynn, T., & Ward, E. (2009). Tobacco control in the United States: Recent progress and opportunities. *CA: Cancer Journal for Clinicians, 59*, 352–365.

Cooper, R., Cutler, J., Desvigne-Nickens, P., Fortmann, S., Freidman, L., Havlik, R., et al. (2000). Trends and disparities in coronary heart disease, stroke, and other cardiovascular diseases in the United States: Findings of the national conference on cardiovascular disease prevention. *Circulation 102*, 3137–3147.

Cornfield, J., Haenszel, W., Hammond, E., Lilienfeld, A., Shimkin, M., & Wynder, E. (2009). Smoking and lung cancer: Recent evidence and a discussion of some questions. *International Journal of Epidemiology, 38*, 1175–1191.

Costenbader, K., & Karlson, E. (2006). Cigarette smoking and autoimmune disease: What can we learn from epidemiology? *Lupus, 15*, 737–745.

Csordas, A., Wick, G., Laufer, G., & Bernhard, D. (2008). An evaluation of the clinical evidence on the role of inflammation and oxidative stress in smoking-mediated cardiovascular disease. *Biomarker Insights, 3*, 127–138.

Cupertino, A., Mahnken, J., Richter, K., & Cox, L. (2007). Long-term engagement in smoking cessation counseling among rural smokers. *Journal of Health Care for the Poor and Underserved, 18*(4), 39–51.

Curry, S., Mermelstein, R., & Sporer, A. (2009). Therapy for specific problems: Youth tobacco cessation. *Annual Reviews in Psychology, 60,* 229–255.

Davis, S., Malarcher, A., Thorne, S., Maurice, E., Trosclair, A., & Mowery, P. (2009). State-specific prevalence and trends in adult cigarette smoking—United States, 1998–2007. *Morbidity and Mortality Weekly Report, 58*(9), 221–226.

Denham, S., Meyer, M., & Toborg, M. (2004). Tobacco cessation in adolescent females in Appalachian communities. *Family Community Health, 27*(2), 170–181.

Dinno, A., & Glantz, S. (2009). Tobacco control policies are egalitarian: A vulnerabilities perspective on indoor clean air laws, cigarette prices, and tobacco use disparities. *Social Science and Medicine, 68,* 1439–1447.

Dino, G., Kamal, K., Horn, K., Kalsekar, I., & Fernandes, A. (2004). Stage of change and smoking cessation outcomes among adolescents. *Addictive Behaviors, 29,* 935–940.

Doescher, M., Jackson, E., Jerant, A., & Hart, G. (2006). Prevalence and trends in smoking: A national rural study. *The Journal of Rural Health, 22*(2), 112–118.

Dorfman, F. (2008). Tobacco and fertility: Our responsibilities. *Fertility and Sterility, 89*(3), 502–504.

Eberhardt, M., & Pamuk, E. (2004). The importance of place of residence: Examining health in rural and nonrural areas. *American Journal of Public Health, 94,* 1682–1686.

Eichner, J., Cravatt, K., Beebe, L., Blevins, K., Stoddart, M., Bursac, Z., et al. (2005). Tobacco use among American Indians in Oklahoma: An epidemiologic view. *Public Health Reports, 120,* 192–199.

Fagan, P., Molchan, E., Lawrence, D., Fernander, A., & Ponder, P. (2007). Identifying health disparities across the tobacco continuum. *Addiction, 102*(Suppl. 2), 5–29.

Ferketich, A., Katz, M., Kauffman, R., Paskett, E., Lemeshow, S., Westman, J., et al. (2008). Tobacco use among the Amish in Holmes County, Ohio. *The Journal of Rural Health, 24*(2), 84–90.

Ferketich, A., Liber, A., Pennell, M., Nealy, D., Hammer, J., & Berman, M. (2010). Clean indoor air ordinance coverage in the Appalachian region of the United States. *American Journal of Public Health, 100,* 1313–1318.

Flouris, A., Vardavas, C., Metsios, G., Tastsakis, A., & Koutesdakis, Y. (2010). Biological evidence for the acute health effects of secondhand smoke exposure. *American Journal of Physiology—Cell and Molecular Physiology, 298,* L3–L12.

Forster, J., Widome, R., & Bernat, D. (2007). Policy interventions and surveillance as strategies to prevent tobacco use in adolescents and young adults. *American Journal of Preventive Medicine, 33*(6S), S335–S339.

Freedman, N., Leitzmann, M., Hollenbach, A., Schatzkin, A., & Abnet, C. (2008). Cigarette smoking and subsequent risk of lung cancer in men and women: Analysis of a prospective cohort study. *Lancet: Oncology, 9,* 649–656.

Gamm, L., & Hutchison, L. (2004). *Rural Healthy People 2010*—Evolving interactive practice. *American Journal of Public Health, 94*(10), 1711–1712.

Gandini, S., Botteri, E., Iodice, S., Boniol, M., Lowenfels, A., Maisonneuve, P., et al. (2008). Tobacco smoking and cancer: A meta-analysis. *International Journal of Cancer, 122,* 155–164.

Gansky, S., Ellison, J., Kavanagh, C., Isong, U., & Walsh, M. (2009). Patterns and correlates of spit tobacco use among high school males in rural California. *Journal of Public Health Dentistry, 69*(2), 116–124.

Hahn, E., Ashford, K., Okoli, C., Rayens, M., Ridner, S., & York, N. (2009). Nursing research in community based approaches to reduce exposure to secondhand smoke. *Annual Review of Nursing Research, 27*(1), 365–391.

Harel-Meir, M., Sherer, Y., & Shoenfeld, Y. (2007). Tobacco smoking and autoimmune rheumatic diseases. *Nature: Clinical Practice: Rheumatology, 3*(12), 707–715.

Hecht, S. (2006). Cigarette smoking: Cancer risks, carcinogens, and mechanisms. *Lagenbecks Archives of Surgery, 391,* 603–613.

Henley, S., Connell, C., Richter, P., Husten, C., Pechacek, T., Calle, E., et al. (2007). Tobacco-related disease mortality among men who switched from cigarettes to spit tobacco. *Tobacco Control, 16,* 22–28.

Horn, K., Dino, G., Kalsekar, R., & Fernandes, A. (2004). Appalachian teen smokers: Not on tobacco 15 months later. *American Journal of Public Health, 94*(2), 181–184.

Hu, M., Davies, M., & Kandel, D. (2006). Epidemiology and correlates of daily smoking and nicotine dependence among young adults. *American Journal of Public Health, 96,* 299–308.

Hutcheson, T., Greiner, K., Ellerbeck, E., Jeffries, S., Mussulman, L., & Casey, G. (2008). Understanding smoking cessation in rural communities. *The Journal of Rural Health, 24*(2), 116–124.

Institute of Medicine. (2007). *Ending the tobacco problem: A blueprint for the nation.* Washington, DC: National Academies Press. Retrieved from http://books.nap.edu/openbook.php?record_id = 11795 Jaimes, E., Tian, R., & Raij, L. (2007). Nicotine: The link between cigarette smoking and the progression of renal disease. *American Journal of Physiology—Heart and Circulatory Physiology, 292,* H76–H82.

Jefferis, B., Lowe, G., Welsh, P., Rumley, A., Lawlor, D., Ebrahim, S., et al. (2010). Secondhand smoke (SHS) exposure is associated with circulating markers of inflammation and endothelial function in adult men and women. *Atherosclerosis, 208,* 550–556.

Jemal, A., Thun, M., Ries, L., Howe, H., Weir, H., Center, M., et al. (2008). Annual report to the nation on the status of cancer, 1975–2005, featuring trends in lung cancer, tobacco use, and tobacco control. *Journal of the National Cancer Institute, 100*(23), 1672–1694.

Julvez, J., Ribas-Fito, N., Forns, M., Garcia-Esteban, R., & Sunyer, J. (2007). Maternal smoking habits and cognitive development of children at age 4 years in a population-based birth cohort. *International Journal of Epidemiology, 36,* 825–832.

Keppel, K., Pearcy, J., & Klein, R. (2004). Measuring progress in *Healthy People 2010. Healthy People 2010 Stat Notes, 25*(1), 1–16.

Kosecik, M., Erel, O., Sevinc, E., & Selek, S. (2005). Increased oxidative stress in children exposed to passive smoking. *International Journal of Cardiology, 100*, 61–64.

Leone, A., Landini, J., L., Biadi, O., & Balbarini, A. (2008). Smoking and cardiovascular system: Cellular features of the damage. *Current Pharmaceutical Design, 14*, 1771–1777.

Lutfiyya, M., Shah, K., Johnson, M., Bales, R., McGrath, C., Serpa, L., et al. (2008). Adolescent daily cigarette smoking: Is rural residency a risk factor? *Rural and Remote Health, 8*, 875.

Mannino, D., & Buist, A. (2007). Global burden of COPD: Risk factors, prevalence and future trends. *The Lancet, 370*, 765–773.

Martin, J., Mousa, S., Shaker, O., & Mousa, S. (2009). The multiple faces of nicotine and its implications in tissue and wound repair. *Experimental Dermatology, 18*, 497–505.

McMillen, R., Breen, J., & Cosby, A. (2004). Rural-urban differences in the social climate surrounding environmental tobacco smoke: A report from the 2002 social climate survey of tobacco control. *The Journal of Rural Health, 20*(1), 7–16.

Meyer, M., Toborg, M., Denham, S., & Mande, M. (2008). Cultural perspectives concerning adolescent use of tobacco and alcohol in the Appalachian mountain region. *The Journal of Rural Health, 24*(1), 67–74.

Nelson, D., Mowery, P., Tomar, S., Marcus, S., Giovino, G., & Zhao, L. (2006). Trends in smokeless tobacco use among adults and adolescents in the United States. *American Journal of Public Health, 96*, 897–905.

Newman, I., & Shell, D. (2005). Smokeless tobacco expectancies among a sample of rural adolescents. *American Journal of Health Behavior, 29*(2), 127–136.

Northridge, M., Vallone, D., Xiao, H., Green, M., Blackwood, J., Kemper, S., et al. (2008). The importance of location for tobacco cessation: Rural-urban disparities in quit success in underserved West Virginia counties. *The Journal of Rural Health, 24*(2), 106–115.

Phillips, C., & McLeroy, K. (2004). Health in rural America: Remembering the importance of place. *American Journal of Public Health, 94*(10), 1661–1663.

Polendak, A. (2009). Trends in death rates from tobacco-related cardiovascular diseases in selected US States differing in tobacco-control efforts. *Epidemiology, 20*(4), 542–546.

Poole-DiSalvo, E., Liu, Y., Brenner, S., & Weitzman, S. (2010). Adult household smoking is associated with increased child emotional and behavioral problems. *Journal of Developmental Behavior and Pediatrics, 31*(2), 107–115.

Rafalson, L., Donahue, R., Dmochowski, J., Rejman, K., Dorn, J., & Trevisan, M. (2009). Cigarette smoking is associated with conversion from normoglycemia to impaired fasting glucose: The western New York health study. *Annals of Epidemiology, 19*(6), 365–371.

Rahilly, C., & Farwell, W. (2007). Prevalence of smoking in the United States: A focus on age, sex, ethnicity, and geographic patterns. *Current Cardiovascular Risk Reports, 1*, 379–383.

Rayens, M., Burkhardt, P., Zhang, M., Lee, S., Moser, D., Mannino, D., et al. (2008). Reduction in asthma-related emergency room visits after implementation of a smoke-free law. *The Journal of Allergy and Clinical Immunology, 122*(3), 537–541.

Salihu, H., & Wilson, R. (2007). Epidemiology of prenatal smoking and perinatal outcomes. *Early Human Development, 83*, 713–720.

Sargent, R., Shepherd, R., & Glantz, S. (2004). Reduced incidence of admissions for myocardial infarction associated with public smoking ban: Before and after study. *BMJ, 328*, 977–985.

Sarvela, P., Monge, E., Shannon, D., & Nawrot, R. (1999). Age of first use of cigarettes among rural and small town elementary school children in Illinois. *Journal of School Health, 69*(10), 398–402.

Smith, K., Siebel, C., Pham, L., Cho, J., Singer, R., Chaloupka, F., et al. (2008). News on tobacco and public attitudes towards smokefree air policies in the United States. *Health Policy, 86*, 42–52.

Song, H., & Fish, M. (2006). Demographic and psychosocial characteristics of smokers and nonsmokers in low socio-economic status rural Appalachian 2-parent families in southern West Virginia. *The Journal of Rural Health, 22*(1), 83–87.

Stampfli, M., & Anderson, G. (2009). How cigarette smoke skews immune responses to promote infection, lung disease and cancer. *Nature Reviews: Immunology, 9*, 377–384.

Sullivan, S., & Glantz, S. (2010). Local smokefree ordinances are passing in tobacco-growing states. *American Journal of Public Health, 100*(11), 2013–2014.

Swan, G., & Lessov-Schlaggar, C. (2007). The effects of tobacco smoke and nicotine on cognition and the brain. *Neuropsychology Review, 17*, 259–273.

Tamer, A., Yeldiz, S., Yeldiz, N., Kanat, M., Gunduz, H., Tahtaci, M., et al. (2006). The prevalence of neuropathy and relationship with risk factors in diabetic patients: A single-center experience. *Medical Principles and Practice, 15*, 190–194.

Tanriverdi, H., Evrengul, H., Kuru, O., Tanriverdi, A., Seleci, D., Enli, Y., et al. (2006). Cigarette smoking induced oxidative stress may impair endothelial function and coronary blood flow in angiographically normal coronary arteries. *Circulation Journal, 70*, 593–599.

Tesfaye, S., Chaturvedi, N., Eaton, S., Ward, J., Manes, C., Ionescu-Tirgoviste, C., et al. (2005). Vascular risk factors and diabetic neuropathy. *New England Journal of Medicine, 352*, 341–350.

Tong, V., Jones, J., Dietz, P., D'Angelo, D., & Bombard, J. (2005). Trends in smoking before, during, and after pregnancy—pregnancy risk assessment monitoring system (PRAMS), United States, 31 sites, 2000–. *Morbidity and Mortality Weekly Report, 58*(SS04), 1–29.

US Department of Agriculture. (2004). *Measuring rurality: Rural-urban continuum codes.* Retrieved from http://www.ers.usda.gov/briefing/rurality/ruralurbcon/

Weg, M., Cunningham, C., Howren, M., & Cai, X. (2010). Tobacco use and exposure in rural areas: Findings from the behavioral risk factor survey surveillance system. *Addictive Behaviors*, p. 10.

Wewers, M., Ahijevyk, K., Chen, M., Dresbach, S., Kihm, K., & Kuun, P. (2000). Tobacco use characteristics among rural Appalachians. *Journal of Community Health, 25*(5), 377–388.

Willi, C., Bodenmann, P., & Ghali, W. (2007). Active smoking and the risk of type 2 diabetes: A systematic review and meta-analysis. *Journal of the American Medical Association, 298*(22), 2654–2664.

Winickoff, J., Van Cleave, J., & Oreskovic, N. (2010). Tobacco smoke exposure and chronic conditions of childhood. *Pediatrics, 126*, e251–e252.

World Health Organization. (2008). *WHO report on the global tobacco epidemic: The MPOWER package.* Retrieved from http://www.who.int/tobacco/mpower/mpower_report_full_2008.pdf

Yanbaeva, D., Dentener, M., Creutzberg, E., Wesseling, G., & Wouters, E. (2007). Systemic effects of smoking. *Chest, 131*, 1557–1566.

York, N., Rayens, M., Zhang, M., Jones, L., Casey, B., & Hahn, E. (2010). Strength of tobacco control in rural communities. *The Journal of Rural Health, 26*, 120–127.

Index

MPM 260118
Printed in Singapore